Science, politics and the pharmaceutical industry

Controversy and bias in drug regulation

John Abraham

University of Reading

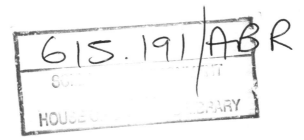

UCL
PRESS

First published in 1995 by UCL Press

UCL Press Limited
University College London
Gower Street
London WC1E 6BT

The name of University College London (UCL) is a registered trade mark used by UCL Press with the consent of the owner.

British Library Cataloguing-in-Publication Data
A catalogue record for this book is available from the British Library.

ISBNs:
1-85728-199-3   HB
1-85728-200-0   PB

Cover photograph by Malcom Watson

Typeset in Baskerville and Gill Sans
Printed and bound by
Biddles Ltd, Guildford and King's Lynn, England

Contents

This book is dedicated to
Lin and Charles

Abbreviations

AAOAC   American Association of Official Agricultural Chemists

ABPI   Association of the British Pharmaceutical Industry

ADR   Adverse Drug Reaction

AMA   American Medical Association

BIRA   British Institute of Regulatory Affairs

BMA   British Medical Association

BOC   Bureau of Chemistry (US)

CRM   Committee on the Review of Medicines (UK)

CSD   Committee on the Safety of Drugs (UK)

CSDIP   Committee on the Supply of Drugs to Insured Persons (UK)

CSM   Committee on the Safety of Medicines (UK)

CTCs   Clinical Trial Certificates

DH   Department of Health (UK)

DHHS   Department of Health and Human Services (US)

DHSS   Department of Health and Social Security (UK)

EEC   European Economic Community

EPA   Environmental Protection Agency (US)

ESR   Erythrocyte Sedimentation Rate

FDA   Food and Drug Administration (US)

FRG   Federal Republic of Germany

FTC   Federal Trade Commission (US)

GI   Gastro-Intestinal

HRG   Health Research Group of Public Citizen (US)

IBT   Industrial Bio-Test Laboratories

IND   Investigational New Drug (US)

IPHAR   Institute for Clinical Pharmacology (Germany)

IRLG   Inter-agency Regulatory Liaison Group (US)

JCP   Joint Committee on Prescribing (UK)

JSN   Joint Space Narrowing

Lilly   Eli Lilly and Company

LM   Leucocyte Migration

MAIL   Medicines Act Information Leaflet

MH   Ministry of Health (UK)

MP   Member of Parliament

NAS   National Academy of Sciences (US)

NCC   National Consumer Council (UK)

NCI   National Cancer Institute

NDA   New Drug Application (US)

NDAB   National Drugs Advisory Board (Ireland)

NHI   National Health Insurance (UK)

NHS   National Health Service (UK)

NPU   National Pharmacists' Union (UK)

ABBREVIATIONS

NRC National Research Council (US)
NSAID Non-Steroidal Anti-Inflammatory Drug
OD Osseous Defects
PAGB Proprietary Association of Great Britain
PEG Pharmaceutical Export Group
PEM Prescription Event Monitoring
PG Prostaglandin
PMA Pharmaceutical Manufacturers' Association (US)
PRO Public Record Office (UK)

PSGB Pharmaceutical Society of Great Britain
SBA Summary Basis of Approval
SPA Society of Public Analysts (UK)
SSRC Social Science Research Council (US)
UK United Kingdom
US United States of America
VPRS Voluntary Price Regulation Scheme (UK)
WDTA Wholesale Druggist Trade Association (UK)
WHO World Health Organisation

Preface

This book is about how medical drugs are tested for safety and effectiveness, and about the efforts made by scientists and governments in the UK and the US to fulfil their public responsibilities to ensure that a safe and effective supply of drugs is made available to patients. By definition medicines should be produced in order to improve the health of patients, and the scientific testing and regulation of drugs are technical, social and political processes on which patients and doctors rely to be confident that a treatment will be beneficial, rather than damaging. Hence, the quality of such processes is vital to any assessment of the adequacy of the systems used to control medicines.

The public pronouncements of government officials generally give the impression that the systems in place for controlling medicines have worked, and continue to work, as well as is feasible. Representatives of the pharmaceutical industry frequently echo that view, although they also complain that too often the benefits of modern medicines are neglected. Critics, on the other hand, argue that the systems for controlling drugs can be improved. They cite estimates of drug injury running into tens or even hundreds of thousands of cases per year in the UK alone, and claim that the regulatory authorities responsible for controlling medicines have been far too slow in removing ineffective drugs from the market.[1]

In this book I focus on one potential problem in drug testing and regulation, namely, the problem of bias. Specifically, I ask if, and how, bias may influence the scientific processes of evaluating the safety and effectiveness of new drugs. This is important because scientific knowledge about drugs is a crucial factor in determining their acceptability to doctors and patients. The research that follows suggests that corporate bias is a significant social and political problem in the testing and control of medicines. It is a problem because that bias may compromise the best interests of patients, who may be exposed to unnecessary medical risks through taking drugs that are either unsafe or ineffective or both. This book demonstrates the scope and depth of the bias: from individual to institution; from animal test to marketing claim. In so doing it scrutinizes the technical and regulatory processes by which corporate bias is expressed.

To acknowledge such bias is in no way to suggest that all the scientists who work in the pharmaceutical industry or the government authorities who regulate them are biased or unprincipled. Nor does it necessarily imply that bias must be deliberate or conspiratorial. Bias may be conscious or unconscious, and in this book I make little or no attempt to determine individual consciousness of bias. It is not being suggested that the scientists discussed have acted in bad faith in any way whatsoever. However, I do make proposals about how the current systems of drug testing and regulation in the UK and the US could be improved by making political changes likely to reduce corporate bias.

To date little systematic research has been undertaken to address the above problems. The social science literature on the pharmaceutical sector is dominated by discussions of the economic effects of regulation on innovation in the industry.[2] Though that work can sharpen understanding of the relationship between regulation and industrial profitability, it tends to ignore scientific knowledge about the effectiveness or toxicity of drug products themselves.

Another (amorphous) branch of literature provides critical surveys of the practices of the pharmaceutical industry and regulatory agencies.[3] Commercial biases in the pharmaceutical industry and government that might adversely affect consumers are foremost among the concerns of that literature. However, those concerns are drawn from an emphasis on industrial policies and regulatory outcomes, which pays little attention to the history and political economy of science-based regulation that may play an important part in defining the basis and boundaries of such policies. It is those historical and political factors that are the particular concern of Chapter 2.

As is discussed in more detail in Chapter 1, sociology of science has made considerable contributions to an analysis of the social processes underlying the development of scientific knowledge. Yet sociological studies containing substantial analysis of the technical content of the scientific knowledge informing drug regulation have remained sparse despite some recent valuable contributions.[4] Thus, in addressing the problem of corporate bias I hope to have extended the boundaries of existing scholarship by conducting a technically detailed micro-sociological examination of the scientific knowledge associated with drug testing and regulation, firmly located in the macro-sociological historical context provided in the second chapter.

Most of the book, Chapters 3 to 7, is devoted to case studies of five non-steroidal anti-inflammatory drugs (NSAIDs). This group of drugs has been chosen because they are very important to both the industry and patients. Since a large and growing population suffers from inflammatory diseases, such as arthritis, there is a large market for anti-inflammatory drugs, especially NSAIDs (see Chapter 3 for more details). As a group, NSAIDs also account for a very significant proportion of the reported cases of adverse drug reactions (ADRs).

There are both intellectual and practical reasons for adopting this case study approach. While some surveys of drug testing and regulation mentioned above are available, only one in-depth analysis of a drug's regulation is cited in the literature.[5] None of those surveys systematically analyzes the scientific knowledge involved in drug testing and regulation, and the one case study, the registration history of cromolyn sodium, remains unpublished and confidential.[6] Consequently, existing research, which touches on possible commercial bias in drug testing and regulation, lacks empirical depth. In taking a case study approach here, I aim to deepen current understanding of such bias. Regarding some of the controversial NSAIDs examined in this book, which were withdrawn because of toxicity, case study research can make an especially important contribution to knowledge. As Dukes, formerly a leading policy analyst at the World Health Organisation's European Regional Office, remarks:

> Some individual instances in which newly marketed drugs have been withdrawn because of serious adverse effects deserve to be investigated. . . . Such work could throw light on the reasons why these problems were not anticipated at the time of registration.[7]

One reason why case studies of individual drugs in the regulatory process have been rarely undertaken is that the data handled by regulatory authorities are highly confidential.[8] The result has been a proliferation of studies, that attempt to judge the performance of various national regulatory regimes by comparing the number of drugs approved with the number of submissions and the number of withdrawals.[9] It is studies of this kind that are often invoked to argue that approval of new drugs in the US lags behind approval in the UK because of American over-regulation. This approach, however, is unsatisfactory because it ignores the way in which scientific knowledge is used in reaching regulatory decisions. Since the best interests of patients are inextricably linked to that scientific knowledge, those studies which neglect it are drastically limited in evaluating the performance of regulatory authorities as patient protection agencies.

Indeed, such studies can provide indicators only of the comparative performance of one national regulatory authority to another, and cannot pronounce on their actions relative to an independent base-line such as the scientific standards in the field, or on the internal coherence of the technical arguments put forward to justify a regulatory decision. Hence, a further reason for applying a case study approach is that it enables sufficient attention to be focused on scientific knowledge so that judgements about the performance of regulatory authorities can go beyond merely declaring that one is a better consumer protector than another, and consider whether both might be good (or poor) consumer protectors, with respect to what is possible on the existing state of knowledge. As Irwin has commented, these questions "call for the study of individual cases in the control of technological risk and not for glib assertions or easy generalizations".[10]

Thus, there are strong arguments for attempting to examine the "black box" of the regulatory process, rather than shying away from it because of the difficulty in obtaining a comprehensive database. Nevertheless, confidentiality rules concerning the regulatory process mean that it is much easier to study regulatory controversies that spill over into the public domain. The cases discussed in this book fall into that category.

The findings in this book are based almost entirely on documentary evidence and interview data collected during fieldwork in the UK and the US, as well as appropriate literature reviews. The public record office in London and the FDA's libraries in Washington DC proved invaluable resources for Chapter 2, while the British Science Reference Library could nearly always supply the required technical literature discussed in Chapters 3 to 7. Publicly available records of product liability cases and relevant Congressional hearings in the US also provided rich sources of information for the case studies, as did the American Freedom of Information Services. I also made use of computer searches and the Science Citation Indices in order to survey systematically the scientific literature relevant to the technical controversies under examination. When I requested access to the files of the British regulatory Committee on the Safety of Medicines (CSM) permission was denied on the grounds that such access would breach confidentiality laws, including those contained within the 1968 Medicines Act.[11] Consequently, the internal workings of the CSM are least well documented in this book but, as I hope will become evident, sufficient data were available to draw some very substantial conclusions about that Committee's actions. In Chapter 8 I draw out some of the implications of the research findings at both the theoretical and practical policy levels.

Thanks are due to many librarians as well as the staff at the FDA and the Public Citizen Health Research Group for their invaluable assistance. I am also grateful to all the people who have encouraged and supported me in my research and writing for this book. These include: Erik Millstone, Lin Creasey, Pauline Sobel, Alan Irwin, Alan Cawson, Daryl Chubin and Justin Vaughan. Much of the fieldwork was funded by the British Economic and Social Research (ESR).

Chapter One

Bias in science and regulation

Any attempt to study industrial and corporate bias in drug testing and regulation raises complex questions about the politics of science. What role have values played in the production of scientific knowledge and regulatory decisions? What is meant by bias, how can it be identified, and whose interests does it serve? Opinions differ and vary according to the institutional context of the scientists in question. Regarding the testing of drugs by industry, representatives of government and industry frequently argue that the effects of any social and political factors in that scientific process are benign, if not beneficial, with respect to patients. Thus, following the thalidomide disaster the British Minister of Health, Enoch Powell, maintained that it was in the commercial interests of any drug company to test its products thoroughly, and thereby to minimize any adverse effects on consumers.[1] Similarly, representatives of industry acknowledge that they have commercial interests in drug development, but argue that those interests coincide entirely with the best interests of patients. For example, Bruce Peck, Director of Regulatory Affairs at Lilly in 1983, declared:

Lilly does not market a drug nor request government approval for its use until extensive and well-controlled scientific studies prove that its benefits far outweigh the risks.[2]

And a senior scientist at Glaxo told a meeting of specialist medics, pharmacologists and clinicians:

I have no doubt the first duty of any research and development organization is to look for, find and develop new medicines which are capable of making substantial contributions to the profit and turnover of our companies. . . . This, however, need not worry any of you because the only way of achieving our objective is to find better medicines for common illnesses.[3]

1

On the other hand, Larry Ramsay, editor of the *British Journal of Clinical Pharmacology*, and a former employee of the drug industry, hypothesized in 1990:

Scientists who work for the pharmaceutical industry get steeped in corporate culture and slip into biases in favour of their own drugs.[4]

As regards the deliberations of government scientists, senior officials have tended to deny entirely the influence of bias resulting from commercial and political factors in regulatory decisions. For instance, on the establishment of the British Committee on the Safety of Drugs (CSD) in 1964, Powell pronounced that it was unthinkable that its members would submit to any influence other than the force of scientific considerations.[5] Furthermore, in 1985 the British Health Minister, then Kenneth Clarke, said of the successor of the CSD:

I have every reason to believe that members of the Committee [on the Safety of Medicines] have maintained the highest level of integrity, objectivity and professional expertise.[6]

Senior scientists themselves seem to take a similar view. In 1990 Adolph Asscher, chairman of the Committee on the Safety of Medicines (CSM), denied that commercial interests affected regulatory decisions because members who declared such an interest in a drug took no part in the Committee's discussions about the product's regulatory status.[7] Similarly, across the Atlantic, in 1974 the Commissioner of the US Food and Drug Administration (FDA) declared the principles on which he believed the regulatory work of the agency was based:

FDA decisions must be based on scientific evidence not personal prejudice. . . . the scientific evidence we use must be sound and must be accurately analysed and evaluated. . . . the arguments used by the agency in decision-making must begin with truthful premises and proceed in a logical and valid fashion to sensible conclusions.[8]

The role and nature of commercial bias in the testing and regulation of drugs is, therefore, by no means self-evident. The purpose of this chapter is to develop a sound theoretical and methodological framework for exploring such matters by examining the strengths and weaknesses of the literature relevant to bias in science and regulation. This is important because unless our empirical investigation of bias in science is informed by a coherent framework it will be analytically weak, lack penetration and fail to provide an adequate basis for social intervention and political change.

The task demands a conceptualization of scientific knowledge and its social context. In particular the concept of interests needs to be theoretically clarified, and the scope of the relationships between scientific knowledge, on the one hand, and industrial and political institutions, on the other, needs to be sketched. I shall do this via a constructive critique of several strands of social and political thought which are relevant to bias in science and regulation, although I do not claim that what follows in this chapter is an exhaustive examination of the field. For example, I make no attempt to articulate the far-reaching critiques of science adduced by environmentalism and feminism.

Sociology of scientific knowledge

Until the 1970s the sociology of science was dominated by the Mertonian tradition. Merton's pioneering work concentrated on the internal social relations of scientific institutions, but accepted that scientific knowledge itself was not susceptible to sociological analysis. Though science could be promoted by the Puritan ethic and directed by external forces, such as the State, scientific *knowledge*, he believed, was generated by an autonomous intellectual ethos, and unproblematically reflected reality.[9] Such a view depended on what some commentators have termed a "positivist conception of science"[10] and an assumption that science could only flourish if protected from political interference. According to Merton:

> The ethos of science involves the functionally necessary demand that theories or generalizations be evaluated in terms of their logical consistency and consonance with facts. . . . Modern science has considered the personal equation as a potential source of error and has evolved impersonal criteria for checking such error. It is now called upon to assert that certain scientists, because of their extra-scientific affiliations are *a priori* incapable of anything but spurious and false theories. In some instances, scientists are required to accept the judgements of scientifically incompetent political leaders concerning matters of science. But such politically advisable tactics run counter to the institutionalized norms of science.[11]

On this view, therefore, science and politics were *ordinarily* not only separate but opposed. Nevertheless, Merton appreciated that bias could enter into science if polluted by politics. Although this Mertonian perspective on science has declined in popularity since the mid 1970s, it still has some committed supporters, such as Bunge and Hammersley.[12]

It was Kuhn's forthright analysis[13] of how social factors influenced, if not determined, the development of concepts and preferred theories in science which drew attention to sociological features of scientific *knowledge*. One of the crucial ways in which Kuhn's analysis of science differed from the Mertonian tradition was that it raised the problem of relativism of truth in science. This has two essential features: any theory can be maintained in the face of any evidence provided scientists make sufficient adjustments to their beliefs; and observations are necessarily "theory-laden" so that what can count as relevant and proper evidence is determined by the theory (or "theoretical paradigm"), which the evidence is supposed to test.[14] Moreover, when scientists switch from one "paradigm" to another that is to be explained by reference to social and psychological factors in the face of anomalies in the "old paradigm" rather than because the "new paradigm" has greater truth-value. Thus, Kuhn states:

> [Scientists] will devise numerous articulations and *ad hoc* modifications of their theory in order to eliminate *any* apparent conflict [with evidence].[15] (Emphasis added)

and

> . . . though the world does not change with a change of paradigm the scientist afterward works in a different world.[16]

Whatever Kuhn intended by these (and other such) remarks he has been interpreted to mean respectively that there are always alternative theories which, consistent with the evidence, might reasonably be adopted by scientists, and that rival scientific theories or "paradigms" are incommensurable (i.e. share no objective point from which they can be judged one against the other).[17] Such interpretations have inspired much of the relativist contemporary sociology of scientific knowledge, whose four main research programmes provide a useful starting point for discussion of the complex issue of bias in scientific knowledge.

The Strong Programme

Researchers following this approach adopt an explicit methodological relativism, stipulating that the sociology of knowledge should be reflexive about its own beliefs, impartial with respect to truth and falsity and symmetric in its explanations of true and false beliefs.[18] Ostensibly the implication of the impartiality and symmetry requirements for the Strong Programme's empirical research is a value-neutral stance.[19] According to Barnes and Shapin, leading advocates of the Programme, one of its major features is that it:

closes no evaluative or political options; it merely ejects them from historical practice. . . . a recognition that explicit, evaluative concerns and commitments are not conducive to good history.[20]

Empirically this research programme has been primarily concerned with analyzing *social history* of scientific knowledge.[21] In so doing, it adopts a "congruence approach", which depends on the identification of an isomorphism between collectively sustained social interests that can be imputed to a social group, on the one hand, and beliefs promoted by individuals affiliated to this group, on the other.[22] For example, Mackenzie suggests that scientific goals (e.g. particular work in statistical theory) are typically sustained by social interests (e.g. eugenics), which may have their origins within or outside science (e.g. the interests of the British professional middle class).[23] Similarly, Shapin argues that by examining the context of use of scientific knowledge one can discover that scientific work may be carried out in order to legitimate a theory that is sustained by social interests.[24] For these reasons Webster and other commentators often refer to the Strong Programme as "the interests approach" in the sociology of scientific knowledge.[25] However, it is important to appreciate that the Strong Programme by no means exhausts an interests approach to scientific knowledge, as will become apparent from later discussions in this chapter.

In its most ambitious forms the Strong Programme aims to locate, and claims to have located, "social causes" of scientists' beliefs, "that is, general laws relating beliefs to conditions which are necessary and sufficient to determine them".[26] Scientists' decisions for preferring one description of a phenomenon (or theory) over another, therefore, are to be explained not by reference to rational reasoning and/or any correspondence to a mind-independent reality, but rather according to the prevailing sociohistorical conditions. Moreover, Bloor, a leading advocate of the Strong Programme seems to argue that such "social causes" can be explanatorily exhaustive.[27] Thus, according to the Strong Programme, scientific knowledge is an entirely social matter, unconstrained by any supracultural real natural world. Such anti-realist perspectives are common to all four "schools" of the relativism which dominate the sociology of scientific knowledge.

The advocates of the Strong Programme rarely deal *explicitly* with bias in science. Indeed, because of their doctrine of value-neutrality and impartiality with respect to truth and falsity, they tend to shy away from assertions about bias. However, the implication of much of this work is that social interests can deeply influence the pursuit of knowledge in certain directions, and that commercial interests, in particular, could have such an influence on science.

The Empirical Programme of Relativism

This research programme, led by Harry Collins, embraces the methodological relativism of the Strong Programme.[28] Moreover, for Collins, the sociologist and the scientist live in different cultures, and the former cannot hope to understand the natural world.[29] In particular, he stresses that producing results acceptable to the scientific community "is the only indicator of successful knowledge transfer between scientists available to a sociologist", and that "there is nothing outside of courses of linguistics, conceptual and social behaviour which can affect the outcome of these [scientific] arguments".[30] Thus, the sociologist cannot make any independent judgements about the status of scientific knowledge.

Based on such "cultural relativism"[31] the Empirical Programme of Relativism examines the production of contemporary scientific knowledge[32] with a focus on *replicability* in science because, argue this Programme's proponents, ultimately scientists will defend the validity of their knowledge claims on the basis of the repeatability of their experiments and/or observations.[33] But, according to Collins, because the reward system in science favours those who discover things first, in practice, few scientists actually undertake replicability experiments.[34]

The major exception to this, however, is in the context of *scientific controversies* when there are sufficient doubts about, and challenges to, knowledge claims to motivate scientists to engage in replicability tests.[35] The programme, therefore, concentrates on contemporary scientific controversies which can bring out "what is hidden in ordinary science".[36] As Collins puts it:

> the salience of alternative interpretations of evidence, which typifies controversies, has acted as a lever to elicit the essentially cultural nature of the local boundaries of scientific legitimacy – normally elusive or concealed.[37]

Some of the findings of this approach have relevance to the problem of bias in science. For example, favoured experimental interpretations were found to have been supported "through selective reporting in the professional journals, management both of professional meetings and of the publicizing of scientists' small errors, [and] magnification of the importance of trivial experiments supporting a popular view".[38] Such findings point to possible ways in which science might be vulnerable to industrial or commercial bias. Nevertheless, Collins denies the sociological significance of bias. Remaining faithful to relativism, he argues that the scientific views on either side of a controversy can be defended indefinitely,[39] and that varying and contradictory opinions should be seen as an unavoidable characteristic of science, rather than as being caused by "incompetence", "eradicable bias" or "fraud".[40]

Constructionism and laboratory studies

If the Strong Programme emphasizes the macroscopic sociostructural level of analysis, then the anthropological and ethnographic studies of scientific practice in the laboratory redress the balance. They focus on microscopic social contingencies as an integral part of the production and content of knowledge, and on the rhetoric of persuasion in scientific writing.[41] This *social constructionist* approach rejects the distinction between social and cognitive aspects of science, and regards the status of any given account as determined not by whether it is true or real, but by how useful it is in the competitive realm of knowledge production.[42] As such, the laboratory studies approach takes an "instrumentalist" as well as a relativist view of science.[43]

In perhaps the best known laboratory study Latour and Woolgar examine science as a process of literary inscription and the transformation of statement types. They attempt to give an account of how a scientific "fact" is generated from the day-to-day contingent acts of laboratory life. For example, the "fact" that a certain drug exists is reported to result from a series of metamorphoses: from a set of separate data points to statements of the form "scientist A suggests the drug X exists", then to the form "it has been confirmed a number of times that drug X exists" and finally when full "facticity" has been reached to the form "drug X can be used as . . . ".[44]

Laboratory scientists were found to be primarily concerned with making things work, rather than with a quest for truth.[45] In the process they engaged opportunistically in consistency-making practices with respect to knowledge claims,[46] and used inscription devices to simplify claims with the purpose of limiting counter-arguments.[47] Knorr-Cetina, an advocate of the social constructionist view, offers the following summary of the findings of laboratory studies:

the constructive operations with which we have associated scientific work can be defined as the sum total of selections designed to

7

transform the subjective into the objective, the unbelievable into the believed, the fabricated into the finding, and the painstakingly constructed into the objective scientific "fact". Laboratory studies demonstrate that scientific products are "occasioned" by the circumstances of their production. "Occasioned" here means that the circumstances of production are an integral part of the products which emerge. Thus we are not just referring to contextual factors that "influence" work which in its core is non-contextual.[48]

This thorough-going context-dependency means that scientific knowledge is viewed as being *arbitrarily* defined by scientists' social practices (e.g. transcription devices), as Law makes clear:

it is first and foremost the text which imposes a structure on the world. . . . The strength of the translation lies in what is selected and how the linkages are built. *But there are no limits to what may be chosen* and how this may be juxtaposed, for the power of the text is a function of the fact that it displays and arrays *whatever* resources may contribute to its strength.[49] (Emphasis added)

The proponents of laboratory studies place heavy emphasis on the importance of scientists' observable social interactions as explanations of scientific knowledge production. They argue that the traditional research methods of interviews with scientists and analysis of published scientific papers and other documentary evidence are limited because they are so removed from "what actually goes on in science".[50]

Accordingly, social constructionists argue that the day-to-day activities of working scientists should be the *origin* of sociological analysis, but there is ambiguity about whether or not this is because such research yields a more accurate account of science. Woolgar and Latour, for instance, warn against using laboratory studies as vehicles for revealing "the true state of affairs", "bias", "interests" or "telling stories about what laboratory life is 'really like'".[51] On this view laboratory studies cannot provide insights into bias in science. On the other hand, Knorr-Cetina seems to disagree, arguing that an inquiry into how knowledge is construed in scientific work can 'inform a structural interest explanation as to whether, when and how interest-based theoretical inclinations have entered laboratory selections'.[52]

Combining this latter argument with some of the findings of Latour and Woolgar suggests that the transformation of statements in the production of scientific papers might be another arena in which commercial bias could become integral to scientific knowledge. However, in his more recent work Latour explicitly rejected the idea that social interests should be invoked to account for scientific practices:

> One might draw the conclusion that if science is not made up of science and led by scientists, it is made up of and led by interest groups. This danger is all the greater since this alternative is exactly the one offered by so called "social studies of science". . . . Fortunately, the danger is not a real one if we can see that all attribution trials should be cleared away, including those which attribute the dynamism of science to social factors.[53]

Clearly, then, there is some tension between the objectives of the Strong Programme and the perspectives of at least some advocates of the social constructionist approach. Nevertheless, the social constructionists share with the supporters of the Strong Programme and the Empirical Programme of Relativism a commitment to anti-realism as affirmed by Latour who claims:

> Since the settlement of a [scientific] controversy is the cause of Nature's representation not the consequence, we can never use the outcome – Nature – to explain how and why a controversy has been settled.[54]

and

> That which is real and that which is not depends on each author or rather, on what each author does with all the articles that preceded his own.[55]

Hence, according to Latour, the natural world may be irrelevant to the judgements scientists make while studying it. For such constructionists, social practices, as with "social causes" in the Strong Programme, are sufficient to account for scientific knowledge.

Discourse analysis

This approach assumes that scientists' discourse is too variable and too dependent on the context of its production for the sociologist to make narrow selections from it in order to "tell" a coherent story about the development of scientific knowledge (e.g. specify connections between actions). Indeed, to do this, argue discourse analysts, is distortive and "fundamentally unsociological in that the socially generated character of discourse itself is denied".[56] In particular, Gilbert & Mulkay suppose that most sociologists' data files contain diverse accounts of action and belief which are "normally suppressed as a result of those sociologists' unreflective commitment to the production of a unitary best account of the area of social life they have chosen to study".[57] Discourse analysts, therefore, do not attempt to go beyond scientists' accounts in order to describe and explain actions and beliefs, but instead investigate how the accounts themselves are socially constructed.[58] Moreover, they argue that the latter is methodologically prior to the former,[59] and that it "constitutes the only approach which holds out a promise . . . of rebuilding the sociological analysis of action and belief on a firmer methodological basis".[60]

Proponents of this approach seek to show how scientists' interpretive procedures vary according to social context, and to describe some of the implicit accomplishments of scientists' discourse.[61] Specifically discourse analysts focus on describing how scientists' accounts are organized to portray their actions and beliefs in contextually appropriate ways.[62] Like the advocates of the other three relativist programmes in the sociology of scientific knowledge, discourse analysts are markedly anti-realist, and reject the possibility of making rational judgements about the relative accuracy of alternative accounts about a real world. For example, Mulkay states:

My conclusion, then, is that neither citation data nor qualitative data can be used to furnish adequate characterisations of action or belief. . . . I hope it is clear that the traditional objective of describing and explaining what really happened has been abandoned . . . one is concerned only with interpreting given documents or recorded utterances.[63]

Similarly, Woolgar, also an active researcher in discourse analysis asserts:

there is no sense in which . . . the phenomenon . . . has an existence independent of its means of expression. . . . there is no object beyond discourse . . . the organization of discourse *is* the object. Nature and reality are the by-products rather than the predeterminants of scientific activity.[64]

To highlight their awareness (i.e. reflexivity) of the ostensible problem of discourse associated with "traditional" sociological descriptions, discourse analysts have experimented with "new literary forms", which involve publishing arguments in the form of conversations between the author and another protagonist, and frequent "reflexions" on the author's previous statements in the text.[65] They have not, however, shown any interest in relating their findings to the possible problem of bias in science, though this does not necessarily mean that it is impossible to detect commercial biases by analyzing scientists' discourse.

The problem of relativism

Adherence to relativism has created difficulties for the sociology of scientific knowledge. This is confirmed by the fact that not only critics, but also supporters of relativism have drawn attention to them. In this and the following section, two distinctly unsatisfactory characteristics of these research programmes in the sociology of scientific knowledge are examined with a view to informing a more valuable sociological approach to commercial bias in scientific knowledge.

Relativist sociology of scientific knowledge is correct to have insisted that it ought to be a reflexive enterprise. Any research is open to reflexivity; we can always ask whether the standards applied to examining some phenomena are also applied to the claims made by those doing the examining. But for a relativism, which is supposedly impartial with respect to the truth and falsity of statements made by scientists, and believes that truth is no more than a social construction, this is particularly problematic because, to be consistent, there can be no criteria for assessing the truth-value of its own claims about scientists' institutional interests, controversial views, laboratory practice or discourse. For example, in reflecting on his own sociology of knowledge Barnes acknowledges:

My own argument can, of course, be applied to itself to show that nothing in particular logically follows from my basic claims.[66]

On this view nothing conclusive can follow from relativist studies in the sociology of scientific knowledge. Collins, aware of this problem, argues against the conclusion that relativist sociology of scientific knowledge is self-defeating because its empirical findings have been interesting and useful.[67] It may well be that those findings are useful, but this response fails to indicate how we could consider any findings interesting or useful in the absence of any criteria of believability, truth or validity in the first place. Collins' argument, therefore, begs the whole question of how relativism can be reflexive without simultaneous self-destruction.

No solution is offered by the discourse analysts' attempt to bolster up the methodology of sociology of scientific knowledge by supposedly retreating from the notion that data refer to an objective reality in favour of analyses that stop at the text. The sense in which discourse analysis offers a *"firmer methodological basis"*[68] is not clear. Collins, for example, notes that the study of discourse as a topic is not qualitatively different from other sociological methods with respect to actually selecting data; it provides no guarantee of reducing the variability of accounts; it merely selects data differently and often provides more of it.[69] Nor is it obvious how discourse

11

analysts' claim to methodological priority can be consistent with a relativist philosophy which asserts that "belief systems [presumably including sociological methodologies like discourse analysis] cannot be objectively ranked in terms of their proximity to reality or rationality".[70] Indeed, as Doran[71] and Gieryn[72] contend, discourse analysts want to proclaim the truth value of their own work, therefore, apparently unselfconsciously taking a contradictory stance.

In an attempt to stave off the evident self-refuting character of relativist sociology of scientific knowledge, Mulkay claims that relativists are not committed to the claim that "we cannot discriminate between different forms of knowledge with a view to their relevance or adequacy in regard to a specific goal".[73] Rather he argues that they support epistemic, but not judgemental relativism. The former asserts that knowledge is historically and culturally relative and rejects any notion of absolute truth, while the latter denies the possibility that there can be any rational grounds for preferring one belief to another.[74] Similarly, in an attempt to defend social constructionism, Cozzens attests that it claims only that "the sciences do not produce absolute truth, not that they do not produce a form of knowledge that is better than others *for some particular purpose*".[75] (Emphasis in original)

The criteria of "relevance", "adequacy" and of being "better", however, remain mysteriously elusive and are relative to a "specific goal" or "some particular purpose". These arguments imply that different goals entail different criteria of relevance and adequacy, and in the absence of any objective criteria, such as truth-value, common to different goals, cannot be distinguished from judgemental relativism. If truth-value is one such criterion, then the relativist commitment to impartiality, with respect to truth and falsity, need not and cannot be maintained; but if not, then the collapse into judgemental relativism cannot be prevented nor fail to be comprehensive. Thus, the position of Mulkay and Cozzens is little more than a re-statement of the problem they attempt to tackle. Moreover, it is clear that some in the relativist camp do subscribe unreservedly to judgemental relativism. For example, Latour states:

> cognitive abilities, methods, adjectives and adverbs do not make a difference among beliefs and knowledge because everyone on earth is as logical or as illogical as anyone else.[76]

As Sismondo notes in his review of constructionism, such relativism is also analytically deprived because it denies the possibility of error or misrepresentation.[77]

A further problem of reflexivity, which afflicts the Strong Programme and the Empirical Programme of Relativism, is the view that the methodology of the sociology of scientific knowledge should be rooted in an idealization of science, which pursues knowledge from a position of value-neutrality.[78] This is problematic because, as Millstone points out, one lesson of the sociology of knowledge is that the possibility of adopting a position of neutrality is limited and not necessarily desirable.[79] It follows, therefore, that the findings of the sociology of scientific knowledge about human beliefs are incompatible with its own methodology if the latter are to be based on the suspension of value-judgements.

Another approach, taken by Woolgar, is to accept that reflexivity poses insurmountable problems for relativism, and to surrender the possibility of criteria of validity for knowledge claims:

> We might as well admit that the problem is both insoluble and unavoidable, and that even efforts to examine *how* it is avoided are doomed in that they entail an attempt to avoid it! . . . the fact that all our analyses are essentially flawed is better celebrated than concealed.[80] (Emphasis in original)

Similarly discourse analysts are pessimistic about their contribution to knowledge since, rooted firmly in relativism,[81] they believe it is unable to provide definitive accounts of participants' texts and utterances.[82] Mulkay, for instance, advocates the dissolution of any boundaries between fiction and the development of knowledge:

> Why not relax and accept that none of us is engaged in describing the social world? We are creators of meanings appropriate to the occasion, like dramatists, novelists and ordinary speakers.[83]

This discourse analysts' retreat from the pursuit of knowledge may be seen as an attempt to make their arguments consistent with their commitment to both relativism and reflexivity. For example, Woolgar reaches his position by criticizing the Strong Programme for (unreflexively) not addressing its own dependence on realist discourse.[84]

Since for relativist discourse analysts, texts can never refer to an independent objective reality, nor form part of such a reality themselves, but merely reflect the construction of the reader, it follows that the meaning attributable to any text is unproblematically arbitrarily malleable according to the whims of the reader. This would make it impossible to fix any meaning to an independent reference point (i.e. the reality to which the text refers) by which agreements and/or disagreements between different readers could be identified and communicated. Consequently, far from facilitating the valuable projects of communication through "new literary forms" and of engaging actively in the world in order to create the possibility of alternative forms of social life"[85] to which Mulkay aspires, the relativism he supports would, if seriously applied, imply that discourse analysts could only talk to themselves.

To summarize the argument so far, attempts to defend relativist sociology of scientific knowledge against the charge that it is self-refuting fail, and only multiply the incoherencies of the position. However, some scholars (e.g. Woolgar and Mulkay) accept that relativism is self-defeating, yet view this as merely a manifestation of the hopelessness of pursuing the goal of systematic knowledge in general. Paradoxically, though, Mulkay and Woolgar do not seem to recognize (at least explicitly) the consequent destruction implied therein for discourse analysis itself.

The problem of internalism
Though Merton and Kuhn differed in their concerns with scientific knowledge, their work shares the characteristic of "academic internalism".[86] Much of post-Kuhnian sociology of scientific knowledge continues this tradition in which modern science is viewed as an autonomous academic research community, rarely influenced by the State, industry or entrepreneurs.[87] Yet as Johnston & Robbins point out, this is an "increasingly idealised, non-existent science".[88] As early as 1969, Ellis[89] noted that *most* scientists worked in industry or government, and that in these sectors they did not internalize the Mertonian and neo-Mertonian[90] ethos of science, but rather took an instrumental careerist view of their scientific work. Subsequently, Blume, Sklair and Johnston & Robbins called for a more broadly conceived sociology of science to investigate the industrialization of the scientific community, and the latter's relationship with political institutions.[91] The importance of these proposals can only have increased as studies such as that by McCain have drawn attention to the commercial instrumentalism within even academic science.[92]

Some research in the sociology of scientific knowledge, particularly the Laboratory Studies approach, has entered the institutions of industrial science but, according to Knorr-Cetina and also Mulkay and Cozzens & Gieryn, the field remains dominated by "methodological internalism",[93] so that the internal practices of the scientific enterprise (whether in academia, industry or government) constitute the focus of inquiry.[94] Consequently, sociology of science has earned a reputation for "avoidance of the roles of professional power and broader structural influences in the constitution of scientific knowledge".[95] This phenomenon is highlighted in the case of discourse analysis which, critics contend, has attempted a "change in sociological focus from scientific beliefs and knowledge to the study of texts for text's sake",[96] and to "incestuous reflexions".[97] Similarly, in relation to controversies, Collins admits:

> Studies of contemporary pure science have rarely looked outside the scientific community itself for explanations of the outcomes of controversies. Only in historical studies have the specific outcomes of debates been explained by reference to wider social and political factors.[98]

Chubin, who notes that sociological studies of science are conspicuously absent from sites of public controversy, remarks fastidiously:

> their scope is oddly confined to "scientific culture"; their thrust eschews the study of disputes that spill into the public domain where ideologies and interest groups clash. If conflicting claims are made by non-experts . . . *and something more than resolution is at stake, such as regulation, then the site is taboo.*[99] (Emphasis added)

Notwithstanding a few exceptions,[100] that progress has been slow in shedding the worst aspects of internalism is confirmed by Nelkin in 1989 who, reflecting on the previous thirteen years of the sociology of science, concludes:

> the concept of "social" is still mainly defined in terms of the inter-actions and discourse among scientists. Moreover, *the field is still turned inward, into itself,* creating its own language with too little reference to the outside world. There are still relatively few studies concerned with [science's] social relations outside the laboratory context. Rare are the studies that focus on the ideologies embedded in science because of its political and economic relationships, and its proximity to centers of power.[101] (Emphasis added)

Marxist science studies

While relativist sociology of scientific knowledge neglects the wider political and economic contexts of science, radical Marxist approaches to science, as typified by the Radical Science Collective, are open to no such criticism. This Marxist tradition owes its origins to the work of Hessen who attempted no less than to locate and describe the "social and economic roots of Newton's 'Principia'".[102] Primacy is given to the *political*

15

economy in such analyses of science. They add to the discussion, therefore, an explicit model of how capitalist societies operate with particular focus on the labour process, capital accumulation and the conflicting interests that arise as a result.

For radical Marxists, scientific knowledge has developed in the context of capitalist industrialization and, as a consequence, is penetrated by ideology – a variably distorted worldview generated by a fetishism with commodity production in capitalist societies:

> The form of thinking which is common to Galilean science and commodity exchange plays an important role in maintaining a given set of social and economic relations. It has an ideological or "socially-synthetic" function. The form of social synthesis prevailing in any epoch depends on the dominant structure of production or, more precisely, on the form of the labour process of production, which, in turn, depends on the stage of development of the productive forces.[103]

Thus, it is argued that the dynamics of science cannot be isolated from the *history* of societal development. Moreover, modern scientific knowledge is responsive to, and reflective of, the prevailing capitalist values. As Slack puts it:

> reorganization of [scientific] theory does not proceed along *any* channels but along particular ones. If certain values are current among those who rule society then certain goals are sought and disciplines are mobilized to achieve them.[104] (Emphasis in original)

More recently, Fisher has extended Slack's model of scientific knowledge production by making use of Gieryn's concept of "boundary work", which incorporates the processes whereby legitimacy and authority come to be attached to knowledge units as a result of capitalist interests.[105] For example, according to Fisher, "boundary work" was done by capitalist interests during the Rockefeller family's involvement with the creation of the American Social Science Research Council (SSRC) in the mid 1920s. The Rockefeller Foundation wished to promote social scientific research geared to the maintenance of social stability and economic efficiency, but wanted those goals to appear to have come from (social) scientists themselves. Thus, argues Fisher, it set up advisory committees of (social) scientists, who were willing to approve of its objectives, and to organize and allocate the Foundation's funding of the SSRC. Consequently, particular kinds of social scientific research were undertaken and the knowledge produced gained significant professional legitimacy and authority.[106]

Like the advocates of relativist sociology of scientific knowledge, radical Marxists reject the proposition that science is essentially neutral in its production and biased solely through its use.[107] Rather, scientific knowledge itself is biased in that it is developed to serve capitalist interests. In its crudest form this thesis has been cast in the slogan "science *is* social relations".[108] (Emphasis in original) On this model science has *no* autonomy; social relations are inseparable from science, facts and nature.[109] Superficially it may seem as though radical Marxist science studies are similar to relativist sociology of scientific knowledge because scientific knowledge is collapsed into social conditions in both approaches. However, the former is, in fact, the methodological converse of the latter. The Strong Programme bases its methodology on an idealization of science and the scientific methodology. It "relativizes everything except science",[110] whereas radical Marxists make science (located in the superstructure) completely relative to *objective* sociohistorical conditions.[111]

It may be noted that the characterization of science found in radical Marxist science studies differs markedly from that contained in the writings of Marx himself, and from what Lukacs referred to as "orthodox Marxism".[112] Marx believed that science provided a valuable methodology for the objective analysis of society,[113] and that science and technology were historically progressive resources used by capitalism.[114] It was on this reading of Marx that the more "reformist" approach to science adopted by Bernal in the 1930s was based. Bernalism recognized the integral role of science in the development of capitalism, but maintained that science was ultimately liberating and, therefore, anti-capitalist.[115] Thus, scientific *knowledge* was accorded a politically neutral status; it could be directed to good or evil. In this respect Bernalism offers little advance on Mertonianism.

On the other hand, one major drawback of adopting the radical Marxist science studies framework is that it is too reductionist because it denies the cognitive autonomy of science throughout history, and because scientists and scientific knowledge in capitalist societies do not always serve capitalist interests.[116] Moreover, empirical case studies are rare within the Marxist camp and, as a result, it remains highly theoretical. Nevertheless, Marxism has the virtue of suggesting how the drive for capital accumulation can bias the development of scientific knowledge. Specifically, it points to the need to relate the study of commercial bias in science to capitalist interests and their historical development.

Risk studies

Risk assessment developed initially as a "scientistic"[117] response by industry, especially the nuclear industry, to the perceptions of environmentalist
and consumer movements in the 1960s that many industrial technologies
posed undesirable and unacceptable risks to (certain sections of) society.[118]
In a similar vein, the strategy adopted by governments was to rely on scientists to define risks as a way of providing a rational basis for technology
policy decisions, which entailed some perceived societal hazards. However, Weinberg's seminal paper on "trans-science" marked the beginning
of an explicit awareness that a different relationship between scientists
and regulators was needed to tackle the inherent problems of risk assessment.[119]

For Weinberg a great deal of risk assessment should be considered
"trans-scientific" because it generates questions "which can be asked of
science yet which cannot be answered by science".[120] The central consequence of this, he argued, is that risk assessment and related technology
policy discussions should involve some wider public, and not merely scientists:

> In so far as public policy involves trans-scientific rather than scien-
> tific issues, the role of the scientist in contributing to the promulga-
> tion of such policy must be different from his role when the issues
> can be unambiguously answered by science. . . . Where science
> and politics meet . . . issues can no longer be settled by scientists
> alone. . . . The issues affect everyone and therefore everyone, in
> some sense, has a right to be heard.[121]

Unlike the dominant perspectives in the sociology of scientific knowledge, contemporary risk control studies share with Weinberg an explicit
concern with the relationship between science and politics in the arena of
regulatory policy.[122] Though Lowrance,[123] Mazur[124] and Ravetz[125] erect a
discrete boundary between an ostensibly value-free risk evaluation, on the
one hand, and value judgements about the acceptability of risk, on the
other, most of the literature focuses on risk assessment as a *socio-institutional
process*, and the way in which it misrepresents social uncertainties as technical ones.[126] Its most frequent complaint is that industrial, governmental
and other official bodies bias discussion about risk regulation by downplaying the pervasive scientific uncertainties involved. The following comment by Linnerooth is typical:

> A highly uncertain decision environment presents untold difficul-

ties to a public institution that must staunchly support its policies and maintain the impression of control. An agency in such an environment will quite naturally attempt to constrain and define the problem in such a way that it has the appearance of being controllable or manageable. In so doing, it is often necessary to frame the uncertainties such that they appear "normal" or "ordinary".[127]

Another common feature of writers on risk is the emphasis on the divisions between experts and lay people in assessments of risk. Expertise is generally associated with scientific rationality about which there is an implicit and sometimes explicit suspicion. Experts utilizing scientific rationality are often presented as short-changing lay groups whose views are supposed to derive from a competing alternative rationality, perhaps of equal validity to that of the experts.[128] That model of competing rationalities has led some sociologists of risk, such as Beck, to conclude that "because risks are risks in knowledge, perceptions of risk and risks are not different things, but one and the same".[129]

This approach is closely associated with the increasingly popular cultural theory of risk. Here political cultures holding different values towards risk (e.g. "egalitarian", "fatalist" and "individualist") are hypothesized to co-exist. Each political culture is tightly bound by its premises which lead to perfectly rational beliefs about risks within their respective frameworks. And according to cultural theorists, such as Schwarz & Thompson, there are no objective criteria by which competing sets of beliefs *between* different political cultures can be judged. We may not conclude that a belief is wrong or irrational, but only that we hold a different view within a different rationality, and, therefore, potentially a different political culture.[130]

For Schwarz & Thompson these plural rationalities give rise to cultural biases towards risk. But because all of these rationalities can be biased, bias is defined to be all-pervasive. Schwarz & Thompson conclude:

> The central message . . . is that all is bias. Our knowing is biased, our acting is biased, our justifying of our actions is biased, and our judging of the actions of others is biased.[131]

Among the social scientists of risk, who advocate social change, there tends to be considerable agreement about the route for reform of risk assessment: institutions, especially regulatory agencies, should be more open to public scrutiny and participation.[132] If implemented, such appeals for change could have dual relevance to bias. First, as Hattis & Kennedy note, bias in *representation* could be reduced:

> . . . risk assessors tend to omit issues that they have decided are too uninteresting, difficult to quantify, speculative, or likely to be "misinterpreted". To prevent this kind of preselection, we should ensure that analysts publicly disclose the choices they make.[133]

And secondly, greater public participation in risk assessment could decrease bias in regulatory *outcomes* thereby enhancing the "social viability"[134] of technology, as Fiorino argues:

> Public participation could inform policy-makers on such generic issues as how to weigh sources of uncertainty in risk assessments, how to compare risks that are distributed broadly to those that are concentrated and socially disruptive, or how to balance scientific uncertainty against the magnitude or irreversibilty of health or ecological effects. The objective should be to inform our [risk assessment] models . . . by engaging people in the reasoning and discussion that defines their role as citizens.[135]

Without question an overriding theme in the burgeoning risk studies literature is the problem of bias in scientific knowledge. Unlike the internalist studies in the sociology of scientific knowledge, risk studies focus on *government* scientists and the political implications of the distinction between scientific expertise and lay knowledge. The bureaucratic scientist, who wants to rationalize social problems into technical solutions, is portrayed as being at odds with the wider public who need scientific knowledge to be demystified and perhaps even deconstructed. It may be said, then, that while relativist sociology of scientific knowledge is sceptical about scientific *knowledge per se*, risk studies are sceptical about scientific *expertise per se*.

Despite the popularity of this school of thought it has major limitations, especially in relation to the conceptualization of bias. There is a tendency to conflate science, rationality and expertise. Consequently, if a group of expert scientists act in an unreasonably dismissive way towards some lay people experiencing certain risks, then risk studies interpret that action as yet another example of the insulated nature of science from alternative rationalities. Consider the following way in which Beck implicates science in increasing risks to the public:

> By turning up the standard of scientific accuracy, the circle of recognized risks justifying action is minimized, and consequently scientific license is implicitly granted for the multiplication of risks.[136]

The key problem with these approaches is that they operate at a level which is too general and undiscriminating. In *some* contexts Beck's claim about scientific standards of accuracy may be true, but in others it is not. For example, in the next chapter I shall discuss how advances in the scientific detection of drug adulteration provided the possibility for stricter regulatory controls which could reduce *risks* to the public. Moreover, scientists do not fit easily into a spectrum of experts versus lay rationalities. Sometimes particular scientists with considerable expertise may be profoundly critical of governmental or industrial scientists. Those critical experts may be allied to certain lay groups and collectively they may draw on the crucial resources of rationality and some aspects of scientific expertise in order to expose the *irrationality* of certain establishment experts who are behaving indefensibly.

Equally, lay perceptions of risk can *sometimes* simply be wrong because those lay people lack certain expertise or knowledge. In such cases we should acknowledge that those perceptions may be irrational and seek to provide the people with the expertise they need in order to make informed judgements, rather than labelling their ignorance as "alternative rationality". Of course, this is certainly not to argue that lay perceptions *per se* should be dismissed or that in most cases lay perceptions of risk are invalid. The crucial point is that the "plural rationalities" approach of cultural theory and cultural bias does not allow for the possibility that critical scientists can utilize expertise to expose the irrationality of claims made by other scientists or that lay people sometimes need rationality and the expertise of science (rather than some alternative rationality) to actually make sense of risks.

Interestingly, Beck does acknowledge the role of critical experts in his discussion of "alternative expertise" and "the scientization of the protest against science",[137] but what is less clear is whether he appreciates the need to distinguish between a protest against science *per se* and a protest against certain aspects of the organization and development of scientists and scientific knowledge. Furthermore, the precise relationship between "alternative expertise" and rationality is not clear in Beck's thesis. Can the "alternative experts" demonstrate the superiority of their claims over those of the establishment experts? Or are they trapped incommensurably within their own rationality? The cultural theory of Schwarz & Thompson suggests incommensurable entrapment:

> Our concern, therefore, should not be with which one is right (for that would be to insist that just one rationality had access to "the truth"), but rather with which is *appropriate* to the task at hand.[138] (Emphasis in original)

Leaving aside the problem of relativism implicit in the above prescription, we should note that it drastically limits the scope and intelligibility of any social and political analysis of science because the *validity* of scientists' claims escapes scrutiny. It follows from the cultural theory espoused by Schwarz & Thompson, therefore, that bias can have no relationship to validity. And since in cultural theory bias is endemic to all beliefs and actions, the concept of bias loses all analytical power within this framework (e.g. to say scientist X is biased tells us nothing more precise than to say that scientist X is alive). Thus, although cultural theory gives considerable attention to the notion of bias, its treatment does not provide a satisfactory framework for empirical investigation.

Finally on risk studies, with a few notable exceptions, such as Irwin's analysis of road traffic safety,[139] little detailed empirical research has been undertaken to document the historical and political factors producing bias in the first place. Important as the government-centred approach is, it is necessary to examine the power structures beyond the State, which influence the context in which government experts operate. This is compounded by an apparent reluctance within risk studies to provide any explicit model of interests in society, of the kind offered by Marxist science studies, within which institutional motivations for suppression of uncertainty or disregard for lay perceptions can be placed, differentiated and understood. The concern with making uncertainty *per se* available to the public fails to specify the precise interests at stake in achieving this goal.

Theories of the State and regulatory capture

I have mentioned that one limitation of risk studies is their inattention to power structures which can *create and sustain* bias. In fact, none of the perspectives considered so far tackles this problem in a way which can be directly related to regulatory institutions and policies. Yet where scientific claims are subject to review by regulatory authorities, as is the case with drug testing in the pharmaceutical industry, the interaction between technical expertise and commercial bias in science cannot properly be understood without an appreciation of the political context in which regulatory decisions are taken. The purpose of this section is to consider some contributions in the literature that can enhance such an appreciation.

Probably the best known theory of regulatory "capture" is Bernstein's "life-cycle" theory of regulatory commissions. According to Bernstein, a regulatory commission is typically established as a result of some compromise legislation designed to protect certain groups against the abuses of the regulated industry. Initially the commission tends to be aggressive and adversarial towards it regulatees, but becomes isolated as its enthusiasts tire and retire. Eventually it is progressively "captured" by, and comes to share the perspectives of, the regulated industry.[140] Judge Lee Loevinger, a former Head of the Antitrust Division of the US Department of Justice succinctly illustrates this model of regulatory authorities:

> Unfortunately the history of every regulatory agency in the government is that it comes to represent the industry or groups it's supposed to control. All of these agencies were fine when they were set up, but before long they became infiltrated by the regulatees and are now more or less run by and for them. More, the agency people consort with this or that representative of some special interest group, and finally they all come to think alike.[141]

From this stage onwards, argue capture theorists, the regulatory authority is biased in favour of industrial interests unless, and until, a scandal highlighting the failures of regulation triggers a new drive for adversary, and consequently, the commencement of a new cycle. Arguments of this genre are often referred to as "public interest" theories because they assume that, at the outset, regulation was established in order to serve the public interest, and that its proper role is to continue to do so.[142] (The "public interest" being the interest of the politically inactive public who nevertheless are deemed to have certain interests which could be reflected by the actions of some organized interest group, such as an industry or a consumer group).

Some traditional Marxist theories of the State stand this view on its head by arguing that regulation is an instrument of working class oppression utilized and propped up by capitalist interests.[143] The State has few, if any, interests of its own: it is used *against* the wider public by private interests. However, modern Marxists argue that the State has some "autonomy" from the capitalist class, and that the people who run it have interests of their own, which cannot be assumed to be synonymous with the interests of the dominant classes in capitalist society.[144] Nevertheless, the main focus of most Marxist theories of the State remains class interests so that the exercise of State power is generally interpreted in terms of class struggle within or outside State apparatuses; the State being seen as in "partnership" with the capitalist class.[145]

Like Marxists, "private interest" theorists[146] have challenged the assumption that regulatory agencies are established to serve the public interest. Stigler, for example, argues that regulation is developed to help certain commercial interests to achieve a monopoly in the market. The direction of regulation is, therefore, heavily influenced by the economic process of supply and demand. However, the industry seeking regulation must be prepared to pay for it by supplying votes and resources to political parties. Regulatory outcomes and attendant biases thus reflect the balance of powers between competing industrial pressures on the State.[147]

Despite the relevance of these theories for a study of regulatory bias, they are subject to a number of criticisms. First, they tend to treat the regulatory agency itself as a "black box".[148] Secondly, as Sabatier suggests, it is not inevitable that regulatory agencies will acquiesce to industrial opposition.[149] Indeed, McGaffrey argues that attempted coercion by private interests can lead to strong reactions within agencies to avoid being coerced.[150] Thirdly, the significant costs and technological changes which private organizations undertake in order to cope with regulation, are not consistent with the view that commercial companies ward off regulation by dominating regulatory agencies.[151] Fourthly, because of divisions within and between industries, they may dominate the regulatory process effectively only when the benefits of a certain policy to sectional interests are concentrated whereas the costs to others are diffuse.[152] Finally, Marxist theories of the State are weak in providing a framework capable of indentifying any bias in regulation other than that related to *class* interests, and, therefore, may be insufficiently discriminating to detect intra-class conflicts of interest and cross-class common interests.

Corporatist theorists, who have recognized some of these problems, assume neither that regulatory authorities merely serve capitalist interests, by capture or otherwise, nor that all interests are reducible to class.[153] Rather, the State has some ultimate powers of coercion, but its precise role is defined in relation to the power of *organized interests*.[154] However, since different groups in society have unequal capacities to organize, the role of the State is biased accordingly. Such "corporate bias"[155] involves regular bargaining between organized interests and the State about the extent of regulation, and goes beyond lobbying and pressure group politics. As Middlemas explains:

> To put it simply, what had been merely interest groups crossed the political threshold and became part of the extended state: a position from which other groups, even if they too held political power, were still excluded.[156]

This kind of interest interdependence can lead to "private interest government" whereby "regulated self-regulation", the devolving of public responsibilities to private interests, is substituted for State regulation.[157] In one sense, therefore, regulatory capture can be thought of as the absolute extreme of corporatism in which the State has yielded virtually all power to the regulated industry.

All these theories of the State are relevant to commercial bias in drug regulation. The role played by government scientists and scientific expertise needs to be conceptualized so as to take account of the constraining influences on the State *vis-à-vis* its relationships with relevant organized interests. As a starting point for investigation corporatist theory has the advantage of not overly prejudging the nature of the regulatory process either in terms of the fundamental interests at stake (e.g. class interests for Marxists) or in assumptions about regulatory authorities in relation to the "public interest". Rather, corporatist theory treats bias as an empirical quantity, whose extent and influence can be documented in particular policy fields (e.g. as in "meso-corporatism").[158]

A synthesis and a framework

Relativism does not provide an adequate philosophical basis for the sociology of scientific knowledge and *a fortiori* for a study of bias in science and regulation since, as Meynell puts it, "when made self-consistent and thoroughly applied [it] destroys itself".[159] However, it does indicate the direction in which a more sound position can be found because, as Lukes has argued, commonly shared standards of truth and of inference together with a common core of beliefs, whose content and meaning is fixed by such standards, must be presupposed before the problem of relativism can be set up in the first place:

> without such a common core, the entire enterprise of interpretation and translation cannot get started: the meanings of beliefs cannot be identified and so questions about the relativity or otherwise of their truth values or rationality cannot even be raised.[160]

This common core provides a "bridgehead"[161] between otherwise radically different belief systems which is justified by the following *objectivist realist* argument advanced by Bhaskar:

> the existence of a common world . . . [and] certain very shared human interests in it, stemming from our nature as biologically con-

stituted beings with a certain innate development . . . facilitate the establishment of a bridgehead between cultures, composed mainly of beliefs about the everyday world geared largely to sustaining a viable mode of material human being.[162]

Such "beliefs about the everyday world" can be thought of as consistent with a *language-learned* correspondence theory of truth (i.e. given that one has learned the meanings of "rat", "cage", "five" etc., then the simple observation that five rats are in the cage is sufficient to conclude that the claim "five rats are in the cage" is true). However, Chalmers[163] and Nagel[164] draw a sharp distinction between this commonsense knowledge and scientific knowledge since, as Bhaskar[165] emphasizes, the latter is not gained *merely* through observations of events, but involves the manipulation of theoretical entities (e.g. magnetic fields).

Beliefs in science, therefore, can be far removed from the observational periphery. Nevertheless, this does not imply the need for a relativist sociology of science. As Laboratory Studies research has shown, the distinction between commonsense and scientific knowledge cannot be so easily retained.[166] Hacking[167] provides an example of this in his discussion of Herschel's experiments using colour filters to study radiant heat. A commonsense truth resulting from the experiment was that Herschel noticed some colours warmed his skin, while others did not. This is something that could be conveyed in any language, and can be regarded as part of a bridgehead in any theoretical dispute between scientists about radiant heat. As Bhaskar puts it, the bridgehead permits the development of a language which acts as a common "a-theoretic intra-scientific auxiliary, in terms of which the conflicting implications of . . . widely meaning-divergent theories can, in the last resort, be spelt out, in the event that the scientific communities are not sufficiently bi-theoretically lingual".[168]

The objectivist realist position, outlined above by Bhaskar and Lukes, therefore, permits and presupposes the existence of at least some truths. In particular, the possibility of meaningful agreement and disagreement depends on a foundation in an agreement (i.e. bridgehead) which comprises truths. Otherwise language could not operate as a means of communication. Whether the bridgehead is a "massive central core of human thinking that has no history", as Strawson[169] maintains, or is historically relative as Bhaskar[170] contends, does not affect the significant consequence of realism that systematic knowledge (of commercial bias in science and regulation) can be pursued with more or less accuracy.[171] Moreover, as Russell,[172] Chubin and Restivo[173] and others[174] have argued, it is neither necessary nor desirable that such knowledge should be sought from a position of supposed value-neutrality or internalism. Millstone's comments are most germane:

> Pursuing knowledge from a non-neutral, committed position is not necessarily incompatible with the discovery of truths. . . . It is not possible to adopt beliefs in total independence of our social condition, so we have to recognize each position as a committed, rather than neutral stance. The choice is not between being neutral or being committed; the question is whether or not to be self-conscious of our commitments, and whether or not we are committed to the right things. If the sociology of knowledge is to be informative and relevant it must be committed intellectually to accuracy and truth. However, some truths are socially more important and useful than others. The sociology of knowledge should be pursued in relation to some broader social objectives.[175]

It does not follow from these arguments, however, that the sociology of scientific knowledge has nothing to offer research into commercial bias in science. As Bartels[176] notes, researchers in the sociology of scientific knowledge have not realized the significance of their own work for the politics of science. Indeed, my previous criticisms of the declared relativist philosophy associated with much sociology of scientific knowledge should be seen in the context of the realism endemic to the *empirical research practised* in the field by the four relativistic schools I have considered. Contrary to the views of Mackenzie[177] and Collins,[178] the previous discussion does suggest that this is because those researchers' mode of argumentation has been severely hampered by an adherence to relativism.

There is no inconsistency, therefore, in arguing that the empirical findings and methodologies of the sociology of scientific knowledge produced in the name of relativism are valuable to an explicitly realist sociology of scientific knowledge because the former's important contributions have been achieved *despite its declared relativism rather than because of it.* Sismondo reaches a similar conclusion about social constructionism when he refers to the "rhetorical role" of anti-realist claims within constructionism – claims which he argues are often ignored or contradicted by the practices of constructionists.[179] A political sociology of scientific knowledge should reject the relativist philosophy that has dominated much of the sociology of scientific knowledge, but embrace a realist reading of the substantive findings therein. The abandonment of relativism, therefore, does not entail the demise of sociology of scientific knowledge.

In fact, Barnes, an enthusiast of relativism, was one of the first to suggest a valuable method for imputing bias by exposing *inconsistencies* between knowledge claims established as standards in the scientific literature and the claims made by certain interest groups. In an uncharacteristically explicit reference to bias, Barnes discusses how social factors, which may provide reasons for departures from "normality" in scientific practice, can be identified by setting institutionalized scientific beliefs against "an unproblematic baseline of normality".[180] As he puts it:

> By recourse to its own normal practice, scientific work can itself be criticized and, if one insists on putting it so, revealed as ideologically determined.[181]

After applying this method to a scientific debate about the adverse health effects of cannibis he concludes:

> There is a strong *prima facie* case for suggesting that social factors making for hostility to cannibis use have biased the popular presentation of our knowledge of its toxic and "harmful" properties.[182]

Chubin has generalized this method of imputing bias in science to inconsistencies in what scientists claim in different contexts:

> Since it is values . . . that researchers bring to bear in the interpretation of data, observing what is claimed, by whom, and to what apparent end . . . should be instructive. This is surely . . . where sociologists of science can bountifully note what scientists do, say they do, and given one's archival data, write about doing. Any emerging gulfs between the written and spoken word, offered in a different setting to divergent audiences, are measures of values and rhetoric in the reconstruction of intellectual and political history.[183]

One of the few researchers to apply this approach in a detailed empirical study is Wynne. He examined the *technical inconsistencies* in a scientific institution's *account of itself* and concluded that the claims it made to superior technical "rigour" over alternative scientific views were "quite false".[184]

The Strong Programme and laboratory studies suggest that scientific knowledge develops in relation to interests and goals, including credibility, promotion and professional recognition. Martin suggests that such interests and goals can create bias by "pushing" science to particular conclusions and not others.[185] Another indicator of bias, therefore, is the inconsistent way in which some arguments are emphasized and others are neglected in the development of scientific conclusions. It is not merely the "pushing" towards the establishment of certainty and facts that is significant, but also the *selectivity* of the pushing process.[186] Contributors to the

Empirical Programme of Relativism and other authors[187] suggest that scientific controversies are a fruitful context in which to examine such bias. In particular, Brante & Elzinga point to the relevance of controversy studies for scrutinizing bias in industrial and governmental scientific activity.[188]

The methodology adopted in this book to investigate bias in drug testing and regulation owes much to the approaches of Wynne, Martin, Chubin and Barnes noted in this section. The study of scientific controversies is extensive in this book, and follows the recommendations of Richards to apply the "controversy method" to the relatively neglected field of contemporary medical science and technology.[189] That analysis focuses on the role of possible commercial bias in industrial and government science by locating and investigating *technical inconsistencies* present in scientists' claims and accounts of their actions. Such inconsistencies may be internal to: an individual scientist, whose claims in different contexts are contradictory; the official view of scientists in a company, who may contradict each other; the scientific field, whose declared standards may be violated by the actions of an individual scientist or institution which generally accepts the standards within the scientific field as legitimate; or a regulatory agency, whose actions may contradict its own scientific standards.

Bias, therefore, should be distinguished from "deviance" or "nonorthodoxy"[190] because in the latter two cases the scientist or institution in question does not accept the prevailing standards of the scientific field as legitimate (e.g. as in parapsychology). Moreover, contrary to the philosophical position adopted by Martin,[191] imputing bias to scientists does not, in my view, necessarily imply a commitment to positivism, in the sense of scientism or value-free science.[192] Nevertheless, in line with the realist position I advanced earlier, it does assume that, given certain socially derived and commonly agreed standards of communication and reason, objective assessments of knowledge claims can be made by reference to those standards. Although scientists sometimes disagree wildly, such assessments are sometimes possible because frequently scientists do agree on some standards. One definition of bias in science, then, is the advocacy/practice of claims/actions that are non-credible because they are inconsistent with the very scientific standards which the advocate/practitioner accepts as legitimate, and are convergent with identifiable interests/values.

For example, toxicologists are universally agreed on the social conventions of arithmetic and counting, although not necessarily statistical techniques. They are also able to agree through enculturation and training on the identification of rats (and even particular strains of rats) as distinct from mice or cages, and on distinguishing a live rat from a dead one. Agreed standards of this kind can be applied by sociologists to provide some objective criteria of validity (truth-value) regarding claims about, say, the number of rats which may have survived a particular experimental test at various points in time. Claims made by toxicologists that depend on inconsistencies with the rules (of counting, rat identification and so on) governing the recording of rat mortality lack validity and credibility, given the cognitive standards of toxicological science. Such inconsistencies are especially, but not exclusively, indicative that there are non-technical reasons for the scientific claims in question. Hence, one might suppose that some form of bias explains the inconsistency, but that supposition would depend on adducing other evidence about the social context of the experiment, including the interests at stake in the results.

It may be noted that objective assessments within scientific standards are not necessarily achieved in a value-free way; they may be pursued from a value-committed, yet no less objective, position. It follows from this that (technical) inconsistencies, though methodologically useful for revealing the role of values and interests in science, are not necessary for such values and interests to be influential, for an entirely consistent set of scientists' claims may derive from a value-committed, interest-laden position. However, inconsistencies in scientists' claims are necessary, though not sufficient, to impute the operation of bias. Thus, to assert bias in science, as I have defined it, is to make a stronger claim than merely to acknowledge a role for values, as cultural theory would have it. Indeed, such a stronger claim is essential if the concept of bias is to offer any substantial analytical power to science and technology studies.

Both Marxist and corporatist theories suggest that regulatory decisions should be interpreted in a wider historical and political context, which defines the demands and goals of the regulatory institution in question. As I mentioned earlier corporatist theory provides a promising methodology for examining empirically specific biases in the interest orientation of State regulation because it neither reduces the interests of the latter to class interests nor conceives of the State as an autonomous entity with fixed boundaries. This raises the question of how "interests" should be conceptualized within an analysis of bias in science.

Notwithstanding the value of corporatist theory for empirical research, I suggest that there is one respect in which the Marxist approach is to be preferred: the specification of *real* interests. Marxism and corporatist theory (including the extreme case of capture) share an implicit "rational action" model of interests in which the "most rational means to a goal are those which give the actor the highest chance of success".[193] For example, the deliberate and systematic pursuit of profit in the case of the capitalist.[194] Hence, rational actors attempt to maximize whatever benefits their own interests. It is in the specification of interests themselves that difficulties arise within corporatist theory which, according to Cawson, asserts that interests are "organized within a framework of opportunities",[195] and that organization is the mobilization of bias whereby some interests are organized into politics while others are organized out.[196] One objection to such a formulation is that the *framework* for identifying interests remains unclear without some evaluative criteria with respect to opportunities, i.e. the framework of opportunities is all-important for giving some order to the identification of interests, yet it remains unspecified. That this presents difficulties is hinted at by two leading commentators on government–industry relations:

> Our primary concern is with the understanding and analysis of the processes of government–industry relations: how the various organizations interact; what goals the key players pursue; how they construct their strategies; and how they influence one another. *Our contention is that there is virtually no systematic ordering of material in this area* . . . [197] (Emphasis added)

A possible response to this problem, advanced by Schwarz & Thompson in the most recent variant of pluralistic cultural theory, is to argue that interest explanations of social action are tautological and, therefore, that "politics of interest" models should be replaced by typologies of "cultural bias".[198] The result, however, is unsatisfactory. In general, they interchange corporatist theory's ambiguity about interests with an over-socialized model of individuals who cling to cultural biases, and an over-voluntaristic view of social groups whose collective commitments are oddly unconstrained by political economy. A corollary to this is that this pluralistic cultural approach lacks a theory of power so that the policy process is effectively reduced to group pressure politics ("political culture") with the government playing a central role in modifying public debate. The possibility that government policy might be constrained or influenced by the international or national economy is overlooked. This seems to be deficient in view of Ronge's hypothesis about government policy-making in the field of risk analysis:

> The political system is by no means autonomous in choosing its

tasks and ends. . . . There are not only general but also specific informational limits affecting political decision making, which mainly result from the decentralised structure of capitalist economy to which policy-making refers and is bound. . . . Consequently, instead of being primarily concerned as to whether the people will voluntarily accept the decisions made, political decision-makers tend to, and are themselves bound to, force the people into compliance because they are themselves subject to the pressures of economic forces and considerations. . . . safety and risk are at least to a high degree problems of . . . a particular structural relationship between State and economy.[199]

Cultural theorists have criticized "politics of interest" models for assuming that actors pursue self-interest; that rational-purposive goals exclusively determine behaviour and policy decisions; and that the construction of actors' interests may be neglected.[200] However, the critique of interest models marshalled by Schwarz & Thompson depends on a misrepresentation of interest theories. Schwarz & Thompson argue, first, that by focusing on actors' goal-seeking such models disregard goal-setting[201] and, secondly that:

[c]ommon to *all* theoretical statements involving interest politics is the idea that each political actor has a set of preferences and associated goals that *determine* his or her *behaviour*.[202] (Emphasis added)

The first claim is incorrect because the model of interests applied by Crenson's seminal discussion of non-decision-making specifically considers how government influences agenda and, therefore, goal setting,[203] and the second is false since it is precisely Lukes's thesis that because of the way society is structured people's "behaviour" can itself be against their own (real) interests.[204]

Whatever the potential merits of cultural theory in *supplementing* interest theories, the former is not yet sufficiently well developed to offer a satisfactory alternative to, or a credible critique of, the latter. Rather, the most valuable theoretical refinement would seem to be to apply certain Marxist approaches to sharpen the definition of interests found in corporatist theory. For example, the Marxist framework is particularly important because it recognizes that a frequent consequence of powerlessness is ignorance (and "ideology"), which can, in turn, lead individuals or social groups to be oblivious of, or to miscalculate, their real interests. In short, the distinction between real interests and perceived interests is indispensable; otherwise the concept of interests becomes vacuous.

To take account of the factor of powerlessness and the concomitant situations when people's behaviour may be against their own interests, Lukes argues that interests should also be related to what people *would* want were they able to make the choice.[205] The relevance of the complex issue of the specification of interests to the study of regulatory organizations is illustrated by Hancher's inconclusive condemnation of capture theorists:

> an almost instinctive belief that "private" influence over regulatory processes is illegitimate pervades this literature. The very idea of "capture", moreover, is based upon the assumption that there is a sphere of public regulatory authority which ought to be inviolate from private influence. . . . If regulation is assumed to be an activity in which some ideal of the public interest is pursued at the expense of the private, any evidence that private interests influence the regulatory process or derive benefit from it, is treated as an indication that the purpose of the activity has been distorted.[206]

It is only possible to make sense of Hancher's criticism if it is underpinned by a model of the relationship between "the public interest" and private interests. Hancher is inconclusive in her above criticism because, while challenging the boundaries of public and private interests assumed by some capture theorists, she neglects to offer an explicit framework of interests by which actions or decisions can be judged to be in the public or private interest or both. The crucial question is how "the public interest" is assumed or defined *at the outset*, and how this is related to the actual practices of regulatory organizations. The issue then becomes whether or not the influence of "private" interests conflicts with "the public interest" as defined by how "the public" would act in its own real interests were it to have the choice.

In this book, therefore, I appreciate the need for an explicit model of interests. That interest model recognizes behaviour and interests as conceptually distinct. Interests are *presumed* rather than demonstrated. But, given the existing knowledge about capitalist enterprise and consumer opinions, it is not unreasonable to presume (self) interests of profit maximization for pharmaceutical companies, and of good health for patients. That is, pharmaceutical companies in capitalist societies have real commercial interests in marketing their drug products profitably, and patients have real health interests related to the therapeutic value of a drug – they take medicines *in order to improve their health* even if that is not always the consequence. (This, of course, excludes people who deliberately wish to harm themselves through use of medical drugs.)

The model further presumes that "rational" companies and consumers will pursue those respective interests. However, whether actors actually pursue those interests, and how successful they are in so doing, are empirical matters. It is not assumed that all individuals within industry will always act so as to maximize the commercial interests of their companies, but it is reasonable to suppose that those individuals have significant, though not necessarily overriding or exhaustive, interests in the commercial survival of their employing institutions. In some cases the professional values and/or interests of some medical scientists in the pharmaceutical industry may conflict with the best commercial options for their company. How individuals respond to such situations is an empirical question which can be settled by examining their actions. In this sense the interests of individual scientists cannot be "read off" from the interests of their employing institutions. It is, therefore, possible to examine whether scientists' actions converge with certain pre-defined interests without *assuming* that actors pursue self-interest.

I also presuppose that the actions of drug regulatory authorities, and of the individual regulators and scientists whom they employ, can be related to the commercial interests of the pharmaceutical industry and the health interests of patients. Nevertheless, the precise form (convergence, divergence, conflict and so on) of this relationship is an empirical question. This does not assume that other institutional interests are absent. It is possible that regulatory authorities have distinct interests that are relatively autonomous of commercial and/or patients' interests. Schwarz & Thompson are particularly concerned that interest models fail to take account of social legitimation as a contributory factor in the decision-making process. Certainly it is wise to appreciate that public policy institutions, such as regulatory authorities, *may* have to be sensitive to socially legitimating their decisions. However, the need of regulatory authorities for social legitimacy can be readily subsumed within an interest model which incorporates that need into the regulatory authorities' institutional interests.

To conclude, it follows from the interests model outlined above that patients' real interests are related to the way that the science of drug testing and regulation defines standards of drug safety and effectiveness, which, in turn, can be related to bias in science. Examination of commercial bias in drug testing, therefore, can provide the empirical detail required to identify extremely specific real interests of patients regarding particular drugs or regulatory activities. Indeed, that is one of the aims of Chapters 3 to 7. However, by necessity such empirical data must be based on the *general presupposition* that it is in patients' real interests that the drugs made available to them are maximally therapeutic and minimally hazardous.

The fact that some pharmaceutical companies may propose raising the safety standards of drugs through regulation shows that the interests of industry and patients *can* sometimes converge, but it does not dissolve all divergence or conflicts of interests with patients unless it can be shown that the regulatory developments resulting are those which patients themselves would desire when expressing their real interests. In so far as regulators compromise those real interests, then *regulation as patient protection is being distorted*, but as corporatist theorists rightly argue, the extent to which regulatory activity is actually intended to protect patients is an empirical question. Hence, for a discussion of regulatory bias to be intelligible, the definition of interests cannot be *entirely in flux*. Contrary to what some corporatist approaches imply,[207] there must be some "givens", with respect to interests, in order to structure empirical enquiry and subsequent analysis. It is to that empirical enquiry that I now turn.

Chapter Two

Partial progress?
The development of American
and British drug regulation

This chapter traces the history of drug regulation in the US and the UK from the nineteenth century up to the early 1980s. Particular emphasis is placed on Government–industry relations and the political economy of the pharmaceutical industry in order to examine the extent to which corporate involvement and bias have been embodied in the regulatory policies of both countries. In so doing, the research presented in this chapter will help us to explore the explanatory relevance and significance of theories of regulation to the pharmaceutical sector (e.g. the corporatist, capture and Marxist theories discussed in Chapter 1).

There are two related reasons for undertaking this historical exploration. First, an historical account of drug regulation provides essential insights into the nature of regulatory authorities and the contextual factors that may affect their decisions. For example, in the US, within what legislative frameworks must the main drug regulatory authority, the Food and Drug Administration (FDA), operate and how did these come about? In the UK, what assumptions about the drug approval process underpinned the instalment of the Committee on the Safety of Drugs (CSD) and the Committee on the Safety of Medicines (CSM)? The importance of such contextual understanding cannot be overstated, with respect to the UK, where the precise bases of regulatory decisions are highly secret.

Secondly, the existing literature leaves scope for improvement. Though much has been written about US drug regulation, it is extremely fragmented. Liebenau, whose main concern is the historical development of the medical industry dedicates little more than a dozen pages to drug regulation.[1] In two books on quackery in the nineteenth and twentieth centuries, Young devotes only a couple of chapters to legislation affecting the control of drugs.[2] By contrast, Marks discusses exclusively drug regulation, but his work virtually ignores developments before the 1950s, and attempts no more than a detailed description of the modern drug laws.[3] Only Temin's *Taking your medicine* offers an overview of drug regulation from its beginnings to 1980.[4] However, the analysis to be found there makes only summary use of the many Congressional investigations into the pharmaceutical industry and the FDA. In particular, Temin ignores a major series of investigations into the internal working of the FDA, which reveal significant ways in which the agency has interpreted its regulatory task.

Frequently the literature on the history of British drug regulation constitutes little more than a cursory chronological listing of major legislation. There is a dearth of literature examining the development of British drug regulation. Nevertheless, a computer search of published literature and a manual search of the index to theses from 1950 did reveal a number of sources of varying substance. Unfortunately almost all these sources share one major drawback, namely, that their accounts of regulatory development centre around the use and hazards of medicines.[5] The result is that the political and economic contexts of regulation remain largely unexplored. Even Penn's substantial thesis on the subject falls short in these respects.[6] One exception is Whittet, but his account of "drug control in Britain from World War I to the Medicines Bill of 1968" includes only a few pages on negotiations between Government and industry over the National Health Service (NHS) drug-testing scheme.[7] The other exception is Stieb, who provides an extensive account of drug adulteration in Britain, but his analysis is confined to the nineteenth century.[8]

This chapter, then, aims to integrate the existing documentation into a more coherent whole, and, where necessary, to extend the research undertaken to date so that the case studies in later chapters can be seen in their proper historical context.

Drug adulteration in the nineteenth century and early legislation

In the nineteenth century drug adulteration was defined as "any procedure that produces an alteration in strength or purity, or both, from the avowed standard of a drug, whether through intent or neglect".[9] As the Industrial Revolution swept across Britain in the early part of the nineteenth century, and across the US a few decades later, the foundations for extensive urbanization were laid. Prior to this period community rules were able to provide checks against drug adulteration because invariably the vendor was known personally to the customer. For example, in 1630 a resident of Massachusetts Bay was whipped and fined five pounds for selling a "water of no worth nor value" as a cure for scurvy.[10] Similarly, in England during the Middle Ages the craft guilds, of which apothecaries were a part, had exercised some control over adulteration practices by setting standards of quality, inspecting shops, confiscating substandard goods, and punishing offenders in order to prevent "unfair" competition between guild masters. In addition, since 1540 the Royal College of Physicians had been empowered to inspect local apothecaries' shops for "faulty wares".[11]

Urbanization, however, created sufficient distance between producer, physician and consumer that these traditional controls collapsed.[12] As the British and American Governments of the early nineteenth century did not provide replacements through State controls, drug adulteration rose dramatically. In his startling *Treatise on adulterations* of 1820 Frederick Accum concluded that in England and Wales "nine tenths of the most potent drugs and chemical preparations used in pharmacy [were] vended in a sophisticated [i.e. adulterated] state".[13] Meanwhile, in the US, the patent medicine business, renowned among the drug trade for their adulterative practices, flourished.[14] Contrary to what their name suggests, patent medicines were rarely patented. Rather they depended on secret formulae to protect their markets.[15]

Industrialization in Britain and the US brought considerable hardship to the labouring classes, who worked long hours for low wages, and were forced to live in unhygienic crowded slums. Such conditions led to fearful kinds of ill-health such as tuberculosis, typhoid, yellow fever, and even cholera.[16] For the drug trade, however, the declining state of health promised new and fruitful markets as people were drawn to anticonsumptive syrups and "Egyptian cures" for cholera.[17] In both countries the patent medicine business co-existed alongside the pharmaceutical firms, which were later to form the basis for the modern pharmaceutical industry. Most of these firms started life as apothecary shops, and grew into family companies before becoming the large corporations of the mid twentieth century. Apothecary shops might sell syrups, emulsions, tonics and all standard pharmaceutical preparations. Frequently the druggist also sold many patent medicines. The apothecary was manufacturer, compounder and retailer, and in some cases a physician too.

In Britain, some of these, such as Allen & Hanbury, were doing business as early as the mid eighteenth century,[18] but in the US similar developments did not unfold until the nineteenth century whence Smith, Kline & French, Wyeth Laboratories, Warner-Lambert, Merck, Sharp & Dohme, Parke Davis, Eli Lilly, Upjohn, Squibb and Pfizer owe their origins.[19] Unlike the patent medicine makers, these companies concentrated on selling higher quality medicines to doctors. Such drugs became known as "ethical" pharmaceuticals, a term which initially meant "honest", but was later defined as medicines advertised only to the medical profession and not directly to the public.[20]

In the early part of the nineteenth century none of these elements of the drug trade showed an interest in combating adulteration. Despite his efforts, Accum's work had no direct impact on the control of adulteration, not only because his methods were crude and scarcely used by most apothecaries to check for drug quality,[21] but also because the political climate in Britain did not favour social reform that extended the regulatory powers of the State. The old Tory orthodoxy remained in power virtually uninterrupted from 1783 to 1830. It held that Government should, as far as possible, leave society how it found it. This anti-reformist view commanded substantial support, if only because there was a common fear that social change could lead to uprisings similar to the French Revolution.[22]

Furthermore, the rise of the *laissez faire* doctrine of liberalism, theorized by Adam Smith in 1776, and successfully championed in Government by Jeremy Bentham during the 1830s and 1840s, viewed legislative interference with private business as abhorrent.[23] Though the American Government acted in 1848 to protect the evolving pharmaceutical industry at home by passing the first federal drug law, which was intended to prevent the importation of "adulterated and spurious drugs",[24] State intervention to control domestic drug adulteration in the US also remained minimal.

The 1850s, however, marked a turning point in Britain. The Chartist opposition to industrial capitalism was in retreat. It had been outmanoeuvred by the Anti-Corn Law League which, organized by manufacturers, had managed to convince significant portions of the working classes that their ills were not due to their exclusion from the franchise, or to the gruesome conditions of the factories, but rather to the high price of bread.[25] The 1850s also marked the beginning of a quarter of a century of unmistakable economic prosperity in Britain. The Great Exhibition of 1851 was a symbol of the international superiority of Britain's enterprise and expertise in terms of manufactured goods, trade, capital, engineering and design.

This was a time when substantial sections of the working classes for the first time tasted the fruits of industrial capitalism as wage increases more than kept pace with inflation.[26] Trade Unions, such as the Amalgamated Society of Engineers, developed among the skilled craftsmen who were "eminently moderate men, and as firmly convinced of the inevitability of the capitalist system as any employer could be".[27] People were ready to listen sympathetically to officials, such as the organizers of the Exhibition, when they asserted that progress and welfare did not lie in Utopian demands, but rather on individual effort at work.

Consequently, extra-parliamentary political agitation withered and the public increasingly looked to the House of Commons for legislative change. The parliamentary parties, in turn, vied to win public support for their legislative programmes. By the late 1860s legislative reforms, including ones to regulate trade, were gathering pace.[28] It is in this context that the campaign to control drug adulteration in Britain can be seen as classic political activity of the period.

In 1850 the English physician Arthur Hill Hassall was the first to realize full and systematic application of microscopy to the detection of adulteration.[29] Microscopy made possible the detection of adulteration in many organic substances for which chemical tests remained unavailable,[30] and probably carried greater significance for the fight against adulteration than any other single instrument. However, Hassall's endeavours might have been confined to one isolated article had it not been for the support of Thomas Wakley, editor of the *Lancet*, who offered Hassall the opportunity to publish his detailed reports of microscopic examinations of drugs in the journal between 1851 and 1854.[31] Of equal importance was the campaigning of John Postgate for Government control of food and drug adulteration. He gained the support of Birmingham MPs, one of whom was to chair the 1855 and 1856 House of Commons Select Committee on Adulteration of Food, Drinks, and Drugs. Hence, this Committee was able to turn to Hassall for substantive testimony and scientific evidence, as well as using the debate generated by Wakley's *Lancet* as a foundation from which to build further testimony.[32]

The Committee heard how chloroform, opium, scammony and other drugs were adulterated.[33] Many witnesses, including physicians, chemists and druggists testified that drug adulteration was extensively practised, and advocated legislation to discourage it.[34] On the other hand, some druggists, such as Jacob Bell, editor of the *Pharmaceutical Journal*, maintained that adulteration was an old custom no longer employed – at least not in "respectable houses in the trade".[35] Nevertheless, as the Committee concluded, the weight of the evidence indicated that adulteration still widely prevailed.[36] Moreover, all were agreed that competition to meet the demand for low priced medicines was the cause of adulteration.[37] Yet so powerful was the ideology of *laissez faire* that Bell felt able to argue that market forces could be relied on to put an end to adulteration:

> We never saw pure scammony 20 years ago . . . even now we could not obtain a sufficient supply of that which is absolutely pure, but if the demand were to extend, the persons abroad would make it to suit the demand; whatever demand exists the supply follows as a matter of course.[38]

The Committee, reluctant to move forcefully against the ideology of free trade, wished merely to define the boundaries of "honest competition", declaring:

> The great difficulty of legislation on this subject lies in putting an end to the liberty of fraud without affecting the freedom of commerce.[39]

The Committee finally recommended that local authorities should be empowered to appoint inspectors who could examine any food or drug item to check for adulteration.[40] By contrast, the dominant preference among the medical and pharmacy professions was for voluntary control, rather than regulations imposed by Government. That these professions were successful in persuading the Government to accept their viewpoint is evident from the fact that the 1860 Adulteration Act left it up to local authorities whether or not to appoint inspectors, applied only to food and drinks, but not medicines.[41]

The pharmacists' profession, as represented by the Pharmaceutical Society of Great Britain (PSGB), was much more concerned with achieving public recognition and the elimination of unqualified competition than with the control of drug adulteration *per se*. In pursuing that goal, however, the Society became drawn into legislation that would not only advance its professionalization, but also Government regulation of adulteration.[42] After lobbying the House of Commons to restrict those who could compound or sell prescriptions to pharmaceutical chemists, the Society succeeded in establishing the Pharmacy Act of 1868, which extended the 1860 Adulteration Act to medicines.[43]

The British Medical Association (BMA), too, concerned itself almost exclusively with issues of professional advancement in its campaign against quackery.[44] By contrast, the profession of public analysts sought single-mindedly to extend and strengthen legislative control of drug adulteration. Indeed, the successful operation of the anti-adulteration acts depended largely on the appointment and expertise of such analysts. This profession developed after the 1860 Adulteration Act, and in 1874 the Society of Public Analysts (SPA) was formed to exert an increasing influence on the nature of anti-adulteration law.[45]

Meanwhile, in 1861 the US had entered the throes of civil war. Of particular significance for the drug trade was the relentless growth of advertising and journalism during the war period. The population craved for news from the war fronts and the number of periodicals received by each citizen grew almost fourfold between 1860 and 1900.[46] It was not only patent medicine makers who took advantage of this situation to advertise their products more extensively; medical practitioners and pharmaceutical firms also took up vigorous promotion tactics, paying little attention to the problem of adulteration. For, as Liebenau recounts, however much the latter may have disapproved of the patent medicine business, they were soon "forced to follow [its] lead in advertising" because of the pressure of commercial competition.[47] In an address before the Massachusetts Medical Society one doctor despaired at the situation:

> I firmly believe that if the whole materia medica, as now used, could be sunk to the bottom of the sea, it would be better for mankind and all the worse for the fishes.[48]

The modest success of anti-adulteration campaigns in Britain, combined with the growing interest of the "ethical" pharmaceutical industry in the competitive advantages of drug standardization, led to the 1875 Sale of Food and Drugs Act.[49] However, the indecisive nature of the 1875 Act became all too evident when in 1877 it was revealed that 18 out of 32 English, and two out of three Welsh counties reporting took no drug samples, and seven counties took fewer than ten. Moreover, less than one-third of the drug cases in which analysis revealed adulteration were brought to trial because of problems related to the legal definition of adulteration.[50] It was not until 1899, following the advocacy of the SPA, that an Amendment to the 1875 Act gave local government the regulatory authority to enforce the operation of the Act in areas where it had been neglected.[51] Nevertheless, all the legislation concerning the 1875 Act avoided completely the term "adulteration", and so the courts had to rely on the British Pharmacopoeia as the legal standard for drugs.[52]

As with regulatory policy, the pace of change in the British pharmaceutical industry was slow during this period. British firms remained characterized by the traditional practice of importing and refining raw materials and packaging them for distribution to chemists and druggists.[53] By contrast, technological innovations in the US had dramatically amplified the manufacturing capacity of the industry bringing supply abreast of demand as never before. For the first time medicine makers confronted the problem of differentiating their products from competitors in a really acute way.[54] The "ethical" pharmaceutical industry sought to use developments in scientific medicine as a way of differentiating their products as superior to patent medicines, especially in terms of meeting the standards of the US Pharmacopoeia. By the 1890s they were employing medical scientists and running laboratories for quality control, standardization and the search for new drugs.[55]

The new scientific approach to medicine also influenced physicians, who increasingly conceived of science as a method for their disciplines.[56] Also physicians, competing for patients and anxious to demonstrate the efficacy of their prescriptions, came to rely more heavily on the Pharmacopoeias and more specific drugs with measured doses, thus augmenting the demand for standard preparations.[57] Consequently, a close relationship based on mutual interest evolved between the big pharmaceutical companies in the US and American physicians; the latter could extend their professional power since only they had the knowledge to prescribe the new science-based drugs, while the large high technology firms created a unique prescription market, in which they had a clear advantage over other medicine makers. Hence, the possibility emerged that State regulations could reduce competition by driving out small producers who lacked the technical facilities and expertise to meet the new regulatory requirements.[58]

This was also a period when the commercial advantages of large-scale business became especially conspicuous in the US.[59] The emergence of big business meant that private economic enterprises, in general, functioned on a much enlarged geographical scale. The railroads and the possibility of rapid communication created by telegraph services enabled companies to seek and co-ordinate markets nationally across many state boundaries. As firms expanded their distribution, they needed to centralize in order to plan effectively for new markets. Such centralization and consolidation swelled the industry's interest in product standardization through State control because federal regulation promised to diminish the economic importance of inconsistencies in state laws.[60]

As the century drew to a close, problems of domestic and international trade also afflicted drug manufacturers in the US, and these provide further reasons why substantial sections of the American pharmaceutical industry became less opposed to State intervention. On the domestic front the trade faced the problem of how to maintain a standard price that could be shielded from unscrupulous dealers. Internationally, not only Britain, but also Germany had established laws to control drug quality. American medicinal products, therefore, appeared unattractive, even substandard, on both the domestic and world markets. To rectify this situation the US pharmaceutical industry experimented with self-regulation through trade associations. However, these associations failed because, like similar cartels in other industries, a few producers nearly always refused to join or uphold the voluntary agreements. Consequently, firms became attracted to regulatory control backed by federal law.[61]

In addition to industrial interest in State control of drug standards in the US, public outrage towards quackery and adulteration, encouraged by the revelations of journalists and the Women's Temperance Union, reached a peak during this period. In the 1890s the *Ladies Home Journal* banished proprietary medicines advertising from its pages, while Colliers the *National Weekly* lambasted the trade with a regular slot on "The Great American Fraud", which provided detailed discussions of the contents and therapeutic impotence of quack medicines together with the names of the producers.[62] Furthermore, as Accum had done nearly three-quarters of a century earlier in Britain, the American Association of Official Agricultural Chemists applied the latest scientific methods to the chemistry of patent medicines. As they published their results, the cloak of secrecy surrounding the fake remedies was removed with unprecedented exactness, enabling critics to further discredit the industry.[63]

Condemnation of the drug trade began to have some effect as bills to control it materialized in state legislatures.[64] From 1879 to 1905 at least 190 bills related to federal control of foods and drugs were proposed to Congress, though none were passed.[65] One of the most vociferous advocates of federal food and drug regulation was Harvey Wiley, the chief chemist at the Department of Agriculture. He wanted stringent legislation requiring every medicine to have its formula listed on the label. In 1905 Wiley and his allies managed to persuade President Roosevelt to recommend the enactment of a law "to regulate interstate commerce in misbranded and adulterated foods, drinks and drugs".[66]

Adding to the pressure, the American Medical Association (AMA) sent a petition supporting such regulation to each senator.[67] The following day an anti-adulteration Bill expressing Wiley's concerns was introduced into Congress by Senator Heyburn, and passed in a compromised form by the Senate in February 1906. Meanwhile, a socialist writer created a public outcry when he published *The Jungle*, a book which exposed the filthy conditions of meat production and processing in the US. This added momentum to the campaign for pure food and drug legislation, and in June 1906 the Heyburn Bill was ratified by the House, and signed into law as the Pure Food and Drugs Act.[68]

The initial legislation passed to control drug adulteration in this period was very similar in Britain and the US. In both countries the new laws provided consumers with some protection against the fraudulent claims of vendors, but the compromised 1906 Pure Food and Drug Act meant that, like its British counterpart, the American drug trade retained the privilege of keeping silent about the contents of its wares, excepting certain poisons (e.g. arsenic).[69] That this compromise was a significant victory for the American patent medicine makers is revealed by the editorial of the contemporaneous *National Druggist*, which commented:

let it not be supposed that the law would have been enacted in its present rather innocuous form but for the hard, intelligent and most tactful work on the part of the representatives of the interests it is intended to regulate.[70]

Another characteristic of early legislation common to both sides of the Atlantic was the dependence on the Pharmacopoeias to define official drug standards.[71] For many scientists this situation was, however, less than satisfactory. In Britain the SPA argued that the Pharmacopoeia lagged so far behind scientific methods for establishing purity that it effectively sanctioned adulteration,[72] while in the US the leading science-based manufacturers expressed concern that the regulatory revisions to the Pharmacopoeia did not keep pace with industrial innovations which differentiated the standard of quality drugs from competitors.[73] During the last quarter of the nineteenth century the SPA consistently argued for the drawing up of stringent standards to be used in law. That the legislature did not support their efforts is testimony to the success of the British drug trade in persuading the Government that, on the whole, regulation should be kept to a minimum.[74]

The main difference between British and American drug control was in the institutional approach to enforcement. Congress had charged the Bureau of Chemistry of the Department of Agriculture to police the 1906 Act. Thus, a centralized group of analytical chemists, under Wiley's committed leadership, pro-actively investigated reports of adulteration, and even carried out their own experimental research.[75] By contrast, British regulation depended entirely on the routine sampling of local inspectors; central government having a weak scientific base, and acting only in response to problems raised by the inspectorate.[76] Furthermore, legislative oversight by Congress and judicial review by the courts in the US was to be much more extensive than the efforts by the House of Commons and the British legal system.

Regulatory reforms: 1907–1945

The first five decades of the twentieth century saw far more Government activity in the regulation of drugs than had been evident in the nineteenth century. In Britain this was intertwined with reformist politics which came to dominate the period. As the twentieth century opened, strong competition from overseas was taking its toll on the international standing of the British economy. Domestic prices and profits were falling, while unemployment, poverty and social unrest had become widespread.[77] Moreover, Britain's defeat in the Boer War led to the view in elite circles that the country's fortunes could only be safeguarded by a more active and efficient State. Whereas Britain's commercial command of world markets in the nineteenth century had been accomplished by *laissez faire* principles, under Chamberlain's leadership the new Liberals argued with considerable success that more effective imperialism was required to finance needed social reforms at home. Chamberlain hoped that the formula of imperialism plus social reform would provide the basis for national consensus, thus improving national efficiency and warding off the burgeoning support for the radical labour and suffragette movements. After a landslide victory in 1905, the new Liberal reform programme began in earnest.[78]

At the centre of the Liberal reforms was the 1911 National Health Insurance (NHI) Act. In 1909 Lloyd George, the Chancellor of the Exchequer, introduced the "People's Budget", which, in his own words, aimed "to wage implacable warfare against poverty and squalidness".[79] NHI was made possible by the 1909 budget, but Lloyd George looked upon the scheme particularly favourably because it gave the poor some relief at minimal cost to the State. In effect, people below a certain income level could receive "medical benefit" via a national system of insurance for sickness funded by statutory contributions from the employer, the State and the employed – of which the State paid less than a quarter.[80]

As a consequence of the NHI Act the British Government became the purchaser of many drugs and prescriptions from pharmacists to the tune of £550,000 per year.[81] Such State involvement was accompanied by new Government interest in the quality of drugs. During the First World War the PSGB and others made representations to the Government, arguing that health services were in a chaotic condition and needed the establishment of a Ministry to improve them. In particular, shortages of supply due to the war situation meant that some drug prices for retailers and consumers rocketed.[82] Lloyd George declared his support for the idea, and in 1919 the Ministry of Health was born into a particularly close relationship, and shared sense of purpose, with the PSGB.[83] As an editorial in the *Pharmaceutical Journal* marking the end of the Ministry's first year noted:

> The Advisory Committees are bound to serve as salutary deterrents from bureaucratic tendencies, and the Ministry of Health Committee of the Council [of the Pharmaceutical Society] and the Federation of Medical and Allied Societies, of which the [Pharmaceutical] Society is a constituent member, hold watching briefs for the medical, pharmaceutical, and allied interests likely to be affected by the policy and operations of the Ministry.[84]

As in Britain, industrial workers in early twentieth century America endured filthy living conditions and appalling dangers at work,[85] but because organized labour was much weaker in the US, there was less pressure for social reform. In 1914 Woodrow Wilson was elected President promising a "New Freedom", which entailed minimal regulation of industry and a rejection of substantial social reform.[86] Rather, business was encouraged to develop codes of ethics, philanthropy and paternalism towards its employees. For the next fifteen years *laissez faire* and welfare capitalism were to be the watchwords in the US.[87]

With the onset of the First World War, both Britain and the US were cut off from their traditional supplies of German synthetic chemicals; a situation which stimulated significant growth of the domestic fine chemical industries, including pharmaceuticals.[88] As Tweedale has noted, pharmaceutical firms found that international conflict was by no means detrimental to profits and, in fact, the drug industries found their products very much in demand during the war.[89] While the war might have brought parallel fortunes to the American and British pharmaceutical industries, this was not true of their respective governments.

Superficially the British and American Governments confronted similar problems of post-war reconstruction. Labour and suffragette movements had made considerable gains during the war and their support was growing. Employers, on the other hand, were determined to recover control of the industrial sector through the abolition of all wartime regulation. In the US the result was a wave of industrial disputes and strikes in 1919, which involved 20 per cent of the workforce.[90] Yet by the early 1920s post-war social dislocation had subsided in the US, whereas the shadow of the war hung over Britain for the next decade. The British suffered more than one million war dead compared with the 112,000 American war victims.

For the US the First World War had accelerated the Fordist modelling of mass production and Taylorist ideas of scientific management, as the nation's industries thrived on supplying the Allied war machine with virtual immunity from attack.[91] For these reasons, having begun the century in debt, the US emerged from the war as the major creditor on international account.[92] In the 1920s Americans saw the first excursion into mass affluence: from 1922 to 1928 industrial production rose by 70 per cent and *per caput* income by 30 per cent;[93] and by 1929 two-thirds of families had electricity and 40 per cent had radios.[94] No pressing need for Government regulation of industry seemed evident. By contrast, in Britain unemployment never fell below 9 per cent of the labour force during the 1920s, and the State was active in managing a depleted economy.[95]

In 1920 the British Government was faced with a grave political and economic situation. Not only had it incurred a huge national debt through financing the war, but the onset of a severe recession was accompanied by industrial unrest and rising unemployment.[96] The Government responded by making cuts in public spending and implementing a budgetary clampdown. It was in this context that the Treasury became concerned about the efficiency of drug services. In Autumn 1920 the Ministry of Health asked the Committee on the Supply of Drugs to Insured Persons (CSDIP) to advise it on the "arrangements for securing that the drugs for insured persons supplied by chemists are of proper standard, quality and quantity".[97]

In 1921 the CSDIP expressed "grave doubt" that the expenditure on the insured was being well spent because the Insurance Committees, which had been established by the 1917 Insurance Act to oversee the supply of drugs to insured people, had no special staff for checking that the drugs supplied were of proper quality.[98] Moreover, the CSDIP concluded:

where reports were submitted by Insurance Committees, the results of the tests made were somewhat disquieting. . . . Certain additional machinery will be necessary if an effective check in the matter of drug supply is to be secured. While much can undoubtedly be done by testing medicines actually dispensed, no provision has hitherto been made for the sampling of crude drugs, medicines and appliances found on the stock shelves of the chemist.[99]

Based on their findings the CSDIP recommended two major extensions of drug testing for regulatory purposes. First, the empowerment of inspectors with special pharmaceutical knowledge to enter insurance chemist's premises and sample stocks of drugs. And secondly, the establishment of a centralized Pharmaceutical Section of the Ministry of Health with £10,000 worth of annual funding in order to control and co-ordinate local arrangement for drug testing.[100] On 18 February 1921 Sir Arthur Robinson, the Minister of Health, responded by agreeing that the CSDIP had revealed "a serious state of affairs" but he expressed reservations as follows:

The doubts which I feel about it are to some extent political, and based on the present general position of the Ministry which makes it wise to avoid ground of public controversy if we can. It seems to me that the chemists would be likely to raise an outcry against inspectors with such extremely wide powers as those proposed . . . this would be a real case of an "inquisition" and we might have difficulty maintaining it. Is there no way out?[101]

The Ministry's particular desire to avoid public controversy at this time is explained by the crisis which faced the Government as a whole, and it had a profoundly dampening effect on regulatory reforms of drug testing. Almost four months later the CSDIP proposed compromise measures involving only half the annual expenditure of the original and confidential discussions with the representatives of chemists before making any formal proposals, with a view to minimizing objections from the pharmacy profession. The weak nature of the drug testing finally adopted is all too obvious from the Committee's later comment:

We are all in favour of a not too ambitious scheme being launched at the outset, and we recommend that amended proposals of a tentative character should be put forward . . .[102]

Nevertheless, even the compromised scheme represented the first systematic testing of dispensed medicines in Britain.[103]

The social dislocation of the First World War also had a direct impact on British drug regulations. In 1917 the Defence of the Realm Regulations, designed to reduce the prevalent use of addictive drugs by soldiers desperate for a "high" during the war, stipulated that the supply of drugs such as cocaine, morphine and opium should be limited to those for whom a physician had prescribed them.[104] These regulations were consolidated in 1920 by the Dangerous Drugs Act much to the dislike of the drug trade.[105] Under the existing Pharmacy Act chemists could sell any of these addictive drugs to a member of the public whom they knew and could do so repeatedly without committing an offence.[106] For the Government, this represented a troublesome social problem as evidenced by the police's "intensified campaign" in 1922 to eradicate the extensive trafficking in "habit-forming drugs".[107] Consequently, the PSGB's argument that protection of the public from powerfully addictive drugs could be allowed to rest with the professional integrity of the pharmacists was rejected by the Home Office.[108] This marked the beginning of *prescription-only* drugs in Britain, and the view that at least some drugs should be sold only under a doctor's instructions.

Following the collapse of the coal market and the general strike of 1926,[109] the British Government was again looking to make budgetary savings. In 1927 the Chief Medical Officer of the Ministry of Health reported with concern that every year since 1921 there had been a considerable increase in the cost of medicines *per caput* for insured persons because of extravagant prescribing by doctors treating patients receiving medical benefit. In an attempt to curb such extravagance the Ministry encouraged Insurance Committee Panels to make doctors justify prescribing a medicine for which there was an equally efficacious but less expensive substitute.[110] However, in order for this policy to be workable common standards of drug efficacy needed to be sharpened. Otherwise, with almost immeasurable licence, doctors could defend expensive prescribing on the grounds of superior therapeutic effectiveness. Consequently, in February 1929 the Minister of Health appointed a Committee to advise on the definition of drugs supplied to insured persons.

By the end of the year the Committee had produced two reports categorizing 165 preparations known to be prescribed into those which were sometimes drugs, those that could never be deemed to be drugs, and those whose composition remained undisclosed, i.e. patent medicines. The Committee advised that doctors who prescribed from the second category should have to pay the cost of the preparation and could be disciplined by the Insurance Committee. As regards patent medicines, the judgement of the Committee was that "the prescribing of such substances is most undesirable, and we are of the opinion that only the most exceptional circumstances could justify a practitioner in prescribing them".[111] Thus, for the first time in Britain a central authority defined, if very crudely, some drug standards according to efficacy.

While the British entertained cost-cutting during the 1920s, many Americans displayed an inordinate desire to get rich quickly. All that changed with the Wall Street crash in 1929, the harbinger of the Great Depression of the 1930s. Unemployment grew rapidly as industry after industry laid off workers by the million. By 1933 nearly 13 million people in the US, one-quarter of the labour force, were unemployed,[112] and even by 1937 as many as one-third of the population went hungry.[113] Drug adulteration increased as the bankrupt turned to quackery in search of an income, and the more intense competition in shrinking markets engendered waves of false advertising.[114]

Many inside and outside the American Government blamed abuse of corporate power and the extremely unequal distribution of wealth during the 1920s for the crash and ensuing depression.[115] In 1932 President Franklin D. Roosevelt responded by setting in motion a ream of legislation lasting the rest of the decade. There was to be a "New Deal", in which Government would play a much greater role in regulating business for the collective interest, and in the provision of social welfare.[116]

It was as part of this reform period that Rexford Tugwell, Assistant Secretary of Agriculture, campaigned for tougher laws to control drug adulteration and advertising.[117] In general, the pharmaceutical industry was sanguine about its performance under the 1906 Act. The industry's sales increased by a factor of six over the first 20 years of the Act's existence.[118] Whereas the advertising expenditures of patent medicine makers reached $70 million in 1929, the average fine paid by offenders under the first 30 years of the Act was a mere $67.[119] The Federal Trade Commission (FTC), which regulated drug advertisements, saw its role as promoting competitive conditions in the trade, rather than consumer protection.[120]

With the backing of President Roosevelt and Walter Campbell, the FDA Commissioner, Tugwell, organized the drafting of a new Bill, which sought to relieve the Government of the burden of proving fraudulence by defining a drug as misbranded "if its labelling bears any representation, directly or by ambiguity or inference, concerning the effect of such drug which is contrary to the general agreement of medical opinion".[121] Under

Tugwell's Bill advertisements for drugs were required to meet the same standards of truthfulness as labelling.

As the Tugwell Bill went before Congress in 1933 it was greeted with public apathy. A popular, if mistaken, feeling that the 1906 Act had tackled the problems of drug adulteration prevailed.[122] Indeed some newspapers, which had backed Wiley's campaign, were initially hostile to the Tugwell's Bill because he proposed to extend controls over advertising. The drug trade also mobilized against the Bill. The United Medicine Manufacturers of America advised its members to "line up with other organizations, such as the Drug Institute, Proprietary Association, National Association of Druggists, and others, to make a mass attack on the Bill".[123]

Such industrial antagonism wielded powerful influence; every Congressional district had manufacturers, wholesalers and retailers concerned with foods and drugs.[124] Opposition came from the most "responsible" elements of the industries to be regulated. Some claimed that it would decimate drug advertising within five years and wipe out self-medication. Campbell, on the other hand, argued that the Bill (now sponsored by Senator Copeland) aimed merely to make self-medication safe. However, opposition was too strong and the Bill failed to make much progress in Congress during 1933. Over the next two years Copeland returned to Congress with compromised bills but industrial resistance, especially to the proposal to substitute the FTC for the FDA as the authority that would regulate food, drug and cosmetic advertising, was still sufficient to prevent legislation, even though some of the large manufacturers were fatalistically preparing for the Bill to be passed.[125]

All sources are agreed that the public's lethargic approach to drug regulation changed when news broke of how Elixir Sulfanilamide had killed some 107 people. Though sulfanilamide was a widely used medicine, in October 1937 an ostensibly respectable drug company marketed the medicine in liquid form using the solvent diethyl glycol, but neglected either to test the resulting compound for toxicity in animals, or to name the solvent on the label. Most of the deadly compound had in fact been prescribed by doctors. The incident brought into sharp focus the fact that existing legislation did not require the testing of drugs for safety. In the wake of this incident Copeland re-introduced a much modified Bill which now excluded any proposals for FDA control of drug advertising. This Congress approved and in June 1938 President Roosevelt signed The Food, Drug, and Cosmetic Act into law.

Undoubtedly one direct result of the Elixir Sulfanilamide tragedy was that the 1938 Food, Drug and Cosmetic Act required manufacturers to test any new drug for safety, and to report the results to the FDA. This created an entirely novel class of drugs. Previously there had been no distinction between new and old drugs, and no need for manufacturers to get governmental permission to market a drug. The agency was also authorized to remove from the market any drug it could prove to be unsafe. Hence, the 1938 Act reflected the view that the Government should assure consumers that they would not be physically harmed in their search for medication, even if this meant the Government making *pre-market* choices on behalf of consumers. It was also a first step in creating a prescription-only class of drugs in the US because certain drugs were exempt from labelling requirements if they bore the warning: "Caution: To be used only by or on the prescription of [a physician]".[126]

Meanwhile, the British pharmaceutical industry, which had benefited from favourable protectionist policies and the mass production of insulin of the 1920s,[127] entered the 1930s with an optimistic economic outlook, and began to develop the large-scale manufacturing and experimental research facilities, so characteristic of its American counterpart at the beginning of the century.[128] Accompanying this was American-style corporate organization. Due to the expansion and increasing concentration that had attended the industry's success in the 1920s,[129] in 1929 many British manufacturing and wholesale firms had amalgamated to form the Wholesale Druggists Trade Association (WDTA), whose purpose was to advance the interests of its members with respect to legislation affecting the drug trade.[130] However, by the mid 1930s the industry suffered from an overproduction of drugs and a declining demand on the home market as the effects of the Great Depression hit Europe, and as public health legislation began to have long-term positive effects on the health of the nation. Moreover, prices and profits in the drug trade were dwindling because of the operations of small distributors who were able to undercut the prices of the mainstream manufacturers and retailers by employing unqualified staff for low wages.[131] Under these conditions drug adulteration persisted and even grew during the 1930s with small-scale enterprises apparently using "sheds" or "backyards" as premises and "oddments of apparatus and utensils valued at a few shillings" as plant.[132]

In response, in 1934 the National Pharmacists' Union (NPU) and the WDTA established a joint committee to find a means of "checking the all-too-free sale of drugs . . . by unqualified and untrained vendors . . . and controlling the innumerable wholesale channels through which the goods reach these vendors".[133] Nevertheless, the patent medicines business continued to flourish with the assistance of intense advertising.[134]

Such trends persisted despite repeated condemnations of the adulterative practices in the trade. In 1909 the BMA had exposed the fraudulence of the "secret remedies" in the patent medicine business, and criticized the Inland Revenue and the existing Medicine Stamp legislation for helping to give credibility to "secret remedies" by encouraging their sale under the Inland Revenue Stamp.[135] Manufacturers and others, who took advantage of the "known, admitted and approved" exemption from stamp duty, were forced to reveal the composition of their drugs, but secrecy could always be bought with a stamp.[136] Thus, a situation obtained, in which the Government had a vested interest in maintaining "secret remedies".

Moreover, in 1914 the Select Committee on Patent Medicines published a report advocating remedial Government action.[137] It recommended that (a) there should be a law governing the advertisement of patent, secret and proprietary medicines; (b) there should be a special Commission with the power to permit or prohibit the sale and advertisement of any such medicine; and (c) an exact and complete statement of the ingredients of and therapeutic claims for such medicines should be furnished to the relevant Government department.[138] A Government Bill to give effect to these recommendations was introduced shortly after the First World War, but did not pass into law due to strong opposition organized by the press, who derived substantial income from the advertisement of proprietary medicines.[139]

It was not until the 1941 Pharmacy and Medicines Act that the Government legislated against the sale of "secret remedies". However, as the origins of this legislation show, it was not derived primarily from a concern to protect consumers' interests, but rather from the conflicts of interest within the drug trade with respect to tax exemptions and related privileges. In fact, as Ministry of Health correspondence reveals, the Government specifically wished to avoid greater tate regulation of proprietary drugs:

> As I understand the Chancellor's letter, the present proposal is to have an enquiry into the taxation aspects of the problem only and no doubt this is right since it would hardly be practicable to introduce legislation (which would probably be controversial) for the control of proprietary medicines at the present time.[140]

The crux of "the problem" to which the Ministry referred was that, though the Medicine Stamp Acts taxed medicines, exemption was granted to chemists, druggists and doctors who sold medicines that were "known, admitted and approved". Despite this, the chemist was permitted to sell at the "taxed price"; the "unpaid tax" being split between the chemist and manufacturer according to mutual agreement. However, in the mid 1930s Woolworths, non-chemist retailers, began to sell *prima facie* taxable medical articles without stamp duty. When the Department of Customs and Excise instituted proceedings against Woolworths the company retaliated by launching an action against the Attorney-General, who felt that it would be embarrassing for him to defend the Government's position unless he could give an undertaking that the law would be amended to eliminate what he considered an unsatisfactory trading situation.[141] Allowing chemists to receive the "taxed price" from consumers was particularly embarrassing for the Government by 1940, when scarcity due to the Second World War had caused drug prices to rise sharply, and when the Government was raising purchase taxes in order to meet the domestic costs of the war effort.[142]

By 1939, in a Report to the Chancellor, the Customs and Excise Department was declaring "untenable" its position as administrator of the tax, arguing that the existence of the tax did nothing to prevent the public from buying ineffective or deleterious drugs because that required *regulatory control*.[143] Thus, it was in response to wrangles within the trade that the issue of drug regulation returned to the Government's agenda. In January 1941 the Chancellor instituted discussions regarding the Medicines Stamp Duty "to try and get agreement among the interests concerned".[144] Given the Government's goal of achieving a consensus, it was attracted to the idea of introducing strict regulatory control over "secret remedies" because this would remove opposition to the legislation from the medical profession, who stood to gain from the demise of quackery.[145] A month later the PSGB, WDTA, Proprietary Association of Great Britain (PAGB), and the Scottish Pharmaceutical Federation all pledged support for a Bill that repealed the tax and prohibited the sale of "secret remedies", provided that legislation was introduced giving chemists and pharmacists the exclusive right to sell certain classes of proprietary medicines.[146] Despite opposition from the NPU, the Bill was passed into law.[147]

The Pharmacy and Medicines Act met with great approval from Customs and Excise. In a letter to the Secretary of Health, Eady from the

Department was candid about the British Government's perspective on the legislation:

> I doubt whether it could be held strongly that these proposals are contrary to the public interest, though they could scarcely be presented as required by the public interest. What they claim to be is an agreement made among the various interested parties which would enable them to accept the repeal of the Medicines Stamp Duty without making political trouble, and . . . that might appear to the Chancellor and your Minister as an appreciable political point.[148]

Indeed, Beckett at the Ministry of Health described the legislation as no more than that which would "give effect to the agreement between the organizations concerned with the sale of medicines".[149]

The growth of prescription drugs and the emergence of modern drug regulation

Elixir Sulfanilamide was one of a number of drugs whose manufacture had been prompted by the enormous therapeutic success of sulfanido-chrysoidine, a 1935 discovery and the first sulfa-drug. The sulfa-drugs exhibited unparalleled anti-bacterial potency and their diffusion, together with the introduction of penicillin in the mid 1940s, marked the beginning of a significant transformation in the kinds of drugs produced by the pharmaceutical industry.[150] Many companies sought to replicate these therapeutic breakthroughs creating a plethora of equally powerful drugs. Since these drugs could only be sold on prescription, the number of prescription drugs rose dramatically in the post-war period.[151] For example, in the US less than one-third of all medicines purchased in 1929 were prescribed by doctors, but by 1969 this had grown to over four-fifths.[152]

As a result industrial promotion of drugs to doctors intensified, especially where companies were competing to introduce patentable molecular modifications with apparently identical therapeutic effects ("me-too" drugs).[153] Moreover, the large high-technology firms used patents to command high monopoly prices for their drugs. With the decline of drug adulteration[154] on both sides of the Atlantic the post-war period was characterized, therefore, by considerable Government concern about drug prices, albeit with markedly different manifestations.

In Britain, with the introduction of the National Health Service (NHS) by the Labour Government in 1948, the State became even more concerned with the control of drugs. The number of prescriptions under the NHS in 1951 had more than trebled to 220 million compared with the number under the NHI Act.[155] Anxious about the excessive prices of NHS drugs, successive British Governments established various committees to consider how the costs of NHS drugs could be rationalized.

By necessity this had some implications for the regulation of drug standards. The terms of reference of the first such Committee, the Joint Committee on Prescribing (JCP), chaired by Lord Cohen, was set up in July 1949 to consider whether it was desirable to restrict or discourage NHS doctors from prescribing "drugs of doubtful value" or "unnecessarily expensive brands of standard drugs".[156] In 1953 the JCP produced its first main report, which classified approximately 5,000 prospective NHS drugs into those which were: new and of proven therapeutic value, but not standard; proprietary brands of standard prescription drugs; and preparations which, according to the JCP, lacked proof of therapeutic value.[157] The Committee recommended that the first category should be freely prescribable, and that the second should not be advertised directly to the public.[158]

The Ministry of Health felt that the JCP's recommendations did not go far enough and asked the Committee to draw up a list of drugs advertised direct to the public, with a view to prohibiting their prescription under the NHS. Indeed, in the meantime, the Ministry had instigated a review of drug legislation, which claimed that:

a major cause of the proprietary drug Bill is the prescription of duplicate or doubtful medicines following skilful propaganda from the drug firms to the doctors in the service, and in some cases following advertising to the public, which in turn results in pressure on the doctor by the patient.[159]

Furthermore, the review reveals that within the Ministry there was extensive concern about the inadequacies of British drug control, in general:

(i) there is no effective control over the manufacture and sale of duplicate or dubious proprietary preparations (ii) there is no effective control over the advertising of proprietary medicines (iii) the existing provisions for the testing of drugs are inadequate.[160]

The review proposed that there should be stricter control over advertising,[161] and that a register of prescribable NHS drugs should be established, excluding those drugs that the JCP thought lacked efficacy.[162]

Not all these perspectives were uncharted by the pharmaceutical industry. In 1948, when the WDTA changed its name to the Association of the

British Pharmaceutical Industry (ABPI), it altered its constitution in ways which indicated a greater concern for the public reputation of the industry. This included a commitment to exercise its influence to prevent misleading advertisments.[163] Nevertheless, the ABPI was anxious about the Ministry's plans to rationalize drug prescribing because too much standardization of the home trade could damage export potential. Exports were particularly important to the ABPI, not only because manufacturing had become domestic at all stages, but also because in 1950 the Association merged with the Pharmaceutical Export Group (PEG).[164] As the President of the ABPI noted at the ABPI/PEG merger:

> If the well-known branded names of preparations disappear they will no longer figure in the medical journals published here and be circulated widely overseas and this will make it more difficult for the export industry to develop.[165]

These were particularly influential arguments in the post-war period. The UK emerged from the Second World War as one of the world's leading debtor nations with badly depleted export potential and earnings. Nevertheless, the UK economy did recover because of the export boom of the sectors, such as pharmaceuticals, that had done well during that war due to the temporary eclipse of Germany as a competitor in world markets.[166]

The macroeconomic landscape of the 1950s and 1960s, then, came to be characterized by almost full employment and a sizeable Government budget generated by successful export trades. In this context high unemployment seemed to be electorally unacceptable, and both Labour and Conservative Governments of the period adopted Keynesian ideas of economic management, which depended on the maintenance of virtual full employment. To do this, however, they needed to preserve a substantial budget with which to intervene in economic affairs.[167] As the ABPI astutely noted in its 1955–56 Annual Report, these macroeconomic factors had tangible implications for drug regulation:

> the contribution of the industry should be taken as a whole – its help in reducing problems of the Chancellor of the Exchequer by maintaining the value of sterling abroad should be put alongside its ability to deliver the goods for our own Health Service. . . . the two sets of factors are inseparable and complementary.[168]

Such considerations affected the Government's approach to drug regulation. For example, the Drug Requirements Advisory Committee to the Ministry of Supplies declared:

It is in the national interest to produce as many drugs as possible in this country, on grounds of saving of currency by curtailment of imports. Demands for drugs are increasing, particularly for export.[169]

In meetings and correspondence with the Ministry of Health in June 1950 the ABPI and the PAGB argued that it would be undesirable for the JCP to publish a report that classified drugs therapeutically because of the adverse effects on the export trade.[170] One month later the Board of Trade also joined the fray. In a letter to Sir William Douglas of the Ministry of Health, a senior official of the Board of Trade pointed out that almost a third of proprietary drugs were exported, and that the annual rate of export was valued at £4 million. The letter continued:

there is a danger that certifying authorities or other import licencing authorities in other countries may gain access to the Ministry of Health list of "banned" items and may refuse to grant authority to sell or import these proprietary medicines . . . Accordingly, I suggest that very great care should be taken to keep the list strictly confidential and, so far as possible, to avoid any undue publicity being given to the scheme as a whole.[171]

Despite these protests the JCP lists were published, albeit discreetly, for, as Sir Douglas pointed out, no cost-cutting benefit to the NHS could be derived from the reports if they were not circulated to doctors.[172]

By the mid 1950s the Ministry of Health had come to accept the basic philosophy that the export trade of the pharmaceutical industry was so precious that regulation of its affairs was to be avoided.[173] Accordingly, the Government implemented the Voluntary Price Regulation Scheme (VPRS) which was merely a modified version of what the industry had proposed for the regulation of drug prices.[174] However, in 1959 the Minister of Health was forced to admit that the savings from the VPRS had been "a little disappointing", and that the whole question of drug control under the NHS was to be re-examined.[175] That the Ministry of Health remained reluctant to embark on regulatory action is illustrated by the Parliamentary Secretary's comment in 1960 that "unwelcome as restrictions were, there was a duty to safeguard the health of the public".[176]

By contrast, in the US, where consumers paid for medical treatment, Government agencies were less motivated to initiate investigations into the cost of drugs. However, high drug prices and related problems of drug regulation were brought to the attention of the Government via Congressional concern for consumers' interests. In 1959 Senator Estes Kefauver began Congressional hearings, which investigated pricing and other competitive practices in the pharmaceutical industry. The time was ripe for a battle over the shortcomings of the pharmaceutical industry. John F. Kennedy's accession to the presidency marked a new period of reform in the US, in which the administration would at least lend a sympathetic ear to the critics of the drug industry's excesses in marketing and promoting ineffective products.[177] Unlike the discussion in the UK, Kefauver's investigation was to be a very public affair, which applied legislative oversight to probe into the industry's practices more thoroughly than any previous scrutiny.

In the late 1950s Kefauver and his staff discovered that the difference between companies' production costs and the prices they charged to consumers were enormous – sometimes as high as 1800 per cent.[178] On the other hand, most witnesses from the industry testified before the Kefauver committee that high profits were required to offset the amount of research needed to obtain a marketable product, especially since only a small number of such endeavours were successful. However, this view was not universal among industrialists.[179] For example, when Kefauver asked Dale Console, a former medical director at Squibb, whether much of the industry's research led to the marketing of useless drugs, he replied:

> I think more than half are in this category. And I should point out that with many of these products it is clear while they are on the drawing board that they promise no utility. They promise sales.[180]

To be sure the industry expended considerable effort and capital on the advertising and promotion of drugs. In 1958 an average of 24 per cent of the gross income of the country's 22 largest manufacturers went on advertising and promotion.[181] Drug company officials retorted that advertising and similar promotional activities made it possible to inform physicians quickly on new drug products.[182] Yet the quality of this promotion also received criticism. The Kefauver committee heard how drug companies had diluted the seriousness of the adverse effects of major drugs on package inserts (i.e. labelling) and on advertisements.[183]

After the hearings Kefauver and his staff drew up a Bill, which proposed that the FDA should licence all drug manufacturers, and require them to meet strict quality control standards. Furthermore, advertisements were to contain explicit warnings about a drug's adverse effects and a statement of its efficacy. It also argued that manufacturers should be required to demonstrate that all the drugs which they sold were not only safe, but also effective.[184]

In general, the Pharmaceutical Manufacturers' Association (PMA) and the AMA resisted the Bill. The AMA, concerned about its advertising revenues, opposed the efficacy requirement, which even the PMA and the AMA's own Council of Drugs supported.[185] Thus, the AMA's chairman, Hugh Hussey argued that only the individual physician could determine the efficacy of a given drug in the treatment of a given patient, but a spokesperson from the AMA's Council on Drugs disagreed:

> The average practising physician . . . just does not have the time, the facilities, the skill, nor the training to be an expert in the determination of drug efficacy.[186]

In his 1962 State of the Union speech President Kennedy recommended improvements in the drug laws "to protect our consumers from the careless and the unscrupulous".[187] Nevertheless, in committee stage on 9 April 1962 Kefauver's Bill was shorn of its compulsory licencing amendment by Congressional opposition. Moreover, on 8 June, unbeknown to Kefauver, a secret meeting with White House backing took place between the pro-industry senators from Kefauver's subcommittee, senior Government officials and representatives of the PMA. The purpose was to work out a compromise drug Bill which could be passed quickly. The compromise Bill neglected advertising entirely and contained a weakened efficacy requirement, which permitted a drug once approved as effective in one field to be used in some other fields without further testing.[188]

The impact of Kefauver's hearings, however, was felt well beyond Congress, and for this reason considerable industry opinion shifted towards support for legislation that would restore public confidence in drug products. As Harris explains:

> Perhaps the most compelling reason for believing that a drug Bill would be enacted was that opposition within the industry had weakened. Since March, the value of shares in the 22 largest pharmaceutical companies studied during the drug hearings had fallen anywhere from 10 per cent to as much as 60 per cent, with an average drop of about one-third. Surveys showed that people were reducing their consumption of drugs; even sales of aspirin had dropped. Some elements within the industry actually wanted a Bill – though not a strong Bill – to help assure consumers about the safety of drugs.[189]

Similarly, in Britain pressure for the reform of drug regulation was mounting. At the beginning of 1960 the Hinchliffe Committee recommended that all new drugs should be subjected to "independent" clinical trials, and that the Government should set up a clinical trials committee to "organize clinical trials of new drugs".[190] In the same year the Working Party on Medicines Legislation of the Advertising Inquiry Council recommended that some administrative instrument should be established in order to review the trial and testing of every new drug, and the PSGB urged that control of medicines should be vested with the Ministry of Health.[191] Moreover, the industry itself began to see some advantages in rationalizing the legislative patchwork over therapeutic classes which had emerged since the Second World War. In 1959 the ABPI advocated the creation of an "independent" voluntary trust to vet new drugs.[192] It was in this context that news broke of the thalidomide disaster.

It has been estimated that 8,000–9,000 mothers who took thalidomide bore deformed children, about 400 of them in the UK.[193] However, in the US, Frances Kelsey, a medical officer at the FDA, had delayed approval of thalidomide because of her concerns about its safety. By this time European physicians had discovered a cause and effect relationship between ingestion of the drug during pregnancy and phocomelia (the congenital absence of the upper arm and/or upper leg).[194] Consequently, support for reform of drug regulation rocketed, especially in the UK, where focus on improving the *safety* evaluation of drugs sharpened.

The *Pharmaceutical Journal,* not renowned for radical criticism of the British drug regulatory system, carried an editorial stating:

> It is hard to imagine a more difficult choice than that which faces a manufacturer who has to decide whether or not to withdraw a profitable drug from the market on the basis of the evidence that, on the one hand the drug may be dangerous to a small number of patients and, on the other has valuable properties. So difficult must the choice be that it is questionable whether the manufacturer should be the one to make it.[195]

Lord Cohen was prompted to remark at a symposium in April 1962 that in the previous year more than half of the drugs which had been issued, had not been correctly clinically tested, and that there was ample evidence of manufacturers supplying biased and unreliable information to physicians.[196] In Parliament, too, the safety of drugs came to be extensively debated with some MPs advocating that new drugs should be issued under a positive system of licencing with the Medical Research Council made responsible for testing new drugs, while others suggested the FDA as an exemplary model for emulation.[197]

Furthermore, the British pharmaceutical industry became concerned that the thalidomide experience might have detrimental effects on the consumption of drugs generally. In May 1962 the ABPI set up a Study Group to examine arrangements for the toxicity testing and clinical trials of new drugs. Within a few months it concluded "that to give greater assurance to the medical profession and the public, an independent body should be set up to review and offer advice on the evidence on safety submitted by manufacturers".[198]

In the US the President was provoked to recommend that Congress should support the Oren Harris's House Bill, which gave the FDA the power to withdraw immediately from the market a drug which was an "imminent hazard to public health".[199] Nevertheless, even though the thalidomide disaster created international anxiety about the regulation of drug *safety*, the US already had substantial safety regulations in place, and the most significant American reforms which came in the aftermath of thalidomide related to drug *efficacy*.

By mid August the Kefauver Bill was still being discussed in semi-secret meetings between senators, representatives of the drug industry and Government. On the question of efficacy the industry representatives insisted that the law should require only "substantial evidence", whereas the Government wanted it to require "preponderant evidence". Ultimately a compromise was reached whereby the law would require only "substantial evidence" of efficacy, but that would consist of "adequate and well-controlled investigations, by experts qualified by scientific training and experience to evaluate the effectiveness of the drug involved".[200] Finally, Congress passed a combination of these Harris and Kefauver Bills, which was signed into law as the Kefauver–Harris Amendment to the 1938 Food, Drug and Cosmetic Act in October 1962.[201]

The new laws entailed the transfer of regulatory jurisdiction over prescription drug advertising from the FTC to the FDA, requirement of proof of efficacy of all new and old drugs, disclosure of information about contra-indications on the label, and the keeping of records by drug companies on the adverse effects of all their drugs.[202] The agency also gained the authority to withdraw approval already granted to drugs if they were considered unsafe or lacked "substantial evidence" of effectiveness. Hence all approved drugs including those approved for sale before 1962 would have to meet the new effectiveness standard.[203]

After 1962 the FDA required the sponsor of a drug to supply an Investigational New Drug (IND) form that was to contain information on drug standards, pre-clinical studies on animals and cell tissue and proposed clinical investigations on humans. The IND form also included an agreement that the drug's sponsor would notify the FDA if adverse reactions were seen, and submit annual progress reports to the agency. Provided the agency had no objections to the details in the IND then the sponsor could move on to a further three phases of drug testing: (1) studies of toxicity, metabolism, absorption, elimination, dosage range and other pharmacologic actions in healthy volunteers; (2) limited clinical trials designed to test the safety and efficacy of the drug in the sick; and (3) extensive trials carried out by practising doctors as well as clinical investigators. On completion of these three phases the sponsor could submit its New Drug Application (NDA) containing all the data relating to the safety and efficacy of the drug in question.[204]

The US Drug Efficacy Study

It was not until 1966 under the leadership of Commissioner James Goddard, somewhat of a critic of the pharmaceutical industry, that the FDA decided to undertake a Drug Efficacy Study of those drugs approved and marketed between 1938 and 1962.[205] Since there were over 4,000 of them, the agency contracted the National Research Council (NRC) of the National Academy of Sciences (NAS) to carry out an initial evaluation in an advisory capacity.[206]

The NRC's conclusions were rather disconcerting. The industry's evidence in support of therapeutic claims was frequently found to be wanting. Approximately 2,000 of the 4,000 reviewed were cleared as "effective", whereas 760 were categorized as "ineffective as a fixed combination". About 600 were banned from the market and the remainder were classified as "probably effective" or "possibly effective".[207] So pervasive was the shoddiness of industry's efficacy data that nearly every major manufacturer was affected by the NRC's list of "ineffective" drugs.[208]

When the FDA tried to remove "ineffective" drugs from the market the drug industry resisted in the courts. Perhaps the most famous example of this is Upjohn's opposition to the FDA's decision in 1968 to withdraw approval of the company's combination product, *Panalba*, which delivered sales of about $9 million per year.[209] Upjohn claimed that the drug's widespread use should qualify as evidence of its effectiveness and demanded a hearing on the matter. The FDA Commissioner, Herbert Ley, who was

Goddard's chosen successor, refused. The agency won its case by stipulating that "adequate and well controlled investigations" had to include a formal test with explicit objectives, selection procedures for both subjects and control groups, observation and recording methods, and statistical analysis.[210]

It was not only the courts to which Upjohn resorted in its attempt to keep *Panalba* on the market. On 5 May 1969 Upjohn representatives met with Secretary Finch of the Department of Health, Education and Welfare, Commissioner Ley's superior in the Nixon Administration. Four days later Ley was told officially that Finch had decided that Upjohn, whose Director made contributions to the Nixon Campaign, must have a hearing on *Panalba*. This information was leaked to Congress, and later that day staff of Congressman Fountain's Committee demanded to examine the agency's files on *Panalba*. This embarassing oversight prompted Finch's office to reverse his decision, but Fountain made it a painful experience by requiring the Commissioner and the Secretary to come before his committee and put the whole sorry episode before the public.[211] The trade press strongly suspected that it was this incident, along with the banning of cyclamates (lucrative food additives for Pepsi-Cola, another major contributor to the Nixon Campaign fund), which prompted Ley's unceremonious removal from office a few months later.[212]

Ley was replaced by the "industry-friendly" Charles Edwards, following a review of FDA organization which had been ordered by Finch. Subsequently, the FDA became sluggish in exercising its powers. Thus, in 1972 the American Public Health Association and the National Council of Senior Citizens sued the FDA for taking so long to remove ineffective drugs from the market. The courts upheld their complaints and ordered the FDA to complete implementation of the NRC findings within four years, and to deal with drugs already judged to be ineffective during the next year.[213] However, in 1980 critics claimed that as many as 607 prescription drug products, which had been judged to lack adequate evidence of effectiveness, remained on the American market.[214]

Thus, even the weakened definition of efficacy established by Congress was not adequately enforced by the FDA, though some attempt to do so was made by Commissioners Goddard and Ley. Moreover, there is some indirect evidence that commercial bias in the Executive arm of the US Government may have contributed to the FDA's failure to remove from the market drugs considered to be ineffective by the agency's own scientific advisers. Though not conclusive without a detailed examination of the scientific evidence, this is strongly suggestive of regulatory bias contrary to the interests of patients.

The British Committee on the Safety of Drugs

The response of the British Government to the thalidomide disaster was contradictory; accepting, on the one hand, that new legislation was needed to require the testing of all new drugs, while simultaneously arguing that it was against the commercial interests of any drug firm to market a drug whose effects had not been subjected to the most relevant tests known.[215] Nevertheless, in June 1962 Enoch Powell, the Minister of Health, asked the Joint Subcommittee of the Standing Medical Advisory Committees under the chairmanship of Lord Cohen to consider the testing and regulation of new drugs. It was to give crucial advice on the whole institutional framework for drug safety regulation in the UK.

Despite Cohen's previous remarks about the problems of bias in the industry's drug testing, in November 1962 this Committee advised: (a) that pre-clinical toxicity testing of drugs should remain the responsibility of individual firms because "the industry, as a whole, discharges that responsibility effectively within the limits of contemporary knowledge of methods of testing"; (b) that the suggestion of a central drug testing authority was "neither desirable nor practicable"; and (c) that there should be an advisory body to review the evidence and offer advice on the toxicity of new drugs.[216] Powell, accepted (a) and (b), and awaited more detailed advice on (c). Significantly the ABPI was to co-operate with the Cohen Subcommittee in consideration of the composition of the proposed advisory body.[217]

It is not difficult to find plausible reasons for Powell's interest in consulting closely with the industry. The Ministry of Health was the industry's sponsoring department,[218] and the National Economic Development Council had just noted the importance to the British economy of the fast growing sectors, such as pharmaceuticals. For its part, the industry wanted some regulation to help raise the standing of its products at home, but did not want a regulatory system too critical of its brand name products that were already established exports.[219] It was in this context that the Cohen Subcommittee sat down in consultation with the ABPI to advise the Ministry of Health on the kind of regulatory body which should set the tone for modern drug safety control in the UK.

The ABPI argued that the advisory body should be constituted as a

Trust independent of the industry and the Government, comprising professional and trade associations.[220] The Cohen Subcommittee was divided on the nature of the proposed advisory body. Two pharmacists on the Subcommittee believed that the Government should have been told that the situation required comprehensive legislation.[221] In its Final Report the Subcommittee reached a compromise between this view and the industry scheme by proposing that the Ministers of Health should immediately, and without legislation, appoint a Committee on the Safety of Drugs (CSD), which would depend on the *voluntary* co-operation of the industry. The Cohen Subcommittee also argued that public opinion would require (a) that the CSD should be entirely independent of industry and (b) some type of formal machinery for the safety evaluation of drugs.[222]

Accepting the advice of Cohen's Subcommittee, the Health Ministers appointed the CSD with Sir Derrick Dunlop as chairman, and Powell pronounced that its membership was of such eminence that it was unthinkable that they would submit to any influence but the force of scientific considerations.[223] Yet members evidently held strong views about industrial drug testing. For example, in 1962 Professor Wilson, who had been a member of the Cohen Committee, and who was later to be appointed to the Medicines Commission of drug regulation, and to the chair of the CSD's successor, the Committee on the Safety of Medicines, *assumed*:

If a drug is shown to be harmful to animals, its use in Man is not contemplated, . . . and every reputable pharmaceutical firm and clinical investigator ensure to the best of current knowledge that all the appropriate investigations have been done before the drug is given to Man.[224]

Within its terms of reference the CSD was to invite reports on toxicity tests from the manufacturer, consider whether drugs should be put to clinical trial, obtain reports of such trials, and take into account the safety, efficacy and adverse effects of drugs.[225] In 1963 the Cohen Committee had recommended that a central registry of adverse reactions should be set up to act as an "early warning system" once a new drug had been marketed.[226] The CSD, therefore, initiated the yellow card system, which has continued ever since.[227] This provides doctors with cards on which to voluntarily report to the British regulatory authorities any suspected adverse drug reaction.

The Committee began operations on 1 January 1964, and the ABPI and PAGB undertook not to market or submit to clinical trial any new drug against the advice of the Committee.[228] Two months beforehand, the CSD had pledged that information submitted to it by manufacturers about new drugs would be treated as confidential to the Committee; ostensibly to ensure that the development of new drugs of therapeutic value was not hindered. Thus, before it had even begun regulatory activity the Committee sealed itself off from public scrutiny.[229] The industry was content with these arrangements, especially because they provided it with valuable time and experience with which to gain strategic influence over the regulatory process and any forthcoming legislation.[230]

Meanwhile the infrequent public announcements about the CSD and its staff's activities showed that there was certainly room for improvement in the manufacturers' standards of safety. For example, in its first year the CSD received 600 submissions for new drugs. In 99 cases it requested further information, and in 15 rejected the manufacturers' proposals. The number of formal decisions by the CSD to reject the marketing of new drugs was, however, small.[231] Review was deliberately rapid; averaging three months for new chemical entities and one month for novel reformulations.[232] As the CSD commented in its annual report for 1966:

> ... it is fully recognized that a Committee such as this might exercise a detrimental effect on pharmaceutical research progress by unduly delaying the introduction of a possibly valuable drug or even by preventing its use altogether.[233]

The ABPI hoped that any forthcoming legislation would emulate the CSD approach.[234] Significantly, in January 1965 Dunlop echoed these views, arguing that while legislation "may well prove necessary and desirable, it is hoped that the Committee's present freedom will not be curtailed by a bureaucratic straitjacket".[235]

Other Government committees concerned with the efficiency of the NHS were not so generous to the industry. In May 1965 the MacGregor Committee of the Scottish and Central Health Service Councils employed the concept of comparative efficacy in recommending that two out of its six categories of branded medicines should require specific justification for prescription under the NHS.[236] The Hinchliffe Committee complained that some manufacturers made advertising claims for their products which were "not justified by acceptable evidence",[237] and the Public Accounts Committee showed repeated concern over promotion expenditure in the industry.[238] Perhaps most significantly, the Sainsbury Committee, appointed by the Government to advise on the relationship between the pharmaceutical industry and the NHS, concluded in 1967 that some of the existing arrangements for promotion, including the extensive employment of manufacturers' medical representatives, were wasteful and lacking in the appropriate responsibility.[239] The Sainsbury Committee recommended the abolition of brand names, the requirement that therapeutic classifications appear on all medicines, and the establishment of a Medicines Commission funded by, but independent of, direct control by the Ministry of Health with wide statutory powers to regulate the quality, safety, efficacy and promotion of drugs.[240]

In response to these kinds of criticisms the ABPI revised its Code of Practice by stipulating that information on adverse effects, precautions and contra-indications should be provided in promotional material, and by prohibiting gifts to doctors, other than promotional aids of little monetary value and relevant to medical practice.[241] With new medicines legislation imminent, the industry sought to give a good impression in the hope that self-regulation of drug promotion would be preserved. As the new chairman of the ABPI's Marketing Practices Committee remarked:

> These steps underline the Association's policy of ensuring accuracy and responsibility in the promotion of medicines in the professions . . . It is important, however, not only that the industry should take these measures, but that it should be seen to be taking them.[242]

Moreover, in a memorandum to the Government the ABPI strongly opposed the idea of a regulatory Commission with substantial executive powers. It disputed the need for external statutory control over advertising with elaborate supervisory machinery in preference to self-regulation, and argued that a statutory system of classifying medicines according to therapeutic value would be damaging to exports. Furthermore, the industry claimed that the abolition of brand names would also be disastrous for exports with consequent reductions in investment in pharmaceutical research at home.[243]

In summary, the CSD was established on the presupposition that industry's drug testing was sound and did not conflict with patients' interests, and that scientists serving on the Committee could not be subject to conflicts of interest. Corporate bias may be considered intrinsic to the CSD because the pharmaceutical industry played such a large part in shaping the Committee's frames of reference. This is confirmed by the extent to which members of the CSD shared the industry's view of regulation as a process by which to clear drugs rapidly for the market.

The British Medicines Act

The Government's 1967 White Paper on forthcoming medicines legislation outlined a product licencing system to regulate the quality, safety, and efficacy of new drugs, but it rejected the Sainsbury concept of an independent Medicines Commission in favour of an advisory one, which was to be appointed by, and ultimately accountable to, the Minister of Health acting as the licencing authority. The Medicines Commission was to advise the Minister on the appointment of expert committees, who would advise the licencing authority on specific aspects of drug regulation.[244] The Government also ignored the Sainsbury Committee's suggestion to abolish brand names.

During the period of drug legislation review in the 1960s, the ABPI and the CSD maintained close liaison. This coincided with some representatives of the Committee responding with remarkable similarity to those of the ABPI on how the Government should regulate drugs. In March 1968 Dunlop, chairman of the CSD, made a telling speech which indicated his approach to drug regulation.[245] He asserted that it should not impose unnecessary restraints on the prosperity of the pharmaceutical industry nor "pontificate" on the efficacy of medicines. A flexible approach, he explained, was to be preferred, and this meant that contacts with companies were informal, good-humoured and often over the telephone, rather than through official communications.[246] As Cahal, the CSD's Medical Assessor explained, the Committee was *dependent* on the industry's co-operation:

> One is often asked how the Committee manages to comply with its terms of reference with so small staff. The answer is "decentralization", which means, since there is nowhere else to which we can decentralize, decentralization to industry.[247]

Such extensive contact with industry, however, was not without impact on the way the CSD conducted itself as Wade, a former member, later explained:

> Looking back I see only one major error in our performance. We were so aware of the enormous co-operation that we received from the drug industry that the main Committee made every effort it could to see that submissions from firms were handled as rapidly as possible – as a result . . . the Adverse Reactions subcommittee and . . . the work of that subcommittee suffered.[248]

On the question of brand names Dunlop argued that their abolition was probably undesirable because it could place the major innovating companies in Britain at a competitive disadvantage overseas. He further noted that the medical profession depended on the industry's wellbeing, and warned:

> *From this point of view alone* we should be very chary of interfering with the reproductive processes of a goose which has laid so many golden therapeutic eggs.[249] (Emphasis added)

As the Medicines Bill was debated in Parliament and outside, the Government's fundamental perspective on the new legislation became clearer. At Committee stage Julian Snow, Parliamentary Secretary to the Ministry of Health, commented that the Government was working towards a "Dunlop type" speed of administration, while the Minister himself assured critics of the Bill that there was no need for clauses to safeguard industrial innovation because some of the members of the Commission would be drawn from the industry, and it was unlikely that the Commission would use its influence to limit the introduction of new products by being unduly exacting in its requirements.[250] The extent of Dunlop's influence in shaping regulations also emerged when Snow revealed that the Bill's clauses concerning clinical trials had been closely modelled on the practices of the CSD.[251]

The Bill also maintained the all-encompassing confidentiality procedures initiated by the CSD; the British Government apparently unmoved by the establishment of the 1966 Freedom of Information Act in the US, which made possible public scrutiny of many agency files.[252] On its second reading on 15 February 1968 the Bill won approval in the House of Commons to become the Medicines Act.[253] In May 1969, a few weeks after Dunlop had been appointed chairman of the new Medicines Commission, the ABPI and the PAGB were invited to have discussions with the Ministry of Health about the Commission's functions, structure and membership.[254] In April 1970 Dunlop outlined the regulatory philosophy he envisaged for the Medicines Commission, namely to find "a happy medium" between the "conflicting objectives" of maintaining the wellbeing of the industry, on the one hand, and the control over the use of powerful drugs in the interests of public safety, on the other.[255] Industrial interests, then, were to form an integral part of the Commission's concerns.

So successful had been the industry in preserving a flexible regulatory approach by Government that Harold Davis, a former chief pharmacist at the Ministry of Health, who had been closely concerned with the new medicines legislation from 1962–7, and Lord Aberdare of the Department of Health and Social Security (DHSS), both felt able to predict that manufacturers would hardly notice the difference when the Medicines Commission took over from the CSD.[256]

Though the Cohen Committee on the safety of drugs had recommended that the CSD should be "entirely independent of industry", members of the latter were permitted to, and did, retain consultancies with pharmaceutical companies.[257] In 1970, however, the DHSS, formerly the Ministry of Health, invited the ABPI to consider a change of policy, whereby persons holding consultancies in the industry would no longer be appointed to the CSD or its subcommittees. The ABPI refused to support such a change and it was never made.[258] Indeed, all the major elements of the regulatory organizations concerned with drug safety and efficacy have exhibited a close relationship with the pharmaceutical industry via direct representation, consultancies or prior and/or subsequent employment.

Several examples may be readily cited. After retiring as chairman of the Medicines Commission in Spring 1972 Dunlop, formerly chairman of the CSD, joined the board of directors of the Sterling-Winthrop Group Ltd, a wholly owned subsidiary of a US pharmaceutical company which sold prescription and over-the-counter drugs.[259] Also the initial 13-person membership of the Medicines Commission contained three fully employed members of the pharmaceutical industry. Though the Medicines Act requires the Health Ministers to appoint at least one person having "wide and recent experience of . . . the pharmaceutical industry"[260] to be a member of the Medicines Commission, it has regularly included more than one representative from the industry. For example, in 1984 the 17-person Commission included five representatives of the pharmaceutical industry.[261]

Perhaps the most dramatic example of the close relationship between the pharmaceutical industry and the British regulatory authorities is the career of John P. Griffin. In 1971 he joined the Medicines Division of the DHSS, having previously been head of clinical research at the drug company Riker 3M. He had worked in the pharmaceutical industry for 14 years and had been a medical director of a company. During his time at the DHSS Griffin was medical assessor to the CSM and to the Medicines Commission. In 1977 he was appointed professional Head of the Medicines Division, a position he retained until August 1984 when he returned to industry by becoming director of the ABPI.[262] As he joined the ABPI

Griffin revealed that the extent of exchange of personnel between industry and the Medicines Division went well beyond his own case:

> . . . all my deputies [at the Medicines Division], principal medical officers, have been in industry. All the superintendent pharmacists that I had working for me, all came from industry. It is equally clear that within the last 12 months I am not the only member of the medical staff of the division to move back into industry.[263]

Given the longevity of Griffin's important position at the Medicines Division his views about the role of the Medicines Division in regulating the industry are significant. These he also revealed on moving to the ABPI, as follows:

> It is abundantly clear to me that the Medicines Division could not function if it did not recruit the expertise that it requires from industry. . . . I have always opposed the development of any attitude which I could only classify as adversarial, and I have resisted any attempts by either the industry, the permanent staff of the Medicines Division, or the committees to adopt an adversarial role. . . . the role of the regulators is in fact to achieve the release on to the market of those products which have had peer review which has shown them as satisfactory for the indications for which they were going to be marketed.[264]

In similar fashion Frank Wells, a member of the Toxicity and Clinical Trials Subcommittee of the CSM from 1977–81 became Director of Medical Affairs at the ABPI on 1 October 1986.[265] Indeed, in 1988 the personal and non-personal interests of the members of the Medicines Commission, the CSM and the Committee on the Review of Medicines (CRM) (established in 1975) in the pharmaceutical industry were published for the first time and are summarized in Table 1.

These references to the closeness between the pharmaceutical industry, on the one hand, and Dunlop, Griffin, Wells and members of the CSM, CRM and Medicines Commission, on the other, do not necessarily imply that the regulatory judgements of those individuals have been biased. Furthermore, there is no suggestion whatsoever that those individuals have acted improperly. Nevertheless, such closeness to industry, combined with the insulation of the regulatory authorities from public scrutiny, may increase the likelihood of conflict of interest and commercial bias in drug regulation.[266] The risk of such bias via conflict of interest and the Government–industry "revolving door"[267] was a major reason for the US Congress passing the 1978 Ethics in Government Act, which prohibited

Table 1   Financial links with the pharmaceutical industry in 1988.

	Personal interests[a]	Non-personal interests[b]	Neither
Med. Commission (n=24)	17	7	5
CSM (n=21)	14	15	4
CSM Subcommittee on Safety, Efficacy and Adverse Reactions (n=18)	12	13	2
CRM (n=17)	7	10	6

a) Defined as consultancies, fee paid work, and shareholding.
b) Defined as payments that benefit department for which member is responsible but are not received by member personally.
Source: Delamothe, T. 1989. Drugs watchdogs and the drug industry. *British Medical Journal* **299**, 19 August, p. 476.

employees of American federal agencies, including the FDA, from joining the industry they were regulating for at least two years after leaving the agency.[268]

Adversary and retreat in British regulatory policy

During the 1970s the industry maintained its strategic influence over the DHSS and its advisory committees on drug safety through close consultation about regulations on data requirements for clinical trial certificates and product licences.[269] Nevertheless, the regulatory authorities did demand increasingly detailed and complex pre-clinical data before granting a clinical trial certificate. In 1977 just over one-third of clinical trial certificate applications were granted without requesting further information compared with 74 per cent in 1971.[270] Furthermore, it was claimed that the average time before clinical testing in the UK was four times that required in several other major Western countries.[271] Consequently, the number of clinical trial certificates issued fell from 170 in 1972 to 87 in 1980, and according to industrial representatives, companies shifted investment in clinical trials to locations outside the UK.[272]

However, neither these controls nor the yellow card monitoring system prevented several thousand patients in Britain suffering serious adverse effects while taking Imperial Chemical Industries' beta-blocking drug practolol (*Eraldin*).[273] At the time that was the biggest drug disaster recorded in the UK, and put the regulatory authorities under close and critical scrutiny.[274] This, then, was a period of searching for more effective forms of regulating drug safety, rather than one of deregulation.[275]

In 1975 the Committee on the Review of Medicines (CRM) was established under the chairmanship of Eric Scowen to comply with the EEC directive requiring all medicines to be reviewed and assessed according to modern existing licencing standards by May 1990. The task involved reviewing the "licences of right" of some 36,000 medicinal products, including over 4,000 proprietary prescription drugs, which had been allowed to stay on the market after the Medicines Act came into force without any independent scrutiny of the evidence for their safety or efficacy.[276] The industry was reluctant to assist a body which threatened to restrict or revoke existing licences. Moreover, to accelerate the review process, the Minister of Health decided that consultation procedures with industry should be bypassed for products which the CRM thought to represent a special hazard. As a consequence the industry and regulatory authority drifted into "an adversarial attitude".[277] In particular, the CRM was challenged in the courts by the industry for recommending the revocation of a licence based on a comparison of a manufacturer's product with other products of the same therapeutic class.[278] Though the CRM had rejected in principle the Health Minister's proposal to categorize the drugs under review into those of first, second and reserve choice, it had in this case introduced the criterion of comparative efficacy in a way which the courts ruled as acceptable.[279]

Extended regulatory activity occurred also in the context of Labour being returned to power under Harold Wilson in the February 1974 General Election with a manifesto containing for the first time proposals to take over sections of the pharmaceutical industry.[280] Yet the pharmaceutical industry was not nationalized in any form. In fact, 1976 marked a change in the general political climate. The Keynesian-inspired system of fixed exchange rates collapsed in 1972 paving the way for rapid and destabilizing fluctuations, while the oil price explosion of 1973 led to a series of balance of payments problems for the Government. To maintain its commitment to public expenditure the Government opted for a programme of major overseas borrowing, which resulted in a severe collapse of sterling. In an attempt to salvage the situation, in 1976 Denis Healey, Chancellor of the Exchequer, obtained a £3.9 billion loan from the International Monetary Fund, but on the condition that the Government reduced its public expenditure and adopted monetarist policies in the form of stringent money supply controls in the economy.[281]

The speech by Prime Minister James Callaghan at the 1976 Labour

Party conference signalled the Government's shift from a Keynesian approach:

We used to think that you could spend your way out of a recession, and increase employment by cutting taxes and boosting Government expenditure. I tell you in all candour that that option no longer exists.[282]

For Labour the necessary monetarist strategy involved less State intervention in the economy. Thus, in November 1976 Callaghan proclaimed:

We must give absolute priority to industrial needs ahead of even our social objectives . . . we must ensure that industry is profitable . . . we must aim at faster growth and high productivity.[283]

Labour not only abandoned any thought of nationalizing the pharmaceutical industry, but also became responsive to complaints from industries in general of excessive State regulation.[284] Throughout the late 1970s the ABPI complained about the extent of the DHSS regulatory activity concerning pre-clinical data submissions for clinical trial certificates (CTCs). Reflecting on the problem of this period the President of the ABPI in 1981 explained the industry's difficulty:

No company . . . can afford to expend more on preliminary testing than it can expect to recover in sales. More and more companies were undertaking preliminary clinical effectiveness trials in overseas countries where the data requirements for such studies were less prohibitively expensive.[285]

Of particular significance, the National Economic Development Council's "sector working party" on the pharmaceutical industry concluded in 1976 that, in order for the pharmaceutical sector to maximize its contribution to a positive UK balance of payments through expansion of direct exports and import substitution, the DHSS should seek to have the minimum impact on the industry's research by ensuring that decisions regarding CTCs be reached within two months.[286] Consequently, the CSM was asked by the Government to examine ways in which its procedures for assessing CTCs could be expedited.[287]

In 1979 the Conservatives were elected with a positive monetarist philosophy and a commitment to reduce State intervention in the economy. By April 1980 Patrick Jenkin, Secretary of State for Social Services, had announced the Government's intention to introduce a clinical trial exemption scheme.[288] Thus, from March 1981 under this scheme an applicant needed only to submit a summary of the data relevant for a CTC to the Medicines Division of the DHSS, who then had five weeks to object to the proposed trials.[289] The clinical trial exemption scheme was much welcomed by the industry.[290] In August 1981 senior representatives of the Medicines Division stated that the clinical trial exemption scheme had become necessary "because early developmental work on new drugs was going abroad to the detriment of British industry"; thus indicating that the regulatory authority had adopted both the industry's interpretation of the effects of the clinical trial certificate requirements and its suggestions for change.[291]

Government regulation of advertising also sounded the retreat. In 1975 the Medicines Division undertook a modest inspection of advertisements and some action was taken on 49 of the 65 unsatisfactory cases considered by its advisers.[292] Two years later, however, the DHSS entered into an agreement with the ABPI, whereby the latter would take over the policing of drug companies' advertisements on condition that its code of practice was somewhat strengthened. The industry, therefore, had, in effect, won self-regulation of advertising, even though the ABPI had refused to undertake a programme of pre-publication scrutiny requested of it by the DHSS.[293]

In short, during the early 1970s the Medicines Division and the CSM extended their regulatory controls in a number of fields, thereby forcing pharmaceutical firms to raise the standards and thoroughness of their drug testing. Such regulations are likely to have improved patient protection, but the industry perceived them as damaging to its commercial interests. Consequently, the Government sought to accommodate the industry's anxieties by increasing self-regulation and accelerating the review process of the Medicines Division and the CSM by reducing the extent of their checks on industry.

Adversary and neutralization at the FDA

Consistent with the assumptions on which the British regulatory authorities were set up, they readily adopted a non-adversarial approach to industry when faced with opposition. However, the FDA's official mission to protect the public from unsafe and ineffective drugs had attracted some scientists who supported adversarial relations with industry. Any retreat from adversary by the FDA, therefore, was likely to be much less smooth than for the agency's British counterpart.

In 1974 Congress heard remarkable testimonies from nine reviewing officers at the FDA's Bureau of Drugs and two physicians who had previously worked in the agency. All were, or had been, responsible for reviewing some part of the NDAs submitted by drug companies. They claimed that when they recommended the approval of a drug their analyses were hardly ever challenged, but that their recommendations for non-approval were sometimes unjustifiably overruled. Furthermore, many of these witnesses testified that when they insisted on the inadequacy of data to support approval they experienced harassment within the agency, and in specific cases were removed from reviewing the particular drug in question.[294] Frequently, the contrary reviewer would be tranferred into an entirely different division within the Bureau, and in some six cases transferral resulted in reviewers having to work in a field which was not their primary area of expertise.[295] So began an episode, which led to the most extensive Congressional investigation of the FDA ever undertaken.

In response to these and many other allegations Alexander Schmidt, the FDA Commissioner, told Congress on the next day that he would carry out an investigation to ascertain their accuracy.[296] In 1975 he undertook an extensive investigation, and in October 1975 reported no improper drug approvals; no bias towards drug approvals; no industry domination of the Bureau; no harassment of employees or pressure to approve drugs by punitive transfers or otherwise; and no arbitrary overruling of anyone. He did, however, acknowledge that many agency employees may have been overruled or transferred, but these instances, he claimed, reflected "administrative and personnel deficiencies not involving the integrity of the drug review process or its managers".[297]

A Review Panel on New Drug Regulation had been established by Congress to oversee the Commissioner's investigation. In May 1976 the Review Panel found the Commissioner's report unsatisfactory:

> . . . the Panel found that the Commissioner's general conclusions favourable to FDA are not supported by the evidence he adduced. The Commissioner concludes his Report with broad statements affirming the propriety of FDA's operations despite the fact that he did not develop an adequate evidentiary basis to support these statements. In fact, the fundamental questions raised by the allegations remain not simply unanswered but virtually unasked by the Commissioner's Report.[298]

For example, the Panel found that, in some cases, the Commissioner had accepted the accounts offered by the Bureau's management, over and above the equally credible accounts of complainants.[299]

Consequently the Panel set about the task of re-investigating four sets of allegations: "undue industry influence"; "improper transfers, details or removals"; "improper use of advisory committees"; and "improper use of medical officer recommendations". This amounted to a re-investigation of almost 20 per cent of the total initially voiced, and was undertaken by the Panel's Special Counsel.[300]

The Special Counsel submitted his report to the Panel in March 1977. This revealed that the Commissioner's investigation had indeed been inadequate as a comprehensive response to the allegations made against the Bureau. The Special Counsel concluded that, although the FDA had not been "dominated" by the pharmaceutical industry during the period under investigation, "inappropriate contacts with drug companies occurred". Furthermore, from 1970 the FDA's management established and sought to implement a deliberate policy of "making the agency less adversarial towards and more co-operative with drug manufacturers, and to neutralize reviewing medical officers who followed a different philosophy". The report identified those reviewing officers who made the allegations against the agency as belonging to "the more adversarial or critical school", whom the management sought to "neutralize".[301] As to the method of "neutralization" the report revealed:

> The program to neutralize the more adversarial reviewers was carried out by various devices, including a *systematic pattern* of involuntary transfers to positions which the incumbents did not want, and, in a few cases removal from the review of particular drugs. FDA management *generally* concealed the truth about the reasons for the transfers from the persons affected.[302] (Emphasis added)

Regarding drug approvals the Special Counsel was limited because he did not undertake analyses of the scientific literature pertaining to the drug approvals related to the investigation. Hence, he was unable to make any substantial judgements as to the bias in the scientific aspects of drug approval decisions. In view of these limitations the Special Counsel's conclusion that "we found no bias towards drug approvals as such" is not very revealing, for it is difficult to see how this re-investigation could have uncovered bias of such a detailed nature.[303] Nevertheless, he did feel able to conclude that "a non-adversarial philosophy *vis-à-vis* drug companies ... brought a kind of pressure to approve drugs on more adversarially inclined reviewers".[304]

The extent to which the FDA's "neutralization" policy reflects the behaviour of the organization in periods other than the early 1970s is not known. It may be noted, however, that several key officials involved in the FDA's neutralization policy either remained in high office or were subsequently promoted within the agency, The Congressional Panel recognized that those officials were very distinguished scientists and it is not being suggested in any way that they were promoted because of their involvement with the neutralization policy. Nevertheless, such promotion does suggest that the perspectives of the FDA management are likely to have remained sympathetic to the non-adversarial approaches underpinning that policy.

Conclusion

The emergence of drug regulation in both the US and the UK is complex. Nevertheless, a substantial amount of the empirical evidence presented in this chapter provides support for "public interest" theories of regulatory capture. Regarding incentives to capture, in both countries key regulatory personnel have assimilated the interests of the regulated industry, and this has affected regulatory policy as illustrated by the rapid approval philosophies adopted by the CSD in the 1960s, the CSM in the late 1970s and early 1980s, and the neutralization strategy at the FDA during the early 1970s. Regulatory capture has been more comprehensive in the UK, however, because of the very large extent to which the British regulatory authorities have depended on the pharmaceutical industry for expertise, both within the regulatory process and via the particularly vigorous operation of the "revolving door".

Another important difference between the UK and the US in relation to capture is that when the FDA finds itself in an adversarial situation with industry, Congressional oversight and judicial review are apt to call the agency to account in public for any disengagement from its regulatory responsibilities. For this reason, the agency's actions have at least to be seen to be defensible, irrespective of industrial interests. This is likely to have imposed limitations on the possibilities for capture of the FDA. By contrast, the British regulatory authorities have operated under conditions of extreme secrecy, which may have facilitated their retreat from adversary with industry.

The adversarial relationship between the FDA and the industry can, however, be overstated. Collier, for instance, characterizes the FDA's regulatory function as "defending the public from the capricious demands of the profit-seeking drug industry".[305] While a superficial analysis of the FDA may represent its relationship with the pharmaceutical industry as adversarial, the evidence suggests that such a representation needs to be qualified by taking account of divisions within the agency. Investigations of the internal workings of the agency during the 1970s suggest a managerial prerogative to suppress such adversary. Moreover, the neutralization policy of the period may have served a long-term purpose in signalling to agency personnel that amicable relations with, and a permissive approach towards, industry are conditions for the maintenance of good relations with FDA management – thus increasing the likelihood of agency capture. There are no comparable data available concerning the internal functioning of the drug regulatory authorities in the UK. However, given the secrecy and industrial influence under which British regulators operate, it is reasonable to suppose that Government scientists who support an adversarial approach to industry are even less tolerated than at the FDA.

Capture theories of the "public interest" type also imply that when first established, and during subsequent periods of public pressure, regulatory reforms have primarily served the public interest, rather than the interests of industry. Similarly, it is frequently claimed by representatives of the regulatory authorities themselves that public concern about the dangers of drugs has motivated the development of regulation, and that such regulation has been fundamentally aimed at protecting patients' health. For example, the FDA's official history of American drug regulation reads:

> Wiley took his campaign public. . . . By the turn of the century, a group of crusading writers had joined the campaign. National magazines . . . aroused public opinion. All this campaigning finally led to the passage of the 1906 Pure Food and Drug Act. . . . The Sulfanilamide tragedy ignited enthusiasm for a new law to ensure the safety of drugs before marketing. In response to this need the Federal Food, Drug and Cosmetic Act was passed in 1938. . . . like the Sulfanilamide episode, thalidomide dramatized the need to strengthen the drug provisions of the 1938 Act. In 1962 the Kefauver–Harris Amendments tightened up the requirements for testing new prescription drugs.[306]

And in the UK, Penn, a representative of the Medicines Division at the DHSS in 1980, states:

> the regulatory agencies are concerned with the safety and protection of the public. I see these agencies as the logical and most re-

cent development and expression of the anxiety long felt by the
public and their elected representatives about the safety of
drugs.[307]

Furthermore, critics of drug regulation have accepted this account of history, as is clear from Braithwaite's assertion that:

The great lesson from the history of regulation in the international
pharmaceutical industry is that massive reforms can occur following a crisis. . . . the world's regulatory systems are a muddle because they were born of hasty reactions to crises.[308]

Undoubtedly drug disasters have contributed to the urgency with which
proposals for reforms were passed into new legislation, but the supposition
that major threats to public health have been the crucial motors of regulatory change is not supported by the available evidence. Drug regulation in
the late nineteenth century in Britain and the early twentieth century in
the US resulted from a culmination of factors, including scientific and
technological changes, which facilitated the detection of drug adulteration, public campaigns for legislative change, and the transformation of
the economic interests of powerful sections of the drug trade. In saying
this, the evidence suggests that the desire of the technologically advanced
firms to support State regulation seems to have been the most crucial factor. The scientific efforts of Accum in Britain and the American anti-adulteration campaigns of the 1880s and 1890s came to nothing in the
absence of significant industrial concern. Moreover, the regulatory reforms eventually implemented by the State did not follow logically from
the real interests of consumers as expressed by the campaigns of Hassall
and Wiley. Rather, those reforms benefited primarily the dominant interests of the drug trade, and consumers only at the margins.

We may conclude that the American and British Governments have
been centrally concerned to negotiate with, and between the interests of
the drug trade. Consequently, so far as patient protection is concerned,
legislation has been consistently weak, compromised and not necessarily
hasty. In Britain, this is evident from the 1860 Adulteration Act, the 1875
Sale of Food and Drug Act, the dilution of the proposals on drug testing
made by the CSDIP, the origins of the 1941 Pharmacy and Medicines Act
and the 1968 Medicines Act, and the ten year delay between thalidomide
and the implementation of the Medicines Act in 1971; and in the US from
the 1906 Pure Food and Drug Act, the 1938 Food, Drug and Cosmetic
Act, and the definition of drug efficacy under the 1962 Kefauver–Harris
Amendments.

The evidence suggests that corporate bias in the moulding of regulation has been more comprehensive in the UK than in the US. The origins of the Ministry of Health indicate that the British regulatory authorities were created into a condition of corporate bias much more than Wiley's Bureau of Chemistry in the US. The Ministry's response to the CSDIP, and to the problem of patent medicines demonstrates such corporate bias in action; consumers' interests were either compromised or incidental. Further evidence that the British Government has not protected consumers' interests is provided by the fact that there is no trace of regulatory reform activity in the Ministry of Health after the Elixir Sulfanilamide disaster, even though the dire implications of that event for consumer safety applied no less in the UK than in the US, where the tragedy occurred.

Scientific and technological developments in the pharmaceutical industry, combined with Government concern over drug prices, were at the heart of the pre-thalidomide debates about regulatory reform. As a consequence, drug standards and promotion were investigated by elements of the British and American Governments. In the UK the dominant approach was to take minimal regulatory action against industrial interests. Where such action was taken the primary motive seems to have been budgetary savings rather than patients' interests *per se*. By contrast, in the US Kefauver's campaigning in Congress was directed towards greater patient protection, and met with considerable success, boosted substantially by the thalidomide disaster. Yet even the Kefauver–Harris Amendment was characterized by corporate bias with drug industry representatives being central to discussions about its final form, such that the definition of drug efficacy compromised patients' interests.

It is also important to appreciate that the improvement of regulatory standards for patients has sometimes lagged behind even industrial support for it because the interests of the industry have changed and divided over time. For example, in the late nineteenth century the major pharmaceutical companies, especially in the US, were among the vanguard of regulatory reform because the existing fragmentary regulations were no longer seen as sufficient to enforce the drug standards which offered competitive advantages to the most progressive firms. These factors explain why in 1908 William Graham, a senior official at Smith, Kline & French, defended the 1906 Act by arguing:

> only competent and reliable firms can now be engaged in the manufacture of pharmaceuticals.[309]

Other less powerful and technologically advanced elements of the trade campaigned to retain the status quo and its attendant adulterative practices, but were unsuccessful. Hence, American and British regulatory developments in the late nineteenth and early twentieth centuries, though compromised to meet the dominant trade interests, did bring marginal benefits to consumers. However, those benefits were more incidental to, than causal of, regulatory change. Clearly there are other examples which support this interpretation. To name one: in the UK the 1941 Pharmacy and Medicines Act brought incidental consumer protection by putting an end to patent medicines, but was motivated by the changing commercial interests of the industry. Further evidence that industrial, rather than consumer, interests conditioned the 1941 Act is provided by the fact that the BMA in 1909, and a House of Commons Select Committee in 1914, both exposed the inadequacies of the existing legislation to protect consumers from the fraudulence of patent medicines, yet no reforms ensued at those times.

Since drug regulation in both countries has often emerged according to the balance of trade interests, its development can be seen as consistent with "private interest" theories to a considerable degree. However, on occasions the State has rejected the demands of the industry in total. The objections of the PSGB to the extension of the 1917 Defence of the Realm Regulations to peacetime were overruled by the Home Office on the grounds of State security. Also in the UK, during the budgetary crisis immediately following the Second World War the Ministry of Health did not revise its plans to publish prescription drug lists designed to rationalize NHS prescribing, despite the fears of the pharmaceutical industry; and the regulatory authorities did instigate the 1975 review of medicines required by EEC Directives. In the US, similar remarks apply to aspects of Goddard's Drug Efficacy Study, especially the prosecution of the *Panalba* case by unilaterally introducing new regulations, despite substantial opposition from industry.

Evidently, the historical study of drug regulation in this chapter suggests that certain interests reside with the State itself, and cannot be merely attributed to the interests of capitalist industry as some Marxist and "private interest" theories of the State suppose. In those instances when the interests of the State and the industry do not converge, the former seem to be related to *other organized interests*. For example, the 1975 review of medicines initiated by the British regulatory authorities came at a time when the State had to respond to specific regulatory demands made by powerful European bureaucracies. In the US, Goddard's Drug Efficacy Study was related to the success of the organized interests in Congress and the American consumer movements, which had been much in evidence during the Kefauver Hearings and immediately prior to Goddard's appointment.

Also among the State's major considerations of regulatory reform have been the management of the national economy as a viable capitalist unit in terms of domestic budgets, balance of payments and social stability. The way in which these three factors have affected drug regulation has varied according to wider social circumstances. The first two have been of little significance for drug regulation in the US because, unlike the situation in the UK, American regulatory policy has been separate from the State's role as a customer or sponsor of the industry. In the UK, balance of payments concerns have generally allowed industrial export interests to dominate regulatory decisions. However, in periods of severe socioeconomic crisis, such as the early twentieth century in the UK and the 1930s in the US, the State has responded to increasing class antagonism, and the demands of organized labour, with a tide of reforms that had indirect effects on drug regulation. During those periods social reform, including some extended drug regulation, was seen by the State as a basis for societal stability, and the State's own interests in maintaining itself are most vivid (e.g. the British Liberal Reforms and the American New Deal), even to the extent of overriding the concerns of the drug trade, as in the case of the 1920 Dangerous Drugs Act in the UK. Marxist theories, which stress class struggle and class bias in their discussions of the role of the State, therefore, seem to have some indirect relevance to the development of drug regulation in the UK and the US, but this is confined to periods of widespread social instability.

The findings contained in this chapter are more comprehensively consistent with corporatist theories than the alternative formulations available. The reason for this is that corporatist theories can accommodate not only the fact that industrial interests have played a key role in the establishment and evolution of regulation, but also the fact that the State under certain conditions defines its own interests independently of the industry.

The uncommon occasions when the State has opted to reject the commercial interests of the industry have led some commentators to mistake such actions for the norm. For example, in an article entitled "Drug famine", Smith criticized the regulatory authorities for failing to approve enough drugs in the aftermath of *Eraldin*. He concluded:

Introduced as they [regulatory agencies] were to prevent epidem-
ics of drug-induced damage, their approach has inevitably been
cautious.[310]

From the evidence in this chapter Smith's account of the actions of the
regulatory agencies may be confidently rejected, with respect to the UK
and the US. In general, the regulatory agencies, especially in the UK, have
adopted a permissive philosophy towards the industry. In the case of drug
advertising in the UK, that philosophy has extended to regulated self-
regulation. Of course, these regulatory authorities have done this within
their legislative prerogative and I am not suggesting that individual regulators have conducted their duties improperly.

As I mentioned previously the Special Counsel's investigation of FDA
bias in approving new drugs was limited by the fact that it did not scrutinize the scientific aspects of the regulatory decisions involved. Indeed, any
argument regarding industrial and corporate bias in drug testing and
regulation is incomplete without such scrutiny. In arguing that industrial
bias is substantial in the regulation of drugs in the UK and the US, this
chapter has relied solely on an examination of the organizational and legislative features of regulation and the statements about and interpretation
of regulation by regulators. To complement that analysis the following
five chapters investigate what industrial and Government scientists *actually do* with the scientific aspects of regulating particular drug products.

Chapter Three

Naprosyn
– reconstructing data

Before discussing naproxen and other non-steroidal anti-inflammatory drugs (NSAIDs) in the following four chapters, some appreciation of the state of scientific knowledge regarding that class of medicines and the arthritic diseases, which they are intended to treat, is required. The purpose of the first two sections of this chapter is to outline briefly the inter-related scientific, technological and commercial dimensions of NSAID therapy.

Development of NSAIDs as a therapeutic class

NSAIDs are one of four main groups of medicines used to treat rheumatoid arthritis and osteoarthritis. The other three are simple analgesics, such as paracetamol, pure anti-inflammatory drugs, such as corticosteroids, and disease-suppressing drugs such as gold salts and penicillamine.[1] The simple analgesics treat only the painful symptoms of arthritis, and have little effect on inflammation while corticosteroids have a powerful anti-inflammatory effect but are extremely toxic. Gold salts and penicillamine are therapies specifically for rheumatoid arthritis and seem to treat not only the symptoms, but actually suppress the progression of the disease. Unfortunately they, too, are very toxic, and only in the more serious cases of arthritis do doctors wish to maintain patients on long-term gold or penicillamine therapy.

By comparison the NSAIDs are relatively less toxic than corticosteroids, gold or penicillamine and, unlike the simple analgesics, exhibit clear anti-inflammatory activity in animal models. In various clinical situations the NSAIDs are reported to relieve the symptoms of arthritis. These are the basic scientific reasons for the NSAIDs having found a place among the

Table 2 A chemical classification of NSAIDs developed by 1983.

(i)	Salicylates – aspirin, sodium salicylate, diflunisal, cholinemagnesium, trisalicylate
(ii)	Pyrazoles – phenylbutazone, oxyphenbutazone, azapropazone, feprazone
(iii)	Indene derivatives – indomethacin, sulindac, tolmetin, zomepirac
(iv)	Propionic acid derivatives – benoxaprofen, fenoprofen, flurbiprofen, ibuprofen, ketoprofen, naproxen, suprofen, fenbufen
(v)	Fenamates – mefenamic acid, flufenamic acid
(vi)	Oxicams – piroxicam, tenoxicam
(vii)	Acetic acid derivatives – diclofenac, fenclofenac.

Source: E.C. Huskisson 1983. Classification of anti-rheumatic drugs. In *Anti-rheumatic drugs*, E.C. Huskisson (ed.), 5. East Sussex: Praeger.

medical profession's anti-arthritic therapies. The NSAIDs themselves can be classified into several groups as shown in Table 2.

Aspirin was the first NSAID to be synthesized and was introduced to the medical profession around 1899.[2] It is still widely recognized as an effective therapy for relieving many of the symptoms of arthritis. However, it is commonly acknowledged that several toxicities, such as epigastric discomfort, nausea and serious gastric erosions may accompany anti-arthritic aspirin therapy. It is thought that aspirin has a direct damaging effect on gastric mucosa, making the latter more vulnerable to injury from acids in the stomach.[3] Half a century passed before Ciba-Geigy's phenylbutazone became available for patients in the UK and the US in the 1950s. However, its use was accompanied by the major, and sometimes lethal, toxic complication of bone marrow suppression, making the drug's widespread and long-term use extremely problematic.[4]

Since then the search for effective treatment of arthritic symptoms with low gastro-intestinal toxicity has continued and, indeed, intensified. Between 1963 and 1982 twenty-three NSAIDs, including indomethacin, were marketed in the UK alone. The continued influx of new products was due to the enormous potential of the anti-arthritic market for pharmaceutical companies. Arthritis and rheumatism accounted for 15.8 million prescriptions in England and Wales in 1980.[5] The total 1981 US retail market for prescription anti-arthritic drugs has been estimated at $525.9 million and in 1979 the total UK market was thought to be around £55.6 million. There are several reasons for this lucrative market.

Arthritic diseases are chronic and incurable, and most types tend to afflict people as they grow older. Hence, they are increasingly common in ageing populations in the West. On current trends in the UK 15 to 20 per cent of the population will be over 65 years of age by the end of the century compared with only 5 per cent at the beginning.[6] Secondly, the rate at which products must be discontinued by doctors because of ineffectiveness or adverse effects can be very high (as many as 15 million new or dissatisfied patients in the US in any one month). And finally, there is little difference perceived between NSAIDs, and so any newcomer has a good chance of penetrating the market if promoted effectively.

Theories of inflammation

The inflammatory process, which is fundamental to arthritis, is poorly understood, and so too is the mode of anti-inflammatory action of NSAIDs. Nevertheless, the logic of attempted scientific innovations within this class of drugs cannot be understood without a brief consideration of key theoretical perspectives on inflammation and mechanisms for its suppression.

Arachidonic acid is present in almost all animal and human cells.[7] Activation or distortion of a cell membrane by some chemical, mechanical, pathological or physiological stimulus can liberate arachidonic acid from the membrane.[8] The arachidonic acid is then converted into a cascade of products via the enzyme pathways known as *cyclo-oxygenase* and *lipoxygenase*. It is some of these products, especially the *prostaglandins*, that are, and have been, believed to play a role in inflammation.

In 1971 Vane, who received the Nobel Prize for his work on prostaglandins, discovered that aspirin and indomethacin strongly inhibited prostaglandin synthesis *in vitro* (i.e. in cell cultures in glass dishes) by suppressing the actions of the enzyme(s) which generated prostaglandins.[9] Consequently, he proposed that inhibition of prostaglandin synthesis might be the mechanism that explained the anti-inflammatory action of NSAIDs. By the late 1970s most NSAIDs had been shown to suppress cyclo-oxygenase, the enzyme which catalyses prostaglandin synthesis, and this was widely accepted as at least one of the drugs' anti-inflammatory mechanisms.[10] However, some of these prostaglandins PGE1 and PGI2 were also known to have the gastro-protective function of inhibiting the production of gastric acid. It has been frequently suggested that the troublesome gastro-intestinal toxicity of NSAIDs is a result of their suppression of cyclo-oxygenase. Conversely, any NSAID that was only a weak inhibitor of prostaglandin synthetase might be expected to exhibit less gastro-intestinal toxicity, according to Vane's theory.

Before Vane's discovery it was known that leucocytes (white blood cells), stimulated by chemical attraction, migrated to sites of inflammation to engage in the digestion of bacteria and other foreign particles. This process could lead to the generation of prostaglandins, and so an additional and related anti-inflammatory mechanism of NSAIDs could be inhibition of leucocyte migration. Two distinctive types of leucocytes, which have received most attention in theories of inflammation, are called polymorphonuclear (*neutrophils*) and mononuclear (*monocytes*). So far as Vane's theory is concerned, both types of cells could be equally implicated in the inflammatory process as mediated by prostaglandin generation. However, in 1967 Weissman focused on the accumulation of neutrophils in inflammatory exudate, and proposed that the *lyzosomal enzymes* secreted by the neutrophils were mediators of various inflammatory reactions.[11] This theory, which implied that inflammatory processes could be *independent* of prostaglandin synthesis, was clearly popular as evidenced by the number of immunologists, rheumatologists and other scientists, who began to give specific consideration to the effects of NSAIDs on neutrophil function.

A somewhat less influential proposition came in 1971 from Di Rosa, Papdimitriou and Willoughby, who suggested that NSAIDs might be active partially through effects on the surface of monocytes.[12] This was based on the finding that, in the rat, phenylbutazone and indomethacin inhibited monocyte, but not neutrophil, migration. Most scientists who hold an opinion on the cellular basis of inflammatory processes have tended to believe that the neutrophils are at least as important as the monocytes in maintaining inflammation in human arthritis, particularly because the neutrophils are the predominant type of leucocyte found in the synovial fluid of rheumatoid arthritic patients.[13] Whatever the majority view, the clinical relevance of all these cellular theories is poorly understood, not least because the vast majority of the relevant studies have been carried out either *in vitro* or in animal models (sometimes called *in vivo*), whose extrapolative validity to human arthritics remains extremely uncertain.

As I mentioned in Chapter 2, since the 1970s before a drug can be approved for marketing in the UK or the US it must have been tested pre-clinically and clinically for safety and efficacy. Pre-clinical tests include long-term tests in animals designed to assess the possible risk of cancer posed by the drug. It is the pre-clinical assessment of *Naprosyn*'s carcinogenicity (cancer-inducing potential) that is the focus of the remaining parts of this chapter.

Assessing the cancer risk – theory and practice

The scientific rationale for carcinogenicity testing of medical drugs is to determine whether the test substance might be expected to cause cancer in humans. By the early 1970s scientists could draw on three types of data in order to assess the carcinogenicity of chemicals to humans; epidemiology, *in vitro* short-term mutagenicity tests with human cells and long-term *in vivo* studies of whole live animals.[14] Unfortunately epidemiological data are of little value in the pre-marketing carcinogenic risk assessment of new drugs for use by humans because such data consist of clinical trials that are short term relative to the long periods which frequently characterize the onset of cancer.[15] Moreover, in so far as such epidemiological data can warn of carcinogenic risk it will be too late for those who have suffered the consequences.[16]

Hence the pre-testing of new drugs has relied heavily on *in vitro* mutagenicity and long-term animal studies. The main limitations of the former are that different types of mutagenicity tests yield inconsistent results, and that some chemicals known to be carcinogenic to animals and/or humans have not been demonstrated to be mutagens (i.e. substances that cause mutations in our genes).[17] These limitations were widely acknowledged among scientists by the early 1970s when it was postulated that mutagenicity tests did not detect all carcinogens because of various epigenetic mechanisms of cancer.[18] Thus, in 1974 the World Health Organisation (WHO) concluded:

> Mutagenicity tests may have value as a prescreening procedure for carcinogenicity. However, for the time being the development of a tumour, verifiable histologically [i.e. through a microscope], in the whole animal must be the ultimate test for carcinogenic activity.[19]

Such was the state of scientific knowledge regarding the value of mutagenicity tests in predicting carcinogenicity during the 1970s and 1980s when many NSAIDs, including *Naprosyn*, were being developed and subsequently subjected to tests for carcinogenicity.

Yet the extrapolation of the results from long-term testing in animals to carcinogenic risk assessment for humans itself has been, and remains, characterized by gross uncertainties. Animal studies may reveal that a chemical is carcinogenic in one species, but not in another, and even if a substance is not found to be carcinogenic in a number of long-term animal tests it may still be carcinogenic to humans. As early as 1954 Barnes & Denz reviewed the methods available for determining chronic toxicity in laboratory animals, and concluded that the extrapolation of the results of these studies to human toxicology had limited validity.[20] The uncertainties of animal carcinogenicity testing have not been reduced since then. Based on a review of the predictive inadequacies of such studies, in 1979 Stevenson commented:

the 1970s may well be characterized as the era in which toxicology created more problems than it solved.[21]

Furthermore, after reviewing 170 reports issued by the National Cancer Institute's Carcinogenesis Bioassay Program between 1977 and 1980, Salsburg reached the conclusion in 1983:

the lifetime feeding study in mice and rats appears to have less than a 50 per cent probability of finding known human carcinogens. On the basis of probability theory, we would have been better off to toss a coin.[22]

Thus, chemical carcinogenicity testing is an extremely uncertain science. Nevertheless, some standards have been developed in order to increase the reliability of the knowledge produced by carcinogenicity studies in animals. As will become evident, the *Naprosyn* case illustrates how far the practice of drug testing can wander from its supposedly scientific principles.

Naproxen is the generic name for *Naprosyn* which is an NSAID manufactured by Syntex in the 1960s. In order to test it for carcinogenicity Syntex contracted Industrial Bio-Test (IBT) laboratories to conduct a 22-month long-term toxicity study in rats between 25 November 1969 and 17 September 1971. Syntex submitted a report of the study to the FDA on 22 March 1972.[23] The drug was approved for the treatment of arthritis (often involving long-term therapy) by the British regulatory authorities in September 1973, and by the FDA in March 1976. The 22-month rat study was the only long-term carcinogenicity study in animals conducted by Syntex prior to approval in both countries.[24] Although the WHO recommended in 1969 that carcinogenicity testing of drugs should be carried out in two species neither the British nor the American regulatory authorities required more than one such test in the early 1970s.

That things were going terribly wrong in the modern post-thalidomide world of drug testing began to come to light when during June 1976

Adrian Gross and Manfred Hein of the FDA's Bureau of Drugs carried out an inspection of IBT laboratories focusing on the 22-month study of naproxen in rats.[25] They found the study "unacceptable" for the following reasons:

(a) many animals recorded as having been weighed alive (some repeatedly) subsequent to the dates of their deaths;

(b) extreme body weight changes on successive weighings for given animals;

(c) extreme variation in body weight within any experimental group and controls at any given weighing;

(d) several animals being listed as having died repeatedly, usually with different versions of gross postmortem findings;

(e) unaccountable discrepancies and corrections in dates of death of the experimental animals in different versions of same record or in different records.[26]

During the inspection Gross and Hein were informed that of the 160 rats in the study the records of 86 (54 per cent) could not be located.[27] Moreover, they found that a significant number of tumours recorded in the animals had not been reported to the FDA or to Syntex.[28]

Gross and Catherine King, another FDA inspector, investigated Syntex's knowledge of the 22-month rat study. On 15 July 1976 they were told by Robert Hill, Assistant Director of the Institute of Clinical Medicine at Syntex, that when IBT first submitted their final report on the study to Syntex he found it unsatisfactory because of discrepancies and omissions of data, most notably a complete lack of data on the histology (microscopic study of tissues) of animals that died during the course of the study.[29] Hill believed that this first final report would have been rejected by regulatory authorities in the US, UK and Canada. Consequently, he required IBT to produce another final report, which they did, and which he thought contained the needed information.[30] It was this second report that Syntex finally submitted to the FDA and probably other regulatory authorities as well.

As a result of their inspection Gross and Hein criticized Syntex for not being more critical of IBT's performance:

it is felt that, particularly in view of the misgivings of Syntex on the initial version of this report Syntex should have been more critical of the performance by their contractor; perhaps if Syntex had carried out even an approximation of the sort of audit and examination of IBT's own laboratory notes as the FDA did, the report on this study would likely not have been submitted as a reliable one.[31]

Immediately after the inspection of IBT the FDA held an internal meeting at which the removal of naproxen from the market pending the completion of new long-term studies was discussed. FDA scientists at this meeting concluded that "since naproxen does not meet our current standards and since its withdrawal would by no means create a therapeutic hardship, the choice of action [to recommend withdrawal to the Bureau Director] seems clear".[32] On 20 July 1976 Frances Kelsey, the Director of the FDA's Scientific Investigations, concurred with Gross and Hein that the 22-month rat study was "unreliable and should not be used in support of claims of safety" for naproxen. Since that was the only long-term study and since the FDA enunciated a policy in 1968 that an adequate 18-month or longer carcinogenicity study in rodents was required in order to approve a drug to be given for six months or longer in clinical practice, Kelsey concluded that the safety of naproxen was no longer supported by adequate toxicological data. She recommended that the agency begin procedures to remove the drug from the market.[33] Two weeks later the Director of the Bureau of Drugs told Syntex that the agency would be publishing a notice of a hearing regarding its intention to remove naproxen from the market, but agreed to a meeting with the company beforehand.[34]

At that meeting Syntex presented a most remarkable re-analysis of the 22-month rat study. Kenneth Dumas, Senior Vice President Director of the Institute of Clinical Medicine at Syntex, informed the FDA that the company had expended considerable effort in reconstructing the report on the 22-month rat study. He maintained that the errors in the IBT report were mostly recording errors, and further argued that the 22-month study was adequate to demonstrate safety when taken in conjunction with the fact that large numbers of patients had received the drug for up to three years.[35] Syntex also argued that the FDA should give less weight to the 22-month rat study because the rat is not an acceptable model for assessing human risk and because withdrawing naproxen would create anxiety in the patients taking the drug. Yet the company simultaneously volunteered to undertake immediately a new long-term carcinogenicity study in rats.[36]

On 30 August 1976 Gross and Hein independently came to review Syntex's reconstruction of the 22-month rat study. According to Gross, Syntex argued that the problematic nature of the IBT study was confined to mistaking some animals' identity for those in adjacent cages during observation and weighing procedures. However, Gross found this explanation inadequate because it could not account for the fact that IBT records on dates of death for experimental animals were internally inconsistent or inconsistent with other records found at IBT, or that many instances of tumours or suspected tumours entered on IBT's records were not reported to the FDA. Thus, Gross recommended that the agency continue to regard the study as of "unacceptable quality".[37] Hein reached similar conclusions and commented:

> The "reworked" 22-month rat study remains unacceptable to demonstrate (i) a lack of toxicity to various tissues after administration of drug over a major portion of the animal's lifetime (ii) that naproxen had or had not a carcinogenic potential. . . . Dates of deaths have not been satisfactorily demonstrated.[38]

Consequently, he recommended that "naproxen be removed from marketing immediately".[39]

Action speaks louder than words

On 4 October 1976 the FDA gave notice of a hearing on the proposal to withdraw naproxen from the market. In response Syntex submitted several volumes of argumentation in support of naproxen's safety and continued marketing. Over three months later Gross and Hein independently reviewed that material. Both reached the conclusion that Syntex's additional submission was not persuasive in rebutting previous evaluations by FDA scientists that the 22-month rat study was fundamentally unreliable.[40] By March 1977 Congress was taking an interest in the FDA's investigations of IBT and questioned the agency's scientists and management about the regulation of naproxen. Acting FDA Commissioner Sherwin Gardner summarized the position as follows:

> The decision reached by the Bureau of Drugs was that the serious errors and discrepancies in this study, which was material to the Bureau's decision to approve *Naprosyn* for marketing, constituted untrue statements in the application. Section 505(e)(4) of the Federal Food, Drug and Cosmetic Act requires that FDA withdraw approval of a new drug application (NDA), if it contains any untrue statement of material fact, whether or not that misstatement was knowing or even negligent.[41]

Moreover, Crout, the Director of the Bureau of Drugs, testified that "a study on the long-term toxicity is essential for the approval of any drug which is to be used long-term in humans".[42] He also testified as to the FDA's interpretation of scientific uncertainty under the law as a matter of policy:

> prior to approval, uncertainty on the safety issue results in no approval. After marketing, the burden shifts to the agency.[43]

However, this does not mean that the FDA as a matter of policy was willing to wait until Syntex completed a new long-term carcinogenicity study before deciding whether or not to withdraw naproxen from the market. According to Crout the FDA were trying to remove the drug from the market:

> Dr Crout: We [FDA] believe that the study needs to be repeated. It is already started. It will be late 1978 before those data are available. The issue is whether the drug will come off the market prior to that. We are attempting to do this . . .
>
> Senator Kennedy: Is it your policy to wait until the repeat study has been done?
>
> Dr Crout: Absolutely not. That is why we are taking action to take it off the market . . .
>
> Dr Crout: As we pointed out repeatedly, we are trying to take it off the market. That is the purpose.[44]

Yet naproxen was never removed from the US market. Instead, the FDA ultimately accepted the suggestion of Syntex; permitting the drug to remain on the market while the company undertook another carcinogenicity test, which proved to be negative and of high quality according to the FDA.[45] Meanwhile the British regulatory authorities permitted Syntex to continue to market naproxen in the UK with a product data sheet (i.e. "label") which made no mention whatsoever of the drug's potential carcinogenicity or the adequacy of its carcinogenicity testing in animals.[46] Such omission can be sharply contrasted with the references in *Naprosyn* data sheets assuring doctors that:

> *Naprosyn* has been shown to have striking anti-inflammatory properties when tested in classical animal test systems. . . . Teratology studies in rats and rabbits . . . have not produced evidence of fetal damage with *Naprosyn*.[47]

Evidently, the results of animal tests that showed the drug in a favourable light could be included in the data sheet, but the carcinogenicity testing in animals by IBT which detracted from the drug's viability was omitted.

Conclusion

A fundamental principle of scientific research is that data collection should be reliable. Assuming the FDA's inspection to be sound, then IBT scientists violated that principle and Syntex managed to use the flawed IBT data to get naproxen approved. More significantly, scientists at Syntex were willing to argue that data, which they had not themselves collected, could be reconstructed *post hoc* on the basis of what IBT scientists *possibly* meant – a sort of reflective guessology. Corporate bias is especially visible here because it involves such wholesale contravention of the scientific standards that are supposed to guide what toxicologists are doing; and because it emerges in order to defend the drug in question from the commercially damaging fate of withdrawal from the market.

The naproxen case study illustrates the importance of the FDA's inspections of industrial laboratories. Without the IBT inspection, for instance, it seems unlikely that the regulatory authorities would ever have become aware of the questionable integrity of Syntex's animal carcinogenicity data on naproxen. Yet, on the assumption that the British regulatory authorities were aware of the FDA's investigation of IBT, then the actions of the regulators on both sides of the Atlantic clearly demonstrate the operation of bias in favour of the manufacturers. The FDA did not remove the drug from the market prior to a repeat carcinogenicity study, disregarding its own regulatory standards and scientists' recommendations. Assuming that the British regulatory authorities were aware of the publicly available FDA inspection of IBT laboratories, then in the UK a regulatory bias operated through the selective emphasis given to commercially advantageous aspects of the pre-clinical testing of the drug. As such the interests of the manufacturers were protected by the regulators and the interests of patients in having adequate information were compromised.

Fortunately, Syntex's subsequent carcinogenicity test was negative and it is not being suggested that the drug has posed a carcinogenic risk to patients. In fact, naproxen is considered to be one of the safer NSAIDs by many within the medical profession. Nevertheless, these comforting findings were not known when the FDA discovered the shortcomings of IBT's carcinogenicity testing of the drug.

Chapter Four

Opren/Oraflex –
the making of a drug disaster

Benoxaprofen, a propionic acid derivative, was developed by Eli Lilly (Lilly) during the 1970s. In the UK it was approved under the tradename *Opren* to treat the symptoms of arthritis, in hospitals in April 1980 and marketed to general practitioners in August/September 1980. In the US it was marketed to all doctors under the tradename *Oraflex* with the same basic indications to all doctors in May 1982. By 5 August 1982 Lilly had withdrawn the drug worldwide following its suspension on 4 August 1982 by the British regulatory authorities on the advice of the CSM, and in the centre of a growing controversy about the drug's safety and efficacy. This chapter examines in detail the production and use of scientific knowledge pertinent to benoxaprofen safety and efficacy by Lilly and the regulatory authorities. Throughout the chapter I refer to the generic name, benoxaprofen, unless wishing to emphasize the use of the drug specifically in the UK or the US, in which case I refer to *Opren* or *Oraflex*, respectively. Similarly, I refer to the drug's manufacturers as Lilly, unless I am specifically discussing the actions of the British subsidiary, Dista Products Ltd (Dista).

Therapeutic effectiveness – pushing results

Lilly promoted benoxaprofen as an exceptionally effective NSAID by reference to its mode of biochemical action and its anti-inflammatory effects in animal and human studies. For example, in the UK Dista ran an advertisement entitled "*Opren*. A brand new anti-arthritic. A brand new way of working" in the *British Medical Journal* on 10 and 24 January 1981, which suggested to doctors that *Opren* promised a new way of life for their arthritis patients, claiming:

Opren represents one of the major significant breakthroughs in the treatment of arthritic conditions since aspirin. . . . *Opren* achieves all this because quite simply it is unique; it has a spectrum of activity completely different from that of other non-steroidal anti-inflammatory agents. *Opren* works at a fundamentally different stage of the chronic inflammatory process of arthritis. Instead of treating the disease only symptomatically by inhibiting the synthesis of prostaglandins, *Opren* can help to break the vicious cycle of chronic inflammation in arthritis. It is perhaps because of this unique process that *Opren* has been shown in experimental situations to actually modify the arthritic process. At long last there's a brand new and very real hope for our arthritic patients.[1]

Dista continued to advertise regularly in the *British Medical Journal* in this fashion until October 1981.[2]

In May 1982 Lilly promoted *Oraflex* to the American press as follows:

Studies conducted with the drug in laboratory animals indicate that benoxaprofen appears to have different activity from that of other drugs currently available for arthritis. These laboratory studies have demonstrated that benoxaprofen reduces bone and joint inflammation. . . . Unlike aspirin and conventional NSAIDs, *Oraflex* is a weaker inhibitor of prostaglandin synthesis. However, laboratory studies show that it is a potent and specific inhibitor of the migrating inflammatory cells that erode the joints of arthritis.[3]

Furthermore, according to Congressional hearings, members of the media were provided with a telephone number, known as the "arthritis hotline". This was still in operation as late as 13 July 1982. On phoning the number one could receive a taped message about *Oraflex*, part of which featured:

Bob Carter: An antiarthritis drug, Oraflex, newly available to the American public, may also limit the actual joint destruction in humans caused by the progression of the disease. To determine its disease retarding qualities, its developer, Eli Lilly and Company, has undertaken one of the most extensive long-term studies of rheumatoid arthritis ever conducted by a pharmaceutical company. In the study, the once-a-day drug has shown to be very effective in reducing arthritis symptoms, but as Dr Gilbert Bluhm, co-ordinator of clinical research at Henry Ford Hospital in Detroit, describes, it has additional potential.

Dr Bluhm: It has clinical laboratory evidence that it may affect the natural progression of the disease in rheumatoid arthritis which, when untreated may go ahead and actually end up destroying joints. There is preliminary clinical data that suggests that it may have this disease modifying potential.[4]

In this section I examine how science was marshalled in an attempt to establish that benoxaprofen was a medical breakthrough.

Mode of action

In 1977 Cashin, Dawson & Kitchen, of the Lilly Research Centre at Erl Wood, England, demonstrated that benoxaprofen was a potent and long-acting anti-inflammatory agent in adjuvant arthritis in rats, as well as two other rat models. However, using the enzyme from ram seminal vesicle they found that benoxaprofen was a poor inhibitor of prostaglandin synthesis compared with indomethacin – a finding somewhat anomalous with Vane's theory. On this basis, they claimed that benoxaprofen could be differentiated from the other NSAIDs.

Brocklehurst & Dawson had also used the ram seminal vesicle model with the same concentrations of arachidonic acid to test the ability of indomethacin, aspirin and paracetamol to inhibit prostaglandin synthesis, with results that did indeed challenge Vane's hypothesis. However, they acknowledged that early studies with the ram seminal vesicle model failed to show *several* anti-inflammatory drugs as inhibitors of prostaglandin synthesis.[5] and stated:

> [w]e cannot conclude . . . that the principal mode of action of AI [anti-inflammatory] drugs is inhibition of prostaglandin synthesis, *or that it is not.*[6] (Emphasis added)

A second way in which Cashin, Dawson & Kitchen attempted to account for the anomalous characteristics of benoxaprofen was to suggest that the drug's anti-inflammatory activity in rats was caused, not by prostaglandin inhibition, but by abatement of leucocyte accumulation at the site of inflammation.[7] On this point, however, they concluded that "the mode of action of benoxaprofen is not yet clear".[8]

Contemporaneously a group of scientists working outside Lilly, Ford-Hutchinson et al., studied the capacity of indomethacin, flurbiprofen and benoxaprofen to inhibit prostaglandin (PG) synthesis and leucocyte migration (LM) *in vivo* in rats.[9] These researchers suggested a distinction between benoxaprofen and the other two drugs, namely, that benoxaprofen only showed inhibition of prostaglandin generation at doses equivalent to that required to inhibit leucocyte migration, whereas indomethacin and flurbiprofen did so at lower doses than those required for inhibition of leucocyte migration. The implication of this distinction was that benoxaprofen's anti-inflammatory activity in various animal studies might be explained equally by inhibition of leucocyte migration as by inhibition of prostaglandin production, whereas indomethacin and flurbiprofen were primarily prostaglandin generation inhibitors.

Nevertheless, Vane and his colleagues interpreted these data as demonstrating that "benoxaprofen is a potent inhibitor of prostaglandin generation *in vivo*" even though it might also have inhibited leucocyte migration.[10] On this view such data were inconsistent with the conclusions of Cashin, Dawson & Kitchen that benoxaprofen was a weak inhibitor of prostaglandin synthesis. Vane's research team also reported that aspirin, flurbiprofen, ibuprofen and phenylbutazone all inhibited prostaglandin generation and leucocyte migration at the doses required to suppress induced inflammation in rats,[11] while Smolen & Weissman challenged the extent to which indomethacin's *in vitro* anti-inflammatory activity could be explained solely by inhibition of cyclo-oxygenase products, such as prostaglandins.[12] These results confirmed that if benoxaprofen did have an exceptional mode of action it was unlikely to be inhibition of leucocyte migration *per se*.

In 1979 Dawson[13] speculated that benoxaprofen was a NSAID with a mode of action unrelated to the prostaglandin system, while Huskisson, a consultant clinical trialist for Lilly based at St Bartholomew's London Hospital, felt able to cite the findings of Cashin, Dawson & Kitchen and to state confidently:

> [benoxaprofen's] pharmacological profile suggested a different mode of action from conventional non-steroidal anti-inflammatory drugs.[14]

Apparently Lilly scientists were sufficiently convinced of benoxaprofen's weak inhibition of prostaglandin synthesis to search for alternative explanations of its anti-inflammatory activity.[15] In 1979 Meacock, Kitchen & Dawson found that the drug significantly inhibited monocyte, though not neutrophil, migration *in vivo* in rats and *in vitro*. They duly concluded that "the inhibition of mononuclear cell migration into the sites of inflammation may be an important contribution to the anti-inflammatory action of benoxaprofen in chronic inflammation".[16]

A few months later in September 1979 at an International Symposium on Benoxaprofen held at Wiesbaden, West Germany, several Lilly scientists provided data in support of the proposition that benoxaprofen might have unusual pharmacological characteristics because of its mode of action.[17] The most important tests constituting such evidence were the comparative studies of leucocyte inhibition reported by Dawson.[18] Yet the extent to which these supported his claim that benoxaprofen exhibited qualities exceptional to NSAIDs is questionable.

For example, in his initial studies aspirin, benoxaprofen, fenoprofen, ibuprofen, ketoprofen and naproxen all significantly inhibited the migration of leucocytes *in vitro* after oral administration of the drugs to an unspecified species. Furthermore, in a rat pleurisy model Dawson could discern no differences between benoxaprofen and other NSAIDs with respect to inhibition of neutrophils. Though benoxaprofen did significantly inhibit the migration of monocytes, so too did ketoprofen and, to a lesser extent, indomethacin. Dawson also studied the differential effect of benoxaprofen and other NSAIDs on leucocyte migration in another rat model producing the results shown in Table 3.

Table 3 shows that benoxaprofen significantly inhibited the migration of monocytes, but not neutrophils. However, ibuprofen also significantly inhibited monocyte migration, though to a lesser extent than benoxaprofen, and substantially inhibited neutrophil migration. Given the prevalent scientific beliefs that either monocytes, neutrophils or both could be involved in contributing to inflammatory activity,[19] ibuprofen's ability to inhibit both could be, as O'Brien,[20] Professor of Rheumatology

Table 3 Differential inhibition of leucocyte migration.

Compound	Conc. mcg/ml	% Change in chemotactic response of leucocytes			
		Monos	p^*	Polys	p^*
Aspirin	100	−10	NS	−2	NS
	200	+8	NS	0	
Benoxaprofen	15	−38	0.01	0	
	30	−56	0.001	+5	NS
Ibuprofen	30	−32	NS	−37	NS
	100	−42	0.01	−28	NS
Indomethacin	5	+11	NS	+10	NS
	10	−11	NS	−1	NS
Naproxen	30	−21	NS	+3	NS
	60	−19	NS	−23	NS
	100	+21	NS	+49	0.05

Key: *= significance value of p using Student's t-test. NS = not significant; mcg = micrograms; ml = millilitres; Monos = monocytes; Polys = neutrophils.
Source: W. Dawson 1980. The comparative pharmacology of benoxaprofen. *Journal of Rheumatology* **7**, Suppl. no. 6, 9.

at the University of Virgina in the US, has argued, of more clinical importance than benoxaprofen's potential to inhibit solely monocytes. Nevertheless, in his summary table of these comparative tests Dawson chose to omit ibuprofen, so that the table showed benoxaprofen as the only inhibitor of mononuclear cell migration. I am not suggesting that Dawson deliberately suppressed the ibuprofen evidence. Nevertheless, his preferred form of presentation of these data introduced a bias favourable to the Lilly thesis that benoxaprofen possessed anti-inflammatory action significantly distinct from other NSAIDs.

Dawson concluded his analysis by using a schema to reinforce the idea of a possible link between benoxaprofen and suppressive therapy capable of retarding the arthritic disease process. On that schema prostaglandin synthetase inhibitors were represented as capable of only symptomatic therapy, whereas regulators of cell function were represented as capable of suppressive therapy also. The schema suggested that since benoxaprofen regulated cell migration it might be capable of suppressive therapy similar to that of gold or penicillamine.[21] Such reasoning was not, however, consistent with the scientific knowledge available from animal studies, particularly with respect to the distinction between prostaglandin synthesis inhibitors, on the one hand, and regulators of cell function, on the other. As early as 1971, Di Rosa, Papadimitriou & Willoughby reported:

> The common property of the non-steroidal anti-inflammatory drugs [indomethacin, phenylbutazone, aspirin and mefenamic acid] was to inhibit the migration of mononuclear cells into the injection site.[22]

By 1976 the combined results of two other groups of scientists suggested that eight NSAIDs decreased the number of neutrophils reaching the site of inflammation.[23] Thus, by the late 1970s there was a significant amount of scientific evidence implying that many NSAIDs, which inhibited prostaglandin synthesis also inhibited leucocyte migration of one kind or another.

Furthermore, the clinical relevance of Dawson's findings was questionable, not only because of the problem of extrapolation of animal data to humans, but also because of the evidence that the neutrophils not the monocytes predominate in the synovial fluid of rheumatoid arthritics.[24] For example, Ropes & Bauer estimated that after four weeks of knee swelling, a rheumatoid arthritic had 1,548 monocytes and 49,020 neutrophils per cubic millimetre of synovial fluid.[25] Applying these figures to Dawson's data in Table 3, 30 mcg/ml benoxaprofen might induce in the inflammatory region a reduction in monocytes of 867 per mm^3, but an increase in neutrophils of 2,451 per mm^3. Although the monocyte reduction might be beneficial to the patient, that might be outweighed by the neutrophil increase. On the other hand, 100 mcg/ml ibuprofen by similar reasoning might reduce the number of monocytes by 650 per mm^3 and the number of neutrophils by 13,726 per mm^3. Notably, neither Lilly nor any other scientists proposed that ibuprofen was anything other than a standard symptom-relieving NSAID.

Despite this, during a symposium on benoxaprofen as part of the 15th International Rheumatology Congress in Paris in June 1981 sponsored by Lilly Research Laboratories and published in 1982, Dawson and co-researchers[26] felt able to state that the most important of benoxaprofen's pharmacological activities in relation to its clinical profile was the drug's regulation of directional monocyte movement. They also asserted:

The relatively weak inhibitory action [by benoxaprofen] on prostaglandin synthetase probably confers clinical benefit with a reduced potential to cause severe gastric side effects.[27]

The highly selective nature of the claims made by Dawson et al. in Paris can be discerned by comparing them with the *Opren* data sheets approved by the UK Licencing Authority between April 1980 and June 1982, which stated:

Opren has a potent and specific action that inhibits migration of inflammatory cells into sites of inflammation. It has been shown to be a weak to *moderately potent inhibitor of prostaglandin synthetase depending upon the tissue and conditions studied.*[28] (Emphasis added)

At the Paris Congress, Dawson et al. were willing to declare that "[b]enoxaprofen is clearly different from the other non-steroidal anti-inflammatory compounds",[29] citing data suggesting that benoxaprofen was a weak inhibitor of prostaglandin synthetase and uniquely able to inhibit monocyte migration among a group of major NSAIDs.[30] Significantly, ibuprofen's ability to inhibit the latter was omitted from the data presented. That does not seem to have been consistent with Dawson's own scientific standards and aspirations about taking account of a broad range of data in this field:

The spectrum or profile of biological activity of a potential anti-inflammatory compound across a wide range of relevant models of inflammation would seem to be essential if laboratory data are to give a clear indication of the value of the compound the clinician is asked to investigate or use. . . . Whereas the basic mechanisms underlying acute inflammation and its transition to the chronic state remain unclear, *the widest range of biological data possible to describe a compound would seem necessary.*[31] (Emphasis added)

In 1982 Higgs & Mugridge produced results which directly conflicted with Lilly's claims that benoxaprofen was unlike other NSAIDs because it was a weak inhibitor of prostaglandin synthetase and a potent inhibitor of leucocyte migration and lipoxygenase products. Using an induced inflammation model in rats these authors found that benoxaprofen inhibited prostaglandin synthetase more than leucocyte migration. That is, it was found to be a selective cyclo-oxygenase inhibitor rather than a lioxygenase inhibitor. As Higgs & Mugridge noted, it was in this sense "similar to conventional aspirin-like drugs".[32]

Two years later Masters & McMillan found that benoxaprofen did not significantly inhibit human leucocyte lipoxygenase *in vitro*, and it was found to share this inability with flurbiprofen, ibuprofen, indomethacin and naproxen.[33] This result further undermined the earlier findings of Lilly's scientists, especially Walker & Dawson[34] and Dawson, Boot, Harvey & Walker.[35] Also in 1984 Vane's research team found that benoxaprofen induced a dose-dependent inhibition of lipoxygenase LTB4 *in vitro*, but that it was ten times more effective at inhibiting cyclo-oxygenase activity. Furthermore, they found that in the rat, *in vivo*, the drug inhibited solely prostaglandin production. They concluded:

in this inflammation model its [benoxaprofen's] activity is indistinguishable from that of conventional aspirin-like drugs such as indomethacin or flurbiprofen. It is likely, therefore, that a major part of the anti-inflammatory activity of benoxaprofen is due to the inhibition of prostaglandin synthesis.[36]

This represented the third finding since 1982 by a group of scientists outside Lilly that benoxaprofen's mode of action was similar to other NSAIDs. Since 1984 the weight of scientific opinion has tended to support rather than challenge this conclusion.[37] By 1988 Greaves & Camp felt able to assert:

Benoxaprofen . . . is not now considered an effective lipoxygenase inhibitor either *in vivo* or in cell free systems *in vitro*.[38]

Anti-inflammatory activity in animals

At the Paris Congress, Lilly scientists also presented evidence relating to the effect of benoxaprofen on induced arthritis in rats. Benslay & Nickander claimed that their radiographic results on bone damage in adjuvant arthritic rats showed that benoxaprofen modified "the experimental disease process".[39] Other comparator NSAIDs used in the study also suppressed bone damage, but to a lesser extent at non-toxic doses than did benoxaprofen.[40] Consequently, the authors freely speculated that this "may be due in part to [benoxaprofen's] reported ability to suppress migration into inflammatory sites".[41] Though Benslay & Nickander argued that experimentally induced arthritis had many similarities to rheumatoid arthritis, just one year later Billingham commented:

> Few workers today feel that adjuvant arthritis is a good model of rheumatoid arthritis, a conclusion reached from considerations of both the appearance and pathology of the disease and the fact that it is very easily inhibited by the aspirin-like drugs (the NSAIDs) which have been found only to inhibit the symptoms of the disease in man.[42]

Furthermore, since the mid 1960s researchers had failed to induce adjuvant arthritis in any species other than the rat, with the possible exception of limited success in the guinea pig and hamster.[43] It could even be argued that the findings of Benslay and Nickander suggested that benoxaprofen was merely a traditional NSAID because paradoxically adjuvant arthritis can be effectively cured by standard NSAIDs, which only afford symptomatic relief in human rheumatoid arthritis, whereas those drugs with remission-inducing characteristics in the human disease (e.g. gold) have been mostly ineffective in the adjuvant arthritis model.[44] And there are good reasons for doubting the clinical relevance of radiological findings of suppression of bone damage in adjuvant arthritis according to Billingham:

> With regard to the bone changes in . . . adjuvant arthritis it is our experience that *all effective treatments prevent these changes* and even allow some reversal of established lesions . . . In animals where spontaneous remission occurs we have also seen some reversal of the bone damage on X-ray. When such changes are drug induced it does not necessarily infer that a similar response will occur during treatment of human rheumatoid arthritis since . . . the bone changes in experimental models are largely outside the synovial cavity, unlike human rheumatoid arthritis.[45] (Emphasis added)

In March 1982 John Harter, the leading medical officer for NSAIDs at the FDA, objected to the rat study by Benslay & Nickander being used to suggest that *Oraflex* could suppress bone damage in arthritis patients because he believed it was irrelevant to clinical efficacy.[46] Senior officials at Lilly and Dista, on the other hand, insisted on interpreting the animal studies of benoxaprofen efficacy much more generously. For example, on this very issue Peck, Lilly's Director of Regulatory Affairs, testified:

Kellogg: Is there any reason to suggest that the studies with the adjuvant arthritic rats demonstrate the same potential to improve the condition of people who have rheumatoid arthritis?

Peck: That's what studies in animals would imply. . . .

Kellogg: Any claim that the drug . . . would produce the same result in people [as in animals] would be misleading unless there had been some study of people with arthritis taking the drug and showing those improvements?

Peck: I have to disagree with you there. I think if you have demonstrated in animals that a particular phenomenon has occurred that it's possible that this could occur in humans. I see no scientific problems with that.[47]

Similarly, Brian Gennery, Dista's Medical Director, took the view that the changes in the adjuvant arthritis in rats "indicate[d] that in the best model of arthritis that we had available benoxaprofen was slowing that disease process down very substantially which could not be demonstrated with other drugs".[48]

The Bluhm, Smith and Mikulaschek paper

One study by Bluhm & Smith, consultants for Lilly, and Mikulaschek, a Lilly scientist, published as part of the proceedings of the Paris Congress, attempted to determine the extent to which benoxaprofen could arrest or retard the progression of rheumatoid arthritis in people, so eliminating the problem of extrapolating animal results to the human disease.[49] Thirty-nine patients with rheumatoid arthritis were given the high dose of 600–1,000 mg benoxaprofen per day for mean duration of 21 months. X-rays of the joints of the patients were taken before and after this period in order to assess the progression of osseous defects (OD) and joint space narrowing (JSN). There were no control rheumatoid arthritic patients, and the effects of benoxaprofen using this method were not compared with other NSAIDs. As Bluhm later explained each patient "served as their own control".[50]

Bluhm et al. acknowledged that their results showed no statistically significant retardation of rheumatoid arthritis by benoxaprofen. However, on the basis of those patients who showed a diminished rate of disease progression by radiological assessment, they concluded:

> Our study of 39 patients with rheumatoid arthritis suggests a trend for benoxaprofen therapy given over a prolonged period to retard the rheumatologic process when measured radiologically by both osseous defect and joint space narrowing rates. . . . Because there is also a trend for this drug to retard or arrest radiological progression, it becomes a promising agent for the long-term treatment of rheumatoid arthritis.[51]

The radiological method employed in this study was to score OD and JSN and, "[a] patient's improvement was determined by a decreased OD and JSN rate during therapy when compared to the pretreatment rate for the same patient".[52] Contrary to the impression given by Bluhm et al., an examination of the data reveals not only that the authors' results were not statistically significant but that, in the case of JSN, the rate, on average, *increased* during benoxaprofen therapy.

Furthermore, the non-significant decrease in the mean OD rate during benoxaprofen therapy compared with the pretreatment observation period was less than the analogous decrease reported during observation. In other words, on average, just being observed was associated with more retardation of the patients' rheumatoid arthritis than being on benoxaprofen therapy. Indeed, O'Brien has argued that the data cannot correctly be interpreted as suggesting that benoxaprofen retarded the progression of rheumatoid arthritis and should have been interpreted as suggesting that the drug had *no* such effect.[53]

Even Huskisson, the consultant for Lilly, who edited the journal in which the paper by Bluhm et al. appeared, stated in January 1983 that the mathematical interpretation of the study was "extremely suspect", and that "the whole design of the study was suspect".[54] Nevertheless, Huskisson said that he published the presentation because it was of "considerable interest".[55] He justified this decision as follows:

> Mangold: If it's suspect how can it be of interest?
>
> Huskisson: These are academics who have done serial X-rays in patients receiving the drug and have drawn certain conclusions from their results. There are various ways in which these conclusions can be challenged and have been challenged both at the symposium and subsequently. And the observations are interesting because they should stimulate . . . further studies properly designed with control groups to see whether these are true observations or not.[56]

In the published journal the challenges to this study at the symposium are conspicuous by their absence. Nor did Huskisson express any clear reservations about the study in his editorial to the journal. Instead, he introduced it as follows:

> No non-steroidal anti-inflammatory has yet been shown to alter the progression of rheumatoid arthritis and the conventional view is that they don't. The observations of Bluhm et al. are, therefore, of great interest and should stimulate controlled studies using parallel groups. The patient could only act as his own control if the rate of progression of the disease was constant over the years.[57]

Despite the many problems with the study, Dawson et al. felt able to cite it to uphold the statement that "a number of findings support the hypothesis that benoxaprofen has a disease modifying effect in man, at least in rheumatoid arthritis".[58] In fact, at a press conference in Lilly's UK headquarters at Erl Wood in February 1981, Bluhm gave a BBC television interview, later to be used by the company as a promotional video, with the following message:

> BBC interviewer: Would you go as far as to say that in your opinion, at this point in time, on the basis of what you've done, you are actually talking about the possibility of modifying the disease?
>
> Bluhm: That's it precisely, what I've tried to tell you.[59]

Thus the Bluhm et al. paper was used to make ambitious claims that were not supported by the data according to the prevalent scientific standards in the field. It is, therefore, a clear-cut case of *technical inconsistency*. Nevertheless, the scientific credibility of that paper was maintained through the sympathetic editing of Huskisson.

Clinical efficacy

In April 1979, Dista applied to the British regulatory authorities for a product licence for benoxaprofen in tablet strengths of 300mg, 400mg and 600mg. As evidence of the drug's efficacy in patients suffering from osteoarthritis and rheumatoid arthritis Dista submitted data from a total of 18 clinical trials, of which 16 were controlled. Fourteen of these trials were based in the UK and four in the US.

Of the 12 controlled UK-based studies, five compared benoxaprofen with placebo and seven compared it with another active propionic acid derivative, except in one case when the comparator drug was indomethacin. In the five placebo studies the number of patients entered varied from 12 to 48 and the duration from 1 to 3 weeks, while in six of the comparator drug studies the former varied from 18 to 40 and the latter from 2 to 4 weeks. By contrast, one trial by Tyson & Glynne comparing benoxaprofen with ibuprofen involved 60 patients and lasted for 4 months.[60]

How far these trials can be relied upon for conclusive results is questionable because their designs had specific shortcomings according to the criteria of Huskisson, one of Lilly's own consultant clinical trialists at the time, and a leading medical researcher in anti-rheumatic drugs. In 1976 at a symposium on "The principles and practice of clinical trials" organized by the Association of Medical Advisers in the Pharmaceutical Industry, Huskisson commented:

> Experience suggests that 12 to 18 patients with active [rheumatic] disease are sufficient to show that a drug like aspirin is superior to placebo, but this is only a crude screening test of effectiveness. Much larger numbers of patients are required to obtain information about variability and frequency of response . . . .[61]

Regarding numbers of patients in trials comparing NSAIDs he further stated:

> any comparison between one propionic acid derivative and another using anything less than about 60 patients would be meaningless . . . I would condemn any [such] study with only twelve or eighteen patients'.[62]

Concerning the duration of such trials he remarked:

> Long term treatment, at least six months, is required to . . . determine whether it [an anti-rheumatic drug] has specific effect on rheumatoid arthritis.[63]

Evidently none of the UK-based clinical trials met Huskisson's criteria on *both* number of patients and duration required to determine a specific effect. Irrespective of duration, if one excludes the benoxaprofen/indomethacin trial because indomethacin is not a propionic acid derivative, then only one of the UK-based comparator drug trials satisfied Huskisson's criterion for number of patients involved; the rest, by Huskisson's standards, were "meaningless". The FDA seems to have supported Huskisson's perspective on this matter, since the agency's Summary Basis of Approval for *Oraflex* did not include an analysis of the UK-based clinical trials, commenting that "several small clinical studies done mostly in the UK . . . were not of sufficient size to be a substantial contribution and did not add to the knowledge of . . . efficacy".[64]

By 1980 the UK-based clinical trials provided little, if any, evidence that benoxaprofen was more effective than established therapies such as ibuprofen. Turning to the two rheumatoid arthritis and two osteoarthritis clinical trials co-ordinated in the US, and reported in 1980 by Gum and Alarcon-Segovia, respectively, these did conform to Huskisson's quantitative criteria of good clinical practice. Undoubtedly these four studies were crucial to regulatory authorities' evaluation of benoxaprofen's efficacy. But there were no spectacular clinical findings. Regarding treatment of rheumatoid arthritis, Gum concluded that "[n]one of the differences in the clinically significant responses between benoxaprofen and aspirin or ibuprofen were great enough to show a statistically significant difference".[65] Similarly, Alarcon-Segovia reported that "benoxaprofen produced improvement similar to that of aspirin and ibuprofen in nearly all measurements of the knees and hips affected by osteoarthritis".[66]

One suggestion made by Gum was that benoxaprofen showed some superior efficacy to aspirin and ibuprofen in treating rheumatoid arthritis because of the small number of patients whose disease deteriorated during benoxaprofen therapy as measured by increased erythrocyte sedimentation rates (ESR).[67] The evidence on which this claim was made amounted to: (a) only 3 out of 39 rheumatoid arthritics got worse (i.e. ESR increased more than before) on benoxaprofen compared with 13 out of 47 on ibuprofen in the benoxaprofen/ibuprofen trial; and (b) only 2 out of 32 rheumatoid arthritics got worse on benoxaprofen compared with 4 out of 37 on aspirin.[68] These findings are noteworthy mainly because of the particular significance attributed to them by Gennery, who considered that they suggested "the possibility of modifying the disease process" by benoxaprofen therapy.[69] This was a controversial position. John Harter, Group Leader for evaluating NSAIDs at the FDA, did not believe that benoxaprofen favourably affected ESR, and took the view that the findings of beneficial effects were "chance occurrence".[70] But even on Gennery's enthusiastic interpretation of Gum's results nothing more than a *possibility* was proposed.

Moreover, the accounts of the clinical trials reported by Gum and Alarcon-Segovia as published in 1980 left much to be desired. It was not possible to ascertain the number or percentage of patients over 65 years old, even though the UK regulatory authorities stipulated in 1976 that the summaries of each individual clinical trial should provide the age distribution of patients and "[w]here possible details . . . of the results of treatment of patients who may be at increased risk . . . e.g. elderly patients".[71] Since the age distribution was so vaguely defined by Gum and Alarcon-Segovia the reports of these trials did not show clearly "comparability of the population studied with the population likely to receive the medica-

111

tion",[72] as the FDA had recommended in its 1977 *General considerations for the clinical evaluation of drugs*. In this same publication the FDA had advised that reports of clinical trials should include a prioritization of the clinical questions to be answered so that the criteria of success and failure were clear from the outset, a rationale for the size of the patient sample, and a statement as to the rationale for the duration of the study. That such requirements were desirable is strongly supported in the medical litera-ture both prior to and after the approval of benoxaprofen marketing in the UK.[73] Yet the accounts provided by Gum and Alarcon-Segovia did not meet them.

Despite these possible criticisms the 18 clinical trials discussed above were sufficient to satisfy the UK Licencing Authority of benoxaprofen's efficacy as reflected in the first *Opren* data sheet of April 1980, which stated that a daily dose of 600 mg of benoxaprofen was effective "[f]or the relief of symptoms of rheumatoid and osteoarthritis",[74] and the second in August 1980, which indicated benoxaprofen for "the treatment of rheu-matoid and osteoarthritis".[75] By contrast, in February 1981 the FDA did not accept the statistical analyses contained in the clinical studies re-ported by Gum and Alarcon-Segovia. The agency's letter of *non-approval* stated:

> The nature of the data presentation and statistical analyses of the data do not allow us to make a definitive evaluation of efficacy . . . of benoxaprofen in the treatment of rheumatoid arthritis and osteoarthritis.[76]

Even after Lilly had re-worked their clinical application to the satisfac-tion of the FDA, in March 1982 Harvey Barnett, the company's Medical Adviser for benoxaprofen's international registration is reported to have agreed with FDA officials that in clinical studies the drug had the same efficacy as other NSAIDs.[77] As for the FDA, Harter believed that benoxa-profen could not be differentiated from other NSAIDs on grounds of effi-cacy,[78] and Rheinstein testified on the agency's behalf that it had found "no clinical evidence and very minimal, if any, laboratory evidence" of benoxaprofen's supposed disease retarding qualities.[79]

In summary, Lilly scientists reported reasonable findings regarding benoxaprofen's capacity to inhibit leucocyte migration and prostaglandin synthesis, and to suppress adjuvant arthritis in rats. However, the main thrust of the company's characterization of benoxaprofen's efficacy was to make the commercially significant claim that the drug was, or was likely to be, more clinically effective in treating arthritis than other NSAIDs.

Lilly scientists, with the uncritical assistance of some consultants, may be said to have *pushed* their data towards that conclusion. Some findings were selectively emphasized and others omitted in a steady trend which supported the thesis that the drug exhibited an exceptional mode of action. The scientific uncertainty, not to say implausibility of positively extrapolating the suppression of adjuvant arthritis in rats to the suppression of the disease in humans was understated. The biased nature of these processes is particularly noticeable when the technical claims being made are inconsistent with Lilly's own scientific data and/or standards.

Scientific standards and carcinogenicity testing

As mentioned in Chapter 3, within the many uncertainties of carcinogenic risk assessment scientists working in various contexts, including regulatory authorities, trade associations, and the WHO have developed standards of good practice by which to evaluate the validity of carcinogenicity testing. In general, of course, it is in consumers' interests that carcinogenicity testing is conducted in a reliable fashion so that informed judgements can be made about the possible risk a drug will pose to consumers. Lilly conducted two long-term animal feeding studies (i.e. of at least 18 months duration) in order to assess the carcinogenic potential of benoxaprofen; one in rats and the other in mice. In this section I examine how Lilly scientists and the regulatory authorities in the UK and the US, handled the results of these two long-term studies in the context of uncertainty and prevailing scientific standards.

Design of the long-term rat study

This study was carried out at Lilly Research Laboratories in Indianapolis from February 1975 to February 1977 in Lilly's Toxicology Division. The type of rat used was a Wistar strain. The dose levels chosen by percentage of the rats' diet were: 0 per cent for controls; 0.003 per cent (i.e. 2.0–2.6 mg/kg) for the low dose; 0.01 per cent (i.e. 6.6–8.8 mg/kg) for the mid dose; and 0.03 per cent (i.e. 20–25 mg/kg) for the high dose.[80] At the time the study was designed Lilly anticipated that the human daily dose would be 100–200 mg, i.e. 1.67–3.33 mg/kg for a person weighing 60 kg. Extrapolating directly from rats to humans on a body weight basis this fell between the low and mid doses of the rat study. In fact, the normally prescribed daily dose when the drug was marketed was 600 mg (i.e. 10 mg/kg for a 60 kg person) and some patients were administered daily doses of up to 1,000 mg (i.e. 16.67 mg/kg for 60 kg person) during clinical trials co-ordinated by Lilly scientists and/or consultants in the late 1970s.[81]

The guidelines for low dosages in long-term carcinogenicity studies have varied, but it may be noted that the dosage regime of Lilly's long-term rat study did not conform to either the 1977 recommendations of the US Pharmaceutical Manufacturers' Association (PMA), of which Lilly was a member, or the guidance notes of the UK Department of Health and Social Security (DHSS) published in 1979.[82] The PMA recommended that it should be at least equal to the intended daily human dose, and the DHSS that it should be 2–3 times the maximum daily therapeutic dose. Taking Lilly's intended human daily dose to be 200 mg (3.33 mg/kg) then the low dose (2.0–2.6 mg/kg) was *less than* the former. Moreover, the low dose was just less than one-third of the actual therapeutic dose (10 mg/kg) that was to be usually prescribed. Though Lilly's Toxicology Division cannot be held responsible for the fact that a daily human dose of 600 mg benoxaprofen was ultimately required for significant clinical efficacy, this fact does cast doubt on the scientific adequacy of the choice of low dose, with respect to the drug's eventual prescription, especially since, as Worden noted in a 1974 review of toxicological methods, the purpose of the low dose is "to demonstrate effects at levels close to those proposed for clinical use, i.e. an attempt to provide 'no effect' evidence".[83]

The long-term rat study was really two "identical" independent studies running concurrently known as R125 and R135. Taking the two studies

Table 4 Survival of male animals in the benoxaprofen chronic/oncogenic rat studies R125 and R135.

	Per cent in diet			
Time interval	0.00	0.003	0.010	0.030
	Per cent survival			
6 months	98.3	97.3	98.7	88.0*
12 months	93.0	86.7	74.7*	64.0*
18 months	73.0	61.3	41.3*	29.3*
21 months	54.8	41.3	26.7*	13.3*
24 months	31.3	26.7	12.0*	6.7*

Key: *Significantly different from ($P < 0.05$) the control, Chi Square, 2×2 contingency table.
Source: E. Lilly 1984. *General commentary on the long-term study on benoxaprofen.* Lilly Research Laboratories, 22nd Feb.

together there were 115 control rats per sex and 75 treated rats per sex per dose, i.e. a grand total of 680.[84] The survival of the rats is shown in Tables 4–6.

It is evident from these tables (especially the third and fourth columns of Tables 4 and 5) that there was a statistically significant dose-related increased death rate among the animals. This has been fully acknowledged by Lilly's Toxicology Division, who stated in 1984 that:

> . . . the two higher doses given induced unequivocal drug-related toxicity in the animals. . . . treatment related toxicity . . . reduced survival in the animals given benoxaprofen.[85]

Lilly's Toxicology Division concluded that the study provided "no evi-

Table 5 Survival of female animals in the benox. chronic/oncogenic rat studies R125 and R135.

	Per cent in diet			
Time interval	0.00	0.003	0.010	0.030
	Per cent survival			
6 months	100	100	98.7	90.7*
12 months	94.8	93.3	86.7*	65.3*
18 months	76.5	74.7	61.3*	42.7*
21 months	62.6	58.7	38.7	32.0*
24 months	37.4	29.3	20.0*	6.7*

Key: *Significantly different from ($P<0.05$) the control, Chi Square, 2×2 contingency table.
Source: E. Lilly 1984. *General commentary on the long-term study on benoxaprofen.* Lilly Research Laboratories, 22nd Feb.

Table 6 Number of rats surviving in studies R125 and R135.

	Per cent benoxaprofen in the diet							
	0		0.003		0.010		0.030	
Month	M	F	M	F	M	F	M	F
1	115	115	75	75	75	75	75	75
6	113	115	73	75	74	74	66	68
12	107	109	65	70	56	65	48	49
15	98	101	60	66	43	58	37	44
18	84	88	46	56	31	46	22	32
21	63	72	31	44	20	29	10	24
24	36	43	20	22	9	15	5	5

Source: E. Lilly 1984. *General commentary on the long-term study on benoxaprofen.* Lilly Research Laboratories, 22nd Feb.

dence of any oncogenic [tumourigenic] potential" and argued that the toxicity, which reduced the rats' survival, was not due to tumour development.[86] Yet this raises questions about the appropriateness of the middle and top doses given to the rats. In 1969, five years before Lilly had even begun this long-term rat study, the WHO outlined the following principles for the testing of drugs for carcinogenicity:

> The highest dose level used should be within the toxic range, but should be consistent with the prolonged survival of a majority of the animals. The lower levels should permit the animals to survive in good health for their natural life span or until tumours develop.[87]

In 1977 the Association of the British Pharmaceutical Industry (ABPI) reiterated these principles by advising that the top dose should "not unduly shorten the life span of the animals" and "produce at most a minimal toxic effect",[88] while in the same year the PMA recommended that the top dose should be "slightly below a toxic dose".[89] Similarly, in 1979 the DHSS exhorted:

> The top dose should produce *minimum* toxic effect.[90] (Emphasis added)

It is particularly significant that Ian Shedden, who was Lilly's Vice-President for Clinical Research and Regulatory Affairs when benoxaprofen was approved and marketed in the UK and the US, was also from 1973–6 a member of the ABPI's Research and Development Committee, which drew up the ABPI's 1977 guidelines on the carcinogenicity testing of drugs.[91] Moreover, that Committee prepared the guidelines in the 1973/74 financial year and, via the ABPI's Scientific and Technical Council, discussed them with the secretariat of the Committee on the Safety of Medicines (CSM) in October 1975.[92] There can be little doubt, therefore, that senior Lilly and DHSS staff concluded that the ABPI guidelines were scientifically legitimate.

Yet arguably the results of Lilly's long-term rat study were inconsistent with all the above recommendations by the WHO, ABPI, PMA and DHSS since, by the company's own admission, not only was the top dose sufficient to considerably affect the survival of the rats, but the mid dose was also unequivocally toxic.

Animal survival in the long-term rat study

A further problem afflicting this carcinogenicity study in rats was that there was an outbreak of chronic respiratory disease which affected about

10–15 per cent of all the rats on test across both sexes and all groups, including controls. All the rats were treated with a penicillin antibiotic in an attempt to control the respiratory disease, and some of them, which developed bone joint disease, had to receive X-irradiation for diagnostic purposes.[93] Indeed, Lilly's Toxicology Division concluded that respiratory infections were a principal cause of death among the control rats.[94]

Many authorities have agreed on the appropriate duration of carcinogenicity studies in rats. In 1969 the WHO commented:

> The experimental period is commonly terminated before the end of the natural life span, but it should not be reduced to less than 2 years for rats.[95]

In 1974, and again in 1979, the UK regulatory authorities recommended that carcinogenicity testing in the rat should be of two years duration as did the PMA in 1977.[96]

Hein completed the FDA's first major review of the two-year rat study on 10 April 1979. He believed that the elevated mortality as early as 12 months into the study should have suggested to Lilly scientists that the high dosed rats might not be able to survive 24 months. In his opinion there was an unusually high mortality rate in the control animals. Though Hein noted a high variety of reported tumours with no apparent greater incidence in the high dosed groups, he found Lilly's data difficult to evaluate because of the high rate of deaths and the uneven numbers of animals available at various points in time between the different groups. He further argued that it might be supposed that the rats most susceptible to the formation of tumours died prior to the end of the 24 months, and were the animals that did not get an opportunity to demonstrate the tumours, which tend to be most evident only in the later parts of the study. Thus, Hein commented:

> The usefulness of this study to make a determination as to whether benoxaprofen is, or is not, a potential carcinogen in rats is severely compromised by the fact that the study had such a high mortality rate even though the initial numbers of animals entered into the study/sex/level may have been adequate.[97]

He concluded his review with the following categorical rejection of the adequacy of Lilly's long-term rat study:

> an inadequate number of animals survived to 18 months and beyond in the high dose group and possibly in the mid dose group to make a reasonable estimate of the carcinogenic potential of the agent since most of the tumours are first observed at 18 to 24

117

months in the rats. To be valid as a carcinogenicity study there must be a reasonable number of animals from each sex and dosage level as is detailed in the guidelines for carcinogenicity studies published by the PMA. . . . In this regard we feel this study was faulty.[98]

On 28 March 1980 William Gyarfus, Director of the Division of Oncology and Radiopharmaceutical Products at the FDA concurred with Hein and told Lilly that the agency had completed their review of the long-term rat study.

Number of species for carcinogenicity testing

Even if Lilly's long-term rat study had yielded a negative result on the basis of flawless design, conduct and analysis, this would not have been an adequate test for carcinogenicity, according to many of the scientific standards which had been established by the late 1970s. Indeed, five years before Lilly undertook the long-term rat study the WHO recommended that long-term carcinogenicity testing should be carried out in *at least two species*.[99] In February 1977 the PMA published its recommendations, which had been under discussion for a couple of years, that such testing ought to be carried out in two species.[100] On this point the PMA and ABPI disagreed, with the latter advising carcinogenicity testing in only one species.[101] However, since the carcinogenicity testing of benoxaprofen was carried out in Lilly's American headquarters, the PMA guidelines are much more relevant to all aspects of the company's animal carcinogenicity programme than those of the ABPI.

Moreover, by 1979 the UK Licencing Authority was also recommending carcinogenicity studies in two species for drugs, which, like benoxaprofen, were to be taken by patients continuously for long periods.[102] One of the major reasons for the growing scientific consensus that carcinogenicity testing ought to be undertaken in two animal species was the limited reliability of the result in a single species. As Stevenson explained in 1979:

It is all too evident that false positives (mistaking a non-carcinogen for a carcinogen) and negatives (mistaking a carcinogen for a non-carcinogen), which would be expected on theoretical grounds anyway, are too common to allow any certainty of a correct conclusion on the basis of a *single* experiment.[103] (Emphasis added)

Nevertheless, Lilly sought approval for benoxaprofen in the UK and the US after having conducted only the single long-term rat study.

UK approval and marketing

Despite the many possible objections to the validity of the long-term rat study discussed above, and despite the many standards implying a need for the carcinogenicity testing of drugs intended for chronic use in two animal species,[104] the DHSS and CSM granted Lilly a product licence for *Opren* in March 1980, and in April and August 1980 approved the first two *Opren* data sheets, which Lilly used to promote the use of the drug to doctors. These *Opren* data sheets did not mention any carcinogenicity evaluation of benoxaprofen in rats; indeed, they made no specific reference to carcinogenicity at all.[105] Unfortunately because of the extensive secrecy surrounding the activities of the DHSS and the CSM it is impossible to be certain about the full extent of their evaluation of Lilly's long-term rat study, but there is no evidence available suggesting that the UK regulatory authorities did anything other than fully accept the company's analysis of the long-term rat study.

US non-approval

By contrast, on 25 February 1981 Marion Finkel, Associate Director of New Drug Evaluation at the FDA, wrote a letter of *non-approval* to Lilly regarding their New Drug Application (NDA) for benoxaprofen. This letter reaffirmed the main criticisms of the two-year rat study previously put forward by Hein and Gyarfus. In particular, Finkel told Lilly:

> You have not provided adequate evidence of freedom from carcinogenicity. Drugs that are intended for long term administration in humans should be carefully evaluated for carcinogenicity. PMA guidelines recommend that two valid studies be done. This has been interpreted as two species with adequate numbers of animals (e.g. at least 50/sex/level), two or more levels, two species, adequate survival of animals and a 24 month duration trial in rats and for mice up to 24 months but at least, 18 months. The long term rat study only, in part meets this standard. We recommend, but do not require, that you carry out a second carcinogenicity trial and submit a protocol and timetable for the second study in your IND.

Thus, a third FDA scientist found Lilly's two-year rat study insufficient as a carcinogenicity evaluation of benoxaprofen. Nevertheless, Finkel took the managerial decision not to *require* a second carcinogenicity study in animals. This decision reflects a very permissive regulatory approach towards Lilly since it was inconsistent with the recommendations of not only the WHO, PMA and DHSS but also those of the FDA's own scientific

119

reviewers of benoxaprofen's carcinogenicity. Indeed, in March 1980 Hein reiterated his rejection of the long-term rat study and warned that "[b]ecause there have been some NSAIDs that have been shown to be carcinogenic in animals . . . benoxaprofen should be adequately tested in animals for carcinogenicity".[106]

By 1 March 1982 Sydney Stolzenberg, another FDA scientist, had completed his review of Lilly's animal toxicology studies on benoxaprofen. At that time no animal study, other than the long-term rat study, had been completed with the primary purpose of evaluating the carcinogenic potential of the drug. Lilly had agreed to carry out a two-year mouse study which was in its 220th day at the beginning of March 1982. Stolzenberg stressed the "great importance" of a two-year mouse study, in addition to the long-term rat study, in order to make a "final evaluation of the long-term safety of benoxaprofen."[107] He found the long-term rat study deficient in the ways mentioned by Hein, Gyarfus and Finkel and concluded:

The two year rat toxicity study does not support the safety of this drug for chronic use in humans.[108]

Lilly's defence of the long-term rat study

Unmoved by the many criticisms of the long-term rat study discussed above, in February 1984 Lilly's Toxicology Division still maintained that it "properly demonstrated the lack of oncogenic potential of benoxaprofen in that species".[109] The Division defended this position by arguing that the low survival rates in the study were typical of the Wistar strain of rat. To support this contention they referred to the survival rates of control Wistar rats in 10 studies carried out in Lilly's laboratories between 1974 and 1978. On the basis of these historical control data Lilly seem to have concluded correctly that the life span of the Wistar rat was of the order of 21 months, and that the number of control rats surviving at 24 months frequently fell below 40 per cent, whereas its life span was, on average, approximately 50 per cent at 21 months.[110] Furthermore, Lilly's Toxicology Division argued that their experience with the Wistar strain of rat suggested that respiratory infections could be expected, and so they took precautions by starting the study with 115 controls per sex and 75 treated animals per sex per dose instead of the usual 50 animals per sex per dose.[111]

The arguments put forward by Lilly, with respect to survival rates, do not, however, meet the objections of the FDA's scientific reviewers. One implication of such arguments is that the rat study could be seen as of 21 months duration instead of 24. Such a retrospective interpretation is generous to Lilly since the company's toxicologists did not terminate the study at 21 months on account of the high animal mortality as recommended by the 1977 PMA guidelines.[112] Thus, the data were not collected in the way that they should have been for a 21 month long-term study. Furthermore, from Table 6 it may be noted that at 21 months the survival rates of the rats did not meet Hein's requirement that 25 animals per sex per dose should be alive. Indeed, his requirements were not even met 18 months into the study.

More pertinent to the adequacy of Lilly's defence of the long-term rat study is the fact that the company's experience with the Wistar rat as having a life span of less than 24 months, and of being prone to respiratory infections, does not detract from the criticism of the study (whether considered as 21 months or not) that it did not meet a wide range of recommended scientific standards including those advanced by no less than four FDA scientists. Indeed, if made consistent, Lilly's defence of the study only serves to demonstrate the inappropriateness of the Wistar strain of rat for long-term carcinogenicity testing. This undermines the study even further, especially in view of the WHO's 1969 recommendation that:

In long-term tests, such as those for carcinogenicity, the health of the animals is of paramount importance.[113]

Moreover, Lilly's argument that they took precautions against the high mortality rate in the Wistar rat merely suggests that the company's toxicologists were aware of the inappropriateness of this type of rat for carcinogenicity testing. As Stolzenberg put it:

it is difficult to understand why this strain with limited longevity was chosen when virtually all guidelines for rat carcinogenicity studies, including those by the PMA and NCI [National Cancer Institute of the United States], suggest carcinogenicity studies of two years or longer in rats and with 50 per cent or greater survival i.e. 25 or more of 50 of each sex per group.[114]

US approval and marketing

In the context of deep reservations among FDA scientists regarding the validity of the long-term rat study, and just seven weeks after Stolzenberg had concluded that the study was inadequate, Finkel wrote a letter of approval for benoxaprofen dated 19 April 1982. In this letter she told Lilly that the FDA had concluded that the drug was "safe and effective for use as recommended in the labelling if it [the labelling] [was] modified".[115] It is significant that in February 1981 Finkel herself had concluded that the long- term rat study was insufficient and recommended that a second species lifetime carcinogenicity study should be carried out.

It seems reasonable to assume that Finkel's February 1981 recommendation was intended to mean that the second carcinogenicity study should be completed before marketing since she had stated that drugs intended for long-term use in humans, such as benoxaprofen, should be carefully evaluated for carcinogenicity. Yet the only lifetime animal carcinogenicity data concerning benoxaprofen available to the agency at the time of FDA approval were derived from the two-year mouse study, still in its first year, and the completed long-term rat study already considered inadequate by FDA scientists. It would have been a violation of virtually all the principles of chemical carcinogenicity testing established at that time to suppose that any interim data emerging from the mouse study, less than half-way through, could have provided the basis for a careful evaluation of carcinogenic risk. In particular, in 1979 the Interagency Regulatory Liason Group, of which the FDA was a member, said of carcinogenicity studies in animals:

> Negative results decrease in value as the exposure and observation periods are shortened, and they become practically meaningless if these periods are shorter than half the life spans of the animals.[116]

In her letter of approval Finkel was clearly aware that the two-year mouse study was not completed and referred to it as "ongoing".[117] However, later in a discussion of the labelling for benoxaprofen she proposed that the label *should* read:

> Long-term studies in mice and rats showed no evidence of carcinogenicity, however the studies were complicated by an epidemic respiratory infection which reduced the number of animals available for long-term evaluation.[118]

After approval this was indeed how the drug was labelled in Lilly's promotion of *Oraflex* on the FDA-approved package insert, and on information brochures sent to doctors in the US.[119] Such labelling was not straightforwardly false, but it did present Lilly's carcinogenicity testing of benoxaprofen in a way which was extremely favourable to the company because neither the long-term mouse study nor the long-term rat study could be expected to show any evidence of carcinogenicity, since the former was only half-completed and the latter was considered flawed by the FDA's own scientists.

Nevertheless, the FDA expressed no doubts about benoxaprofen's supposed lack of carcinogenicity in its official Summary Basis of Approval

(SBA) for the drug in May 1982. In fact, the SBA asserted that "the label-ling adequately indicates toxicity that occurred in animal studies" and that "long-term rat studies did not reveal evidence of tumorigenicity".[120] That the official position of the FDA was that Lilly's pre-marketing car-cinogenicity testing of benoxaprofen was sufficient to grant approval for the drug was confirmed at the highest level by Robert Temple, Director of the Office of New Drug Evaluation at the agency, who testified in April 1983 that, in order to approve *Oraflex* marketing, the FDA must have con-cluded that the carcinogenicity testing of the drug was "sufficient to rule out a major risk".[121]

Lilly's interpretation of the two-year mouse study

This study commenced on 18 June 1981 and was conducted by Lilly be-cause it was requested by the FDA. On 21 December 1983 Lilly repre-sentatives, including the Vice-President of Clinical and Regulatory Affairs, met with several FDA scientists, including Stolzenberg, at the com-pany's request to present preliminary data from the two-year mouse study.[122] Although benoxaprofen had been withdrawn from the market worldwide in August 1982 due to adverse reactions in patients, in the US the drug continued to be prescribed under close clinical supervision to patients who specifically requested it. The drug's potential carcinogen-icity was not, therefore, an entirely academic matter even in 1983.

At this meeting Lilly informed the FDA that they were discontinuing all clinical use of benoxaprofen because data from the two-year mouse study indicated that the carcinogenicity test was positive for liver tumours.[123] Two days later Lilly sent a letter to US physicians regarding this mouse study stating:

> Although hepatic carcinoma was observed in both controls and treated groups of mice, there was an increased incidence in the high-dose treatment groups. The relevance of these findings to hu-man exposure to benoxaprofen is difficult to assess. No increased incidence of tumors was observed in the mice treated with a dose equivalent to the recommended human dose of 600mg per day; the doses that showed the effect were the equivalent of three to ten times the human dose. The mouse liver is a very sensitive organ and frequently exhibits tumors when such a response is not seen in the livers of other species. Furthermore, other toxicologic studies completed prior to the approval of benoxaprofen had not indi-cated benoxaprofen had a carcinogenic effect. These studies in-

cluded a battery of mutagenicity studies all of which were negative. In a two year carcinogenicity study no increased incidence of tumors was observed at any dose level including a daily dose equivalent to the recommended human dose of 600mg per day. . . . The mouse study was only one of many tests that were conducted and it is not possible to directly correlate the findings in mice to possible long-term adverse effects in humans. Nevertheless, we have decided that the prudent course of action is to discontinue the clinical trial program.[124]

Thus, Lilly elected to treat the long-term rat study of benoxaprofen's potential carcinogenicity as a valid negative result, and to use it and various limited negative mutagenicity tests to call into question the significance of their own positive carcinogenicity finding in mice.

On 27 January 1984 Lilly met with the FDA at the company's request to discuss the follow-up to their decision to discontinue all clinical use of benoxaprofen.[125] At this meeting Lilly presented the FDA with the letter they had just sent to doctors, and a report dated 26 January 1984 and entitled "Preliminary analysis of the pathological findings in B6C3F1 mice given benoxaprofen in the diet for two years".[126] This report further developed the idea that the two-year mouse study had very limited implications for humans. For example, it stated that the incidence of "spontaneous" hepatomas (liver tumours) in untreated control mice of B6C3F1 strain can be high, ranging in a number of published studies from 7–58 per cent (with a mean of 32.1 per cent) in male mice and from 0–73 per cent (with a mean of 6.2 per cent) in female mice. The report concluded:

the evaluation of carcinogenic potential requires an examination of the results of all pertinent studies, the findings in the mouse stand in contrast to the findings in other species and in the mutagenicity studies. In the absence of collaborative data from other studies, the findings in the mouse do not constitute sufficient evidence to conclude that benoxaprofen would present a carcinogenic hazard to man.[127]

Evidently Lilly consistently presented the argument that, out of two long-term carcinogenicity studies in animals and a far from conclusive set of negative mutagenicity tests, more than one positive result in a long-term study was required to provide sufficient evidence of a carcinogenic risk. Such a perspective conflicted directly with the following interpretive principles advocated by the US Interagency Regulatory Liason Group in 1979, which embodied scientific standards jointly agreed by the FDA, the

Environmental Protection Agency, the Consumer Product Safety Commission and the Occupational Safety and Health Administration:

> The response to carcinogens in different animal species and even strains is known to vary greatly . . . Present knowledge indicates that a substance that is clearly carcinogenic in one test species is likely to be carcinogenic in other species, that it may take extensive tests in several species to demonstrate this correlation, and that the responsive target tissues or organs and the types of tumors induced in different species may vary greatly. Therefore, although concordance of positive results (even if different tumor types are involved) adds support to an evaluation of carcinogenicity, the finding of negative results in some other species generally does not detract from the validity of a positive result as evidence of carcinogenicity for the test substance. In this respect, positive results supersede negative ones.[128]

On 10 April 1984 Stolzenberg came to review the two-year mouse study. He was not convinced by Lilly's suggestion that the benoxaprofen-related increased incidence of liver tumours in the mice might not have occurred in a less sensitive strain of mouse.[129] Rather, he concluded that the increased incidence of liver tumours in both male and female rats was clearly due to the drug on test, and commented that Lilly had attempted to "minimize the relevance of the tumour findings in mice to assessment of risk of human exposure".[130] Stolzenberg also rejected Lilly's assumption that negative mutagenicity tests were incompatible with the positive result of the two-year mouse study on the grounds that benoxaprofen could be carcinogenic by some epigenetic mechanism. Finally, with regard to Lilly's claim that the tumour findings in the mouse study did not constitute sufficient evidence for a carcinogenic hazard to humans, he accepted that the mouse study could not establish beyond doubt that the drug would or would not cause cancer in humans but, he argued, "this kind of evidence is presently the best we have to reasonably anticipate the possibility of human carcinogenic risk".[131]

FDA's final review

According to the FDA memo of the meeting of 21 December, when the agency and Lilly scientists discussed the two-year mouse study, it was "discovered" that "the package insert incorrectly referred to long-term studies in mice and rats in the Precautions section under Carcinogenesis, Mutagenesis and Impairment of Fertility".[132] This suggests a view within the agency that the FDA actually made a mistake in the labelling they approved, though Lilly seem to have supported that labelling and marketed the drug with it. Nevertheless, the FDA's final review of benoxaprofen makes it clear that the agency's decision to approve the drug would not have been affected even if the "incorrect" labelling had been "discovered" before marketing.

On 18 July 1985 a meeting between Max Talbott of Lilly and John Harter, Senior Medical Officer for NSAIDs at the FDA, took place. The memo of this meeting states:

> Dr Harter will write a final review to be forwarded to Dr Temple attached to the pharmacologist's review of the animal liver studies. His review will state that the findings of the second mouse study, though positive for liver tumours, would not justify non-approval, removal from the market, or further patient follow-up.[133]

Thus, despite a positive result regarding carcinogenicity for the two-year mouse study and benoxaprofen's unexceptional efficacy, senior FDA officials, contrary to the agency's declared risk/benefit policy, were willing to give Lilly the benefit of the doubt by approving the drug under such circumstances, had it not already been withdrawn.

In short Lilly scientists consistently interpreted their own toxicological research in ways which represented benoxaprofen as benign and which coincided with the commercial interests of the company. That these interests may have generated bias is strongly suggested by the company's inconsistent extrapolations to human risk from the long-term rat and mouse studies. Lilly's Toxicology Division vigorously defended the use of a very questionable negative carcinogenicity test as a basis for asserting that benoxaprofen had been shown to be sufficiently free from carcinogenic risk to humans to be put on the market. By contrast, Lilly toxicologists argued in favour of caution in extrapolating to humans the positive carcinogenic result in the two-year mouse study. Moreover, the company's attempt to defend the validity of the long-term rat study and the less than half completed two-year mouse study as bases for concluding that benoxaprofen was safe for chronic human use reveals deeper biases in terms of data interpretation.

Little is known about the review of benoxaprofen's carcinogenicity by the DHSS and the CSM. However, it is clear that, during the 1970s, the UK regulations regarding the carcinogenicity testing of drugs were less stringent than the standards advocated by the WHO, the FDA or the PMA and it is not being suggested that members of the DHSS or CSM behaved improperly with respect to their duties under the Medicines Act. Even so, in approving benoxaprofen for marketing as early as 1980 the British Licencing Authority gave Lilly a substantial benefit of the doubt by not applying the scientific standards which, by 1979, had been established by the DHSS itself. At the very least the British regulatory authorities could have mentioned the problematic nature of the long-term rat study on the product data sheet, assuming they knew about the problems of animal survival and so on.

The four FDA scientists who reviewed benoxaprofen's carcinogenicity repeatedly reached assessments consistent with the prevalent scientific standards. The reviews of three of these scientists, Hein, Gyarfus and Stolzenberg, were consistent with the view that the drug should not be approved until two adequate long-term carcinogenicity studies in animals had been completed. On the other hand, Finkel, acting on behalf of the FDA's management, felt able to give the company the benefit of the very considerable doubts about the drug's safety by not *requiring* Lilly to complete a carcinogenicity test in a second animal species prior to approval.

Neither the labelling nor the Summary Basis of Approval (SBA) for benoxaprofen approved by the FDA can be made consistent with the agency's own scientific evaluation of the drug or with many scientific standards for carcinogenicity testing established at the time of approval. However, approval for the *marketing* of benoxaprofen could have been justifiable in the absence of adequate carcinogenicity testing *if* the drug had been of outstanding clinical effectiveness. Indeed, the FDA had established a risk/benefit policy not to approve a drug found to be carcinogenic in animals unless it conveyed some unique benefit over and above other drugs of its therapeutic class.[134] But, as discussed in the previous section, FDA scientists vigorously objected to the suggestion that benoxaprofen was more efficacious than other NSAIDs; and on 4 August 1982 Frank Hayes, Commissioner of the FDA, testified that the agency had found benoxaprofen "to be about as effective as aspirin and Motrin [ibuprofen]".[135]

Given that the FDA's own scientists acknowledged that benoxaprofen offered unexceptional therapeutic benefits compared with other NSAIDs and that the agency's own scientific reviews and standards pointed to the inadequacy of the carcinogenicity testing of the drug before marketing, it can be confidently concluded that the FDA's management exhibited very substantial bias towards commercial interests in the approval and labelling of *Oraflex*. The enormous magnitude of this bias is confirmed by the FDA's final official verdict that even if the positive carcinogenic result in mice had emerged prior to marketing it would not have prevented approval by the agency.

Photosensitivity and onycholysis – discourse and the fading of truth

Cutaneous reactions were the most common adverse effects of benoxaprofen therapy – accounting for approximately 70 per cent of all those reported.[136] In particular, a very large number of photosensitivity reactions have been associated with benoxaprofen medication. By the end of 1981, 1,072 such photosensitivity reactions had been reported to the CSM[137] – more than any other drug prescribed since 1964.[138] The extent and seriousness of those reactions remain controversial. I do not seek to settle those controversies but rather, in the context of the scientific knowledge at the time, I focus on the responses of Lilly scientists and consultants, and the actions of the UK and US regulatory authorities, as the photosensitivity and onycholysis reactions emerged.

The nature of photosensitivity and onycholysis

Drug photosensitivity reactions are adverse cutaneous responses to the combined actions of a chemical agent and light. Soon after the introduction of the sulfanilamide drugs to antibiotic therapy adverse skin reactions were associated with sulfanilamide in 5 to 10 per cent of the treated patients. The first clue that light was involved in those reactions came from the observation that no untoward effects occurred in hospitalized patients undergoing sulfanilamide therapy.[139]

In the late 1930s Epstein undertook the first well-controlled studies of drug photosensitivity in humans.[140] After an intradermal injection of sulfanilamide followed by light exposure, all six subjects developed a "primary photosensitivity reaction"[141] at the site of injection, consisting of erythema (reddening of the skin) and oedema (swelling due to fluid in the tissues), within one to twenty-four hours. This reaction persisted for a few days. In two of the subjects, however, 10 days after initial exposure an inflammatory urticarial (allergic skin eruption) reaction occurred spontaneously. Subsequent phototesting by Epstein demonstrated that, unlike the "primary photosensitivity reaction" the urticarial reaction could be reproduced within a day of light exposure and further challenge by sulfanilamide. In so doing, Epstein was the first to report *photoallergic* reactions to a drug in the scientific literature.

By the late 1950s the term photosensitivity had come to embrace two different types of adverse cutaneous reactions: *phototoxicity* (i.e. Epstein's "primary photosensitivity") and photoallergy. Clinically a phototoxic reaction is defined as being nothing more than an exaggerated sunburn which, under suitable conditions, such as sufficient dose of drug and light of a specific wavelength, will take place in *all individuals*.[142] The action spectrum for phototoxic drugs includes the sunburning ultraviolet rays UVB (of wavelength 290– 320nm), the far ultraviolet UVA (320–400nm) and visible ranges.[143] By contrast, a photoallergic reaction may be urticarial and eczematous, occur in only a small percentage of those persons exposed to the drug and light, have a long incubation period, recur rapidly on rechallenge of drug and light, subsequent to the incubation period, and not be dependent on specific fixed wavelengths of light.[144] Like phototoxic drugs, photoallergens have been found to have action spectrums in the UVA and UVB ranges.[145]

Most photoallergic reactions are of the type described in the above paragraph. However, the photoallergic reactions to the drugs chlorpromazine and promethazine have been found to cause *persistent* light sensitivity in some patients.[146] Persistent light sensitivity can be distinguished from other photoallergic reactions by two features: sensitivity to light persists for months or even years *without* continued exposure to the photoallergen; and a broad spectrum of light reactivity is manifest.[147] Persistent light sensitivity is an extremely serious adverse reaction since sufferers are, in effect, incapacitated.

Despite some of the differences which have been established between phototoxic and photoallergic reactions, throughout the medical literature scientists have commented on the difficulties of clear diagnosis solely on the basis of clinical examination. Phototoxic reactions can include scaling not unlike eczematous photoallergenicity. Moreover, due to differences in skin pigmentation, in exposure to sunlight, and in the elimination (i.e. excretion) of a photosensitizing drug from the body, the frequency of a phototoxic reaction in a patient population may be so small as to be suggestive of photoallergenicity. Thus, in 1961 Knox exhorted:

> In many instances it is quite difficult to differentiate clinically between drug-induced phototoxic and photoallergic reactions without carefully performed investigative studies.[148]

Twenty years later the situation had changed little, as the comments of Harber and Bickers show:

It is often difficult to differentiate clinically between agents that cause phototoxic reactions and those that cause photoallergic reactions. Indeed, the same drug may cause both types of reactions in human skin. Under ideal clinical *and experimental* circumstances, major differences between the two reactions become evident, however.[149] (Emphasis added)

Sometimes onycholysis (the loosening of toe and/or finger nails from the nailbeds) accompanies photosensitivity reactions, but it can also occur as an adverse drug reaction independently of photosensitivity.

Clinical trials in support of the UK product licence

Clinical trial investigators of benoxaprofen were among the first to publish photosensitivity and onycholysis reactions to benoxaprofen. However, the design of the pre-marketing British clinical trials for adequately detecting and describing adverse reactions to benoxaprofen had significant limitations according to certain clinical standards then available. In 1976 Huskisson, himself a leading consultant clinical trialist on Lilly's benoxaprofen-testing programme in the UK, stated that, for trials with anti-inflammatory drugs:

at least 30 patients in each [treatment] group are required in trials designed to show the incidence of side effects . . . Long term treatment, at least six months, is required to document the side effects and toxicity of a compound.[150]

None of the UK clinical trials met *both* of Huskisson's criteria, with respect to size of patient groups and duration. Seven of the UK clinical trials did not satisfy *either* of Huskisson's criteria of validity.

The published accounts of some of these studies revealed that some patients withdrew from the clinical trials due to skin and/or photosensitivity reactions while taking benoxaprofen.[151] In one study three patients complained of photosensitivity, prompting the clinical investigators to report:

Some patients who had longer exposure subsequently developed erythema in the exposed areas and one woman who was on holiday found this side effect particularly troublesome.[152]

These may be regarded as serious because, as William Shedden, the company's Medical Director in the US has stated:

an adverse effect which causes the patient to discontinue taking the drug is generally also a serious effect.[153]

Indeed, Huskisson's published account of one of his own clinical tests with benoxaprofen refers to "hot flushes" of "moderate severity".

The design of some of the UK trials might also be questioned because the cross-over design used in seven studies may have been inappropriate for a new drug with a long elimination half-life (i.e. the time taken for the concentration of a drug in the bloodstream to fall to half a give concentration), such as benoxaprofen, whose adverse reactions could have been wrongly attributed to the comparator drug when patients switched from the former to the latter. In 1976 Huskisson even suggested that for anti-inflammatory drugs with a long half-life, clinical investigators should consider the option of abandoning the cross-over design in favour of parallel studies.[154]

The four US-based clinical trials submitted to the UK Licencing Authority did satisfy Huskisson's criteria of validity regarding sample size and duration. These were co-ordinated by Walter Mikulaschek, Lilly's Medical Monitor at the company's headquarters in Indianapolis, but published in 1980 under the names of Gum and Alarcon-Segovia. These studies involved comparing over a 28-week period the adverse effects of benoxaprofen with aspirin and ibuprofen in patients suffering from osteoarthritis and rheumatoid arthritis. The design of these trials involved the investigators in attempting to determine whether or not adverse effects were "drug-related".[155] Though Gum and Alarcon-Segovia did list all the adverse reactions recorded, as shown in Table 7, Gum elected to confine his quantitative analyses to "drug-related" adverse reactions stating:

> The overall incidence of drug-related side effects was 24.1 per cent for benoxaprofen as compared to 57.6 per cent for aspirin, which was highly significant in favour of benoxaprofen (chi square $p<.01$).
> There were no statistically significant differences in the number of patients with adverse reactions in Study 1 [the comparison with ibuprofen].[156]

By analyzing only "drug-related" adverse effects Gum increased the risk of underestimating the extent of skin reactions to benoxaprofen because it is more difficult to perceive that adverse effects are related to a new drug whose adverse reaction profile is not well known. As is evident from Table 7, benoxaprofen was associated with a much greater *total* of adverse cutaneous reactions than either ibuprofen or aspirin.

Significantly, Alarcon-Segovia, who elected to analyze all the adverse effects reported, reached the rather different conclusion from Gum that:

> It was apparent that benoxaprofen caused . . . more skin reactions than aspirin or ibuprofen. The latter included photosensitivity,

Table 7 Number of skin reactions recorded in US clinical trials.

| | Rheumatoid arthritis–Gum | | | | Osteoarthritis–Alar.Seg. | | | |
	benox	ibu	benox	asp	benox	ibu	benox	asp
"Drug-related"	7	8	6	1	3	2	5	2
"Cause-unknown"	10	2	9	3	13	1	6	5
Total	17	10	15	4	16	3	11	7

Source: D. Alarcon-Segovia 1980. Long-term treatment of symptomatic osteoarthritis with benoxaprofen: double-blind comparison with aspirin and ibuprofen. *Journal of Rheumatology Supplement* **7**(6), 89–99; O. B. Gum 1980. Long-term efficacy and safety of benoxaprofen: comparison with aspirin and ibuprofen in patients with active rheumatoid arthritis. *Journal of Rheumatology Supplement* **7**(6), 76–88.

Key: asp = aspirin; benox = benoxaprofen; ibu=ibuprofen

pruritis, skin rash and onycholysis. Most of the skin reactions were mild; only one rash was severe enough to require discontinuation of therapy.[157]

The response of the regulatory authorities

Between April and December 1979 the CSM and the British Medicines Division of the UK Licencing Authority considered Lilly's initial application to market benoxaprofen.[158] Having considered the information contained in the clinical trial data, the CSM deferred its decision to obtain further information on adverse effects recorded in some patients. In particular, onycholysis and photosensitivity had been sufficiently conspicuous for the CSM to seek further clarification of these reactions.[159] On 6 December the UK Licencing Authority requested from Lilly further evidence as to the nature, severity and reversibility of onycholysis and photosensitivity.[160] In February 1980 the CSM considered further evidence compiled by Lilly, specifically regarding benoxaprofen safety, and relating to 330 patients in the UK (from the UK clinical trials already discussed) and 1,681 patients in North America.[161]

The North American safety evaluation data on 1,681 patients were published by Mikulaschek in 1980 as a paper entitled "Long-term safety of Benoxaprofen".[162] Much of the data in this paper was derived from the US clinical trials published by Gum and Alarcon-Segovia, combined with open label studies of patients who continued on benoxaprofen beyond the 28 weeks of the double-blind controlled clinical trials. Mikulaschek's analysis shared with that of Gum and Alarcon-Segovia the approach of separating "drug-related" adverse effects from all others. However, unlike Alarcon-Segovia, Mikulaschek listed and analyzed *only* "drug-related" adverse effects; not even signs, symptoms and illnesses classified as "aetiology unknown" were listed. Moreover, Mikulaschek's analysis of "drug-related" adverse effects did not organize the findings according to time period on the drug for each patient – a major limitation given that the review was supposed to elucidate *long-term* safety.

Bearing in mind the comments of Knox[163] and Harber & Bickers,[164] one drawback with the clinical data submitted to the British regulatory authorities was that they did not include any controlled experimental phototesting of benoxaprofen, in order to obtain a more precise characterization of its photosensitivity. The trials submitted relied solely on clinical diagnosis of adverse effects, if and when they emerged. That this was not entirely satisfactory is illustrated by the following remark by investigators Tyson & Glynne about their trial:

Skin changes were classified as those that *seemed* to be photosensitive and those that did not.[165] (Emphasis added)

The determination of the action spectrum of benoxaprofen might have helped to rule out the possibility that benoxaprofen was photoallergic.[166] Moreover, even if it were accepted that the drug was definitely no more than phototoxic, Ferguson et al. have pointed out that information about benoxaprofen's action spectrum was relevant to the selection of the appropriate sunscreening agents, which were most likely to prevent the reaction.[167]

Nevertheless, Mikulaschek's investigation of benoxaprofen did not include any experimental phototesting.[168] Rather, he attempted no more than quantitative estimates of the incidence of photosensitivity and onycholysis derived from clinical observations. Based on his sample of 1,681 patients, Mikulaschek reported that 9 per cent experienced photosensitivity reactions, and that 8.7 per cent developed onycholysis. Of the patients with onycholysis, most exhibited less than half of the nail separating from the nail-bed, but 6.9 per cent of them developed up to two-thirds nail separation. Mikulaschek described most of the photosensitivity reactions as a "mild irritation", but in 0.7 per cent of patients the reaction was sufficient to terminate therapy. Though 0.7 per cent is a small proportion, it has been estimated that benoxaprofen was taken by some 1.5 million people worldwide.[169] Therefore, 0.7 per cent of benoxaprofen consumers could represent 10,500 patients. No details regarding the character of those more severe reactions, which caused patients to end therapy, were provided. Mikulaschek merely stated that "recurrences could frequently be prevented by using ultraviolet sunscreens", but provided no information about those cases for whom, or instances in which, such prevention had not proved successful.[170]

Despite the apparent limitations of the clinical trials and Mikulaschek's safety evaluation data, the CSM advised the UK Licencing Authority that benoxaprofen should be granted a product licence. This advice was accepted and the Licencing Authority granted a licence for use of the drug in hospitals in March 1980, and for use in general practice six months later.[171] As I mentioned earlier in this chapter, in April and August 1980 the UK regulatory authorities approved Lilly's first and second *Opren* data sheets respectively. As with Government-approved data sheets throughout the industry, these were used to provide doctors with prescribing information. Both made the following statements about photosensitivity and onycholysis:

> Photosensitive skin reactions have been seen in some patients. These reactions are generally mild and can usually be prevented by ultraviolet sunscreens. Mild to moderate areas of separation of the nail from the nail bed have also occurred. Such reactions do not usually interfere with *Opren* therapy; however, patients should be advised to avoid prolonged exposure to bright sunlight unless using ultraviolet sunscreens. Rash, urticaria and pruritis have also been noted.[172]

If Mikulaschek's analysis of benoxaprofen safety was less than forthcoming about serious photosensitivity reactions, then the first two data sheets approved by the CSM were uninformative by omission. Although photosensitivity was said to be "generally mild" and "usually" preventable by sunscreens, there was no estimate of the number of cases likely to be more severe, nor any quantitative estimate of how "usual" it was for sunscreens to prevent the reaction. Furthermore, no indication of the reasons why more serious photosensitivity reactions might occur was provided. Even Mikulaschek noted that some patients developed sufficiently severe onycholysis to terminate therapy.[173]

When the FDA came to review the clinical section of Lilly's New Drug Application (NDA) they considered the trials reported by Gum and Alarcon-Segovia to be the four crucial studies on which justification for approval might be based, and, by convention, referred to them as "pivotal studies". By 20 October 1980 Hsu, a mathematical statistician at the agency, had completed his review of them. He concluded:

> The nature of the data presentation and statistical analyses of the data in this submission does not allow us to make a definitive

evaluation of the . . . safety of benoxaprofen in the treatment of rheumatoid arthritis and osteoarthritis at this time. The study results are not acceptable . . . Drug-related and not drug-related SSIs [signs, symptoms and illnesses] should be considered together in a combined analysis as well as considered separately. The incidence of adverse reactions may depend on the duration of study. The incidence of reactions in the first three months of active therapy as well as overall incidence should be examined carefully.[174]

On 25 February 1981 Marion Finkel, Associate Director of New Drug Evaluation at the FDA's Bureau of Drugs, confirmed Hsu's evaluation and added:

the prevalence and severity of certain adverse reactions should be adequately evaluated and described by reanalyses of submitted data or the addition of new data. Two of these that are of special prominence are (i) onycholysis and (ii) photosensitivity . . . compilations of many studies of accumulated SSIs will include short term studies that probably were too short a duration (almost 743 or 39.2 per cent of patients took the drug in studies of less than 30 days) for the recognition of this reaction [onycholysis] and thus dilute its impact. If these two signs [onycholysis and photosensitivity] were related to one another there could be a magnification of the problem. There should be a clinical narrative which would in the example of onycholysis describe any time relationship to drug use, the extent of nail separation, the number of digits affected, the results of withdrawal, etc.[175]

Finkel's letter reveals clearly that the FDA were particularly concerned about the incidence and possible severity of photosensitivity and onycholysis, and so, unlike the CSM, were not convinced of the safety of benoxaprofen based on the initial reports of Gum, Alarcon-Segovia and Mikulaschek.

The incidence of onycholysis and photosensitivity revisited

On 24 and 25 September 1980 Barnett, Lilly's Medical Adviser for benoxaprofen's international registration, visited Lilly's headquarters at Erl Wood, where he discussed the regulatory status of benoxaprofen with Oldfield, a senior member of Dista. Regarding this meeting Barnett noted:

There is some concern in the UK about whether and when to inform the CSM of the latest figures on the incidence of photosensitivity and onycholysis which have been supplied by the United States. The problem is twofold. In the UK equivalent of our rules, it is stated that information from abroad which comes to the attention of the company in the UK relating to adverse reactions that could lead to a serious hazard should be reported to the CSM. It is indeed a question whether the incidence change that has been noted fits this definition. Additionally, however, Mr Oldfield has mentioned that in the course of the EEC procedures there may come a time when a meeting would be held with representatives of each of the countries of the EEC and at such a meeting if information already supplied to Germany and to be supplied to France was discussed, then incidence figures would be much higher than had previously been reported to the CSM. This might cause some embarrassment with and for the CSM. There is a lengthy, drawn out procedure which the CSM might resort to if they considered the hazard serious, ultimately leading to revocation of the product licence. It is doubtful that this latter situation will arise. I left Mr Oldfield with the thought that a decision on informing the CSM need not be made immediately because of the difficulty in deciding which patient populations should be included in incidence figures, and that overall incidence had perhaps not changed that much.[176]

This implies that the incidence of onycholysis and photosensitivity in the US was considerably higher than the company had expected or hoped for – high enough for Lilly scientists to worry about the possibility, albeit small, that the CSM might revoke the licence for *Opren*. Barnett, however, gave the drug the benefit of the doubt and concluded that there probably was not a sufficient increase in incidence to warrant a prompt report to the CSM.

The full significance of Barnett's judgements about the incidence of onycholysis and photosensitivity, however, only emerged in the heat of a controversy following an FDA investigation of Lilly's adverse effects reporting. Early in 1981 Hensley, an FDA scientist at the Clinical Investigations Branch, investigated Lilly's reporting of adverse drug reactions during clinical trials following anonymous complaints from two different sources.[177]

On completing his investigations Hensley alleged that there was a substantial under-reporting of onycholysis and photosensitivity.[178] As a consequence of these findings Hensley, along with Robert Leventhal and two other FDA investigators, interviewed the following Lilly staff on 8 September 1981: Frank Peck, Director of Regulatory Affairs, JoAnn Meuller, Senior Regulatory Reports Co-ordinator, Barnett, formerly Medical Adviser to Regulatory Affairs for the benoxaprofen project, and Mikulaschek. For Hensley, these interviews revealed that: (a) some time prior to NDA submission on 17 January 1980 Mikulaschek ceased his routine review of case reports, and thereafter depended on Lilly's Regulatory Affairs to forward him those containing adverse effects; (b) subsequently, as Lilly encountered adverse effects, such as onycholysis and photosensitivity, with increasing frequency, they decided to cease reporting them in the IND with the rationale, per Barnett, that they were no longer to be considered serious; (c) submission of adverse effect data was deliberately limited to those patients completing clinical trials prior to November 1978; and (d) according to Meuller, just prior to the NDA submission Barnett selected some adverse effects reports, which he considered significant for reporting in a narrative form, but instructed her not to report others, such as onycholysis and photosensitivity, which he felt were less significant because of their frequent occurrence.[179]

Whether these practices were in breach of FDA regulations is unclear because of the scope for autonomous decision-making which the agency apparently awarded scientists in the pharmaceutical industry. At that time the FDA's regulations required sponsors to include in their NDA reports "a full statement of adverse effects and an account of the adverse experiences of each patient".[180] According to Temple, Acting Director of the Office of New Drug Evaluation at the agency, Lilly had complied with those regulations up to their "cut-off point" (i.e. November 1978).[181] However, since Lilly had not submitted their NDA until January 1980, the company's choice of cut-off point meant that data on adverse effects compiled from over a year of clinical trials were not initially reported in the NDA.[182] Though the FDA's regulations did not specify how a company should update its NDA,[183] Lilly was required to continue reporting "fairly serious" adverse reactions and "information that would affect the contraindications, warnings and so forth" in the IND file.[184] In particular, in 1982 Temple testified:

> If there was information indicating that the frequency of these [adverse] reactions was considerably greater than they [the sponsor] had thought to be before, that might reach the level of requiring a further report.[185]

Thus, FDA policy plainly permitted *the sponsor* to decide whether a change of incidence in adverse effects such as onycholysis or photosensitivity was worthy of report. Moreover, while FDA staff had access to the IND file by entering the company's premises, the sponsor was not required to submit the IND file to the reviewing staff at the agency.[186]

Hensley's claims were contested by Lilly and, on the evidence available, we cannot be sure whether all of Hensley's allegations are correct.[187] More significantly the FDA's management does not seem to have been wholly convinced by Hensley's claims, and did not fully endorse them. The final FDA report on Lilly's reporting of these adverse effects, issued by the agency's Office of Compliance, partly exonerated the company:

> 65 adverse effects, primarily onycholysis and/or photosensitivity were not reported to NDA in January 1980 when it was filed . . .. These 65 adverse effects were reported to IND in June 1981 annual report.[188]

Though Hensley believed that these adverse effects had not even been reported in the June 1981 IND submission,[189] Leventhal one of his colleagues in the investigative team, was inclined to believe that the final FDA report was correct.[190] However, Leventhal stressed that, since some of these adverse effects were several years old by June 1981, they were not being reported in a timely manner.[191] This interpretation seems to be supported by a 24 March 1982 memorandum from John Harter, the leading medical reviewer of benoxaprofen at the FDA, which stated:

> The reviewer had "to discover" the higher incidence [of benoxaprofen adverse effects] and then we had to try to decide what "the true incidence" was.[192]

It does not seem possible to come to any firm conclusions about whether Lilly reported benoxaprofen onycholysis and photosensitivity to the appropriate files or whether, as Hensley alleged, the company deliberately withheld adverse reaction reports.[193] But it is certain that senior FDA officials chose to give Lilly the benefit of the doubt on this matter because as late as 3 August 1982, over three months after the FDA had approved benoxaprofen for marketing in the US, Temple stated that he had "no idea" whether Lilly's choice of cut-off point had been a deliberate attempt to minimize the frequency of certain adverse reaction reports.[194]

Even if one discounts Hensley's analysis and accepts that Lilly reported all adverse effects to the NDA and IND before the drug was approved in the US, the reasoning by which Barnett attempted to defend Lilly's reporting practices during his interview with Hensley's investigative team is of interest because of what it reveals about some of the criteria employed by the company in defining the toxicity profile of benoxaprofen. In his report

Hensley recounted the following exchange with Barnett on these matters during the interview on 8 September 1981:

Dr Barnett himself noted that he was "fully cognizant" of his responsibility under the regulations to report any change in incidence of adverse effects, but questioned whether these figures represented a real change. Dr Barnett argued that "10 per cent", (his figure for the occurrence of onycholysis in the FDA) was not really different from 20 per cent (1981 annual report), or at least not significantly different. If it was, he volunteered, "we haven't got a drug". The difference is, of course, a 100 per cent change increase in frequency of occurrence. Further, Dr Barnett argued that it was not really benoxaprofen that caused onycholysis but instead was "the sun" . . . He stated that without the sun photosensitivity and onycholysis would not occur.[195]

Unlike his analysis of Lilly's IND and NDA files, Hensley's account of Barnett's comments at the September 1981 meeting is virtually unchallenged by the available evidence. For example, regarding what Barnett had said, Leventhal testified: "the phrase we wouldn't have a drug does stick in my mind".[196] Peck and Mikulaschek could neither confirm nor deny that the comments Hensley attributed to Barnett were actually made.[197]

In the Borum *vs* Lilly case Barnett declined to answer scores of questions by relying on his Fifth Amendment privileges, which permitted him not to give evidence that might be self-incriminating.[198] Specifically, Barnett refused to answer any questions about the September 1981 meeting with FDA investigators and any statements attributed to him by Hensley thereof.[199] When summing up the trial of that case, the judge professed that, though one could not conclude whether Barnett was guilty or innocent on account of his refusal to testify, one could draw the inference that he committed the acts about which he was interrogated and refused to cooperate.[200] Furthermore, as the plaintiff's lawyer noted, Mueller had not been brought by Lilly's lawyers to deny Hensley's allegations against Barnett, suggesting that no such denial could, in fact, be made.[201]

Given Leventhal's partial confirmation of Hensley's account of Barnett's statements, the apparent inability of Peck or Mikulaschek to recall the meeting sufficiently to confirm or refute Hensley's account, Barnett's refusal to testify for fear of self-incrimination, the failure of Meuller to challenge Hensley's account, and the judge's interpretation of Barnett's decision not to testify, it seems reasonable to conclude that

Barnett had indeed provided the rationale alleged by Hensley. On this assumption there are some far reaching implications for the role of bias in the interpretative frameworks chosen by that Lilly scientist, in order to maintain the safety profile of benoxaprofen as acceptable to the regulatory authorities and the wider profession.

For instance, Barnett, who was responsible for Lilly's IND and NDA files on benoxaprofen, felt able to argue that an increase in the incidence of photosensitivity reactions from 10 to 20 per cent did not represent a "real change". This could then be used as a rationale for not reporting them promptly to the FDA or the CSM, notwithstanding the possibility that those regulatory authorities may *eventually* have received such reports. It may be noted that Barnett's view of "real change" does not seem to have been shared by the FDA or the CSM. Senior scientists at the FDA testified in August 1982 that if there were changes in the frequency of adverse reactions in the course of a clinical trial programme then that would be "important" to the evaluation of the approvability of the drug;[202] and Barnett himself was concerned that, were the CSM to be apprised of the increased incidence in photosensitivity reactions, they might have taken regulatory action against the company. In fact, according to Dista's Medical Director, Brian Gennery, during a meeting with him in July 1982, the CSM expressed alarm at the fact that they had received almost 1,000 reports of onycholysis and photosensitivity reactions to benoxaprofen in the 250,000 patients estimated to be taking the drug – an increase of only 4 per cent,[203] assuming a 10 per cent reporting rate.

The Kligman & Kaidbey study

In the early 1980s Kligman & Kaidbey produced one of the most central and highly cited studies of benoxaprofen photosensitivity. Their research was the first *experimental* phototesting of benoxaprofen. It became a definitive paper on the nature of human photosensitivity reactions to benoxaprofen in the subsequent scientific literature, and played a crucial role in satisfying the US regulatory authorities that the precise character of the drug's photosensitivity had been accurately documented.

In June 1980 Albert Kligman, Professor of Dermatology in the School of Medicine at the University of Pennsylvania, paid a visit to Elizabeth Arden, a subsidiary of Lilly in Indianapolis,[204] during which Mikulaschek invited him to study the photosensitivity qualities of benoxaprofen.[205] Kligman was well known to Lilly because he had regularly engaged in consultancy work for Elizabeth Arden for six years, and had previously researched on other drugs manufactured by the company at its Ivy Laboratories. In fact, Kligman and his wife were, at that time, and at least until 1983, sole shareholders in Ivy Laboratories.[206] Kligman accepted Mikulaschek's invitation and, together with Kaidbey, received a grant from Lilly to undertake the research.[207]

According to Kligman, the purpose of the research was to find out how serious was benoxaprofen photosensitivity; what wavelengths were responsible for it; and in what kind of people it was likely to occur.[208] He was well aware of the significance of the distinction between drug phototoxicity and photoallergenicity, and of the desirability of testing for the existence of the latter:

> While the clinical record does not suggest that benoxaprofen causes photoallergy, *the latter is so serious that the possibility must be explored.*[209] (Emphasis added)

As regards the clinical data on the drug's photosensitivity, which had been collected by Lilly before his experimental investigation, Kligman stated:

> The clinical data leave many questions unanswered . . . . If one looks only at the data given above, *calculation of the risks of photosensitization and estimates of its seriousness are impossible.*[210] (Emphasis added)

In fact, Kligman testified in 1983 that one of the issues in his study was whether benoxaprofen photosensitivity was "due to an allergic change, or was it in the other category, which is a phototoxic change".[211] Thus, Kligman's account of the state of scientific knowledge about benoxaprofen photosensitivity as he began his work on the drug, and of the research problems to be considered during his study, provide further evidence of the limitations of Lilly's knowledge, and that of the CSM, about the nature and, therefore, potential severity of photosensitivity reactions to benoxaprofen when it was first approved and marketed in the UK.

The research conducted by Kligman & Kaidbey led them to judge that photosensitivity reactions to benoxaprofen were phototoxic:

> The conclusive finding is the exhibition of photosensitivity two to three days after starting the drug, far too soon for an immunologically mediated reaction. Another feature strongly supportive of phototoxicity is the capacity to provoke in the laboratory the burning-erythema response in all white subjects tested. It is a characteristic of photoallergy that less than a majority of subjects become photosensitized.[212]

Although these contentions were defensible, they did not imply that benoxaprofen photosensitivity could not have been photoallergic for, as Kligman & Kaidbey noted, there are drugs (e.g. chlorpromazine and sulfanilamide), which are phototoxic *and* photoallergic.[213] This point is of particular significance in view of the fact that Kligman found benoxaprofen's phototoxicity to be of "a unique kind".[214] With this in mind, Kligman and Kaidbey took the reasonable step of testing specifically for benoxaprofen photoallergenicity in 25 subjects. None of these became allergic and Kligman & Kaidbey came to the reasonable conclusion that allergic eruptions from benoxaprofen were likely to be rare.[215] It may be noted, therefore, that their research did not rule out the possibility of photoallergic reactions to benoxaprofen and, in fact, if the drug were to be photoallergic to as many as one per cent of the population a study of 25 subjects might not detect it.

Since Kligman & Kaidbey found no evidence of photoallergic reactions to benoxaprofen during their laboratory tests most of the published discussion of their results focused on an assessment of the drug's phototoxicity. However, the production of the publication raises questions about the appropriateness of the discourse used to represent that assessment.

Though Kligman's studies were ongoing, they were sufficiently complete by June 1981 to present a paper to a benoxaprofen symposium held in Paris. The papers from the Paris symposium were to be published subject to review by Lilly scientists. The following changes were proposed by Lilly's reviewers, although not all were accepted by Kligman:

(1) "Abnormal reactions to sunlight appear to be unusually frequent in patients taking benoxaprofen" was changed by striking out "to be unusually frequent" and inserting "occasionally". Although Kligman did not accept this proposed change because he did not think it accurately expressed his view, he did change his original remark to: "Abnormal reactions to sunlight is a recognized side effect in some patients taking benoxaprofen".[216] Regarding this alteration Kligman testified:

> I ended up . . . and again, in a compromising or in a . . . I think a balanced point of view.[217]

(2) "It is important to emphasize that these [the subjects in Kligman's study] were young adults. Because of more persistent blood levels in the elderly, photosensitivity may not diminish so quickly" was changed by replacing "the elderly" with "some very elderly pa-

142

tients".[218] Kligman did not object to this alteration and stated:

> I don't recall discussing it . . . it's *probably* a reflection of the clinical data Mikulaschek had.[219] (Emphasis added)

(3) "Type 3 individuals [i.e. defined as Caucasoids who rarely burn and tan well] are better off than type 1 [i.e.Caucasoids who always burn and never tan] but need to be apprised that burning-erythema might likely develop in summer" was changed by replacing "might likely" with "could". Kligman had no objections to this alteration because a majority of people taking the drug did not get this reaction.[220]

(4) "Still, given a high enough dose of light, all persons are capable of exhibiting some degree of photosensitivity, particularly burning" was changed to " . . . all persons are at least theoretically capable of exhibiting . . . ". Kligman did not accept this change and the original was the final published version.[221]

(5) "In Philadelphia, light-complexioned individuals will certainly experience phototoxicity after about 30 minutes of noon-day, summer sunlight" was changed to " . . . light-complexioned individuals (Type 1 and 2) may experience . . . " This change was in the final published version though Kligman did not recall discussing it beforehand.[222] He further testified:

> This is a remark that I think now, looking at it in retrospect, I think is too weak and it may have slipped by me. I think I should have remained with the original language. I think I would not accept that statement now. I think the original statement was closer to the truth. This statement should be stronger than it is.[223]

(6) "The risk–benefit ratio does not disqualify the drug" was changed to "the risk–benefit is favourable to the drug".[224] Kligman had no objection to this change although he remarked:

> That's a somewhat stronger statement than the negative way in which I put it . . . I thought at the time that the drug had interesting properties and that the photosensitivity was not so horrendous that it should disqualify the further study with the drug.[225]

According to Kligman, Lilly made no suggestions to alter the tables or the figures and "the substance of the article remained the same".[226] However, when asked if he thought Lilly altered the content of his article, he replied:

Well, this was their way of stating – of looking at the facts and stating them in the *most moderate fashion favourable to the sale of the drug.* I saw – I was aware of that and reviewed every one of those changes and as I've said I accepted some and rejected others.[227] (Emphasis added)

Kligman agreed that the changes (1)–(6) above, four of which were accepted and finally published, had the effect of presenting the scientific findings in a way which was more favourable to benoxaprofen than his original script:

Kellogg: But in each and every case as far as I can see the change sort of waters down what was said previously?

Kligman: Yes.

Kellogg: And that's a fair statement isn't it?

Kligman: Its a fair statement to say that they wanted to keep this as quiescent as possible and I was struggling with trying to say it in such a way which wouldn't scare the hell out of anybody but which would be central to the facts.[228]

The process of suggesting changes certainly had a marked impact on the *interpretation* of the experimental results: Kligman described how a "compromise" was reached over alteration (1); and how, with respect to alteration (5), the final published version did not even reflect his own view.

Turning to the scientific validity of the claim in the paper published by Kligman & Kaidbey, it may be noted that their experimental methods seem to have met conventional scientific standards. However, they made comments that went far beyond the scope of their data. Specifically, they remarked upon the relative efficacy of benoxaprofen and even drew conclusions about its overall risk–benefit ratio:

Benoxaprofen apparently possesses some advantages over other nonsteroidal drugs in the treatment of arthritis. On the balance, the risk–benefit ratio is favourable to the drug.[229]

Kligman & Kaidbey felt able to make these assertions, even though their research did not include any reviews of either efficacy studies of NSAIDs or reports of kidney, gastro-intestinal or liver toxicity associated with benoxaprofen.[230] Kligman acknowledged that he was not an expert on those aspects of the drug.[231] There seems to have been no independent scientific basis for his making such claims about benoxaprofen's risk–benefit ratio:

Kligman: . . . So I had this predicament: as I learned more about benoxaprofen from rheumatologists, I didn't do any of the efficacy studies, *I only know what I heard and what was reported*, they were all saying it was an interesting drug, unusual, and that it might even stop the progression of the disease. *I can't judge the accuracy of those statements*, but it was made many times by figures who are highly esteemed in the field. And for me the judgement that had to be made is here is a drug that produces phototoxic reactions, far greater than with other drugs which are used for the same disease; how serious are these phototoxic reactions in view of the possibility that benoxaprofen is otherwise a very useful drug. I didn't want to exaggerate or frighten anybody with regard to these reactions. I was trying to take the point of view therefore that this is a useful drug and it does indeed produce photosensitivity reactions that the reactions are not of such a character that it should prevent the drug from being tried on a large scale. So *I was struggling with a matter of personal bias.*[232] (Emphasis added)

These extracts also suggest that Kligman allowed his judgement about the photosensitivity of benoxaprofen to be tempered by certain generous statements about the drug's efficacy, despite his own admission that he could not judge their accuracy. The consequence of so doing may have been to permit the perceived benefits of the drug to deflate its risk–benefit ratio, though I am not suggesting that Kligman deliberately introduced bias into his scientific paper.

The contention that Kligman may have been overly sympathetic to benoxaprofen is supported further by his remarks on one of Lilly's promotional videos. Although the Kligman & Kaidbey paper did not contain research on the nature of onycholysis, Kligman claimed that onycholysis was a "minor detail" and recommended that patients be told to "cut the fingernails back and put on some opaque polish to kind of stabilize the nails and *hope it will go away*"[233] (emphasis added). Regarding the incidence of onycholysis he commented:

> The statistics, as I read them, are about 10 per cent and I think that that is overstated . . . . my guess is that it is going to be much lower than that. I'm going to wager that [in] not more than one per cent of cases does separation half way back . . . even cause anyone any concern.[234]

Thus, without any of his own independently collected clinical data, Kligman was willing to assert that the clinical evidence available overstated the incidence of onycholysis. To be precise, Kligman predicted that no more than one-tenth of the cases of onycholysis would involve a nail separation of more than half. Yet Mikulaschek's empirical evidence implied that the figure was likely to be approximately three-tenths.[235] Kligman's minimizing of the incidence of onycholysis seems to have been little more than wishful thinking.

US approval and UK post-marketing experience

During Gennery's meeting with the CSM in July 1981, the large number of yellow card reports on skin reactions associated with *Opren* (over one thousand) was discussed. Well over half of these were onycholysis or photosensitivity reactions. Given that approximately 250,000 patients in the UK had taken *Opren* by that time,[236] a plausible interpretation of those yellow card data was that those reactions could be occurring in as many as 5 to 10 per cent of patients. The reason for this is that doctors' reporting of adverse drug reactions to the CSM is generally estimated to be at most 10 per cent, and Walker & Lumley have provided considerable evidence suggesting that in 1982 less than 5 per cent of adverse reactions to new drugs (e.g. *Opren*) might have been reported on yellow cards.[237] On this latter estimate 1,000 yellow cards could imply 20,000 adverse reactions in reality.

Nevertheless, according to Gennery, the CSM's response to the large number of skin reactions to benoxaprofen reported on yellow cards was not to modify their view of the toxicity of the drug, but rather to conclude that doctors were not listening to the advice given on the data sheet. In line with the CSM's requests, Dista took the reasonable step of sending out a "Dear Doctor" letter, which informed doctors that photosensitivity had occurred in 10 per cent of patients internationally, and reiterated the message on the data sheet about avoiding direct sunlight and using sunscreens to minimize the risk of photosensitivity. In the letter Lilly acknowledged that "a few patients may experience prolonged discomfort".[238]

Meanwhile in the US, despite the apparent problems with accurate reporting of benoxaprofen onycholysis and photosensitivity, the FDA made determinations regarding the risk associated with these adverse effects. In August 1981 Hsu completed a major FDA review, in which he estimated that after six months of taking the drug 10 per cent of patients had developed onycholysis and 15 per cent photosensitivity.[239]

By January 1982 Powell had completed the FDA's Dermatology Review of Lilly's data on controlled light studies with benoxaprofen: the Kligman & Kaidbey study, which he judged to be "excellent and thorough"[240] and a study by Greist & Ridolfo (a direct employee of Lilly). Griest and Ridolfo also concluded that photosensitivity reactions to the drug were phototoxic rather than photoallergic.[241] Unlike Kligman & Kaidbey they studied onycholysis reactions to benoxaprofen. They concluded that both the onycholysis and photosensitivity were manifested by "a hypersensitivity to long-wave ultraviolet light (UVA)" but "not related to a hypersensitivity to light in the sunburn range (UVB)".[242] Moreover, these authors asserted, on the basis of evidence from three patients, that onycholysis could be prevented by regular use of sun-screen-containing nail polish.[243]

Powell disagreed, as is evident from his review of Lilly's proposed package insert for benoxaprofen. Commenting on the "Warnings", he surmised that sunscreens of less than factor 15 broad spectrum might not afford protection, and objected to any assertion in the package insert that opaque nail polish gave protection from onycholysis because, he argued, "it is only an assumption . . . no such polishes were tested".[244]

Overall Powell came to the following conclusions:

> If this drug has *marked advantages over others in its class*, then in spite of the high incidence of phototoxic reactions, I should think the therapeutic gains would justify the risks. This assumes though, that patients take precautions as they are advised to by their doctors. The question whether daily use of benoxaprofen over many years may increase the risk of premature ageing of the skin and carcinogenesis is, I suppose, a moot one.[245] (Emphasis added)

Two points may be noted regarding these conclusions. First, the FDA scientists had determined that benoxaprofen did *not* have marked advantages over other NSAIDs,[246] and, moreover, was not satisfactorily tested for carcinogenicity. And secondly, Powell seems to have been rather dismissive about the increased risk of cancer due to photosensitivity, in view of the fact that in 1979 Valenzeno & Pooler had stressed the medical significance of the positive correlation existing between the photosensitizing ability of drugs and carcinogenicity in an article published in the prestigious and widely read *Journal of the American Medical Association*.[247]

A few days later, on 21 January 1982, the FDA referred the question of benoxaprofen's approval to its Arthritis Advisory Committee. According to Temple, benoxaprofen had been taken to the Arthritis Advisory Committee because "a major question" had to be decided; whether or not the drug should be labelled as a second line treatment (i.e. only to be used if other NSAID therapy proved unsuccessful) because of onycholysis and phototoxicity.[248] Seven members of the Committee attended, namely, Bonnie Hepburn, William Pitts, Kenneth Wilske, Eleanor Vogt, Seymour Geisser, Daniel Hamaty and Norman Gottlieb.[249] The Committee meeting began with a presentation by Mikulaschek, who told the Committee that about 10 per cent of patients had experienced skin phototoxicity and 13 per cent onycholysis. Regarding the former, he claimed that the experimental studies by Greist et al. and Kligman had shown that the activating radiation spectrum lay within the UVA range (320–400nm),[250] and as for the latter, he told the Committee that "use of an opaque nail polish will also be helpful in preventing onycholysis in susceptible patients".[251]

Mikulaschek made no mention of the finding made by Kligman that photosensitivity reactions to benoxaprofen could also occur in the UVB range, even though on 4 November 1981 Kligman wrote to Ridolfo at Lilly stating:

> I have made small changes in the manuscript you submitted to the publisher . . . I wanted to point out that the terminal portion of the UVB probably contributes slightly to the phototoxicity.[252]

Kligman explained the reason for his change as follows:

> We said originally that the portion of the ultraviolet light that produces the reaction is in the UVA region. A refinement developed later as we gained more data to indicate that there was also a small portion of the UVB range which contributed to the reaction . . . *I wanted it to be known that that would be a more accurate statement.*[253] (Emphasis added)

Despite Kligman's wishes, this "refinement" is nowhere to be found in the transcription of the Committee's meeting. Whether this was due to failure of communication or some other reason is not known. More germane, Mikulaschek did not mention an article published in *The Lancet* on 28 November 1981, almost two months before the meeting, by David Fenton et al. who concluded:

> Thus the photosensitivity reactions produced in patients on benoxaprofen are not confined solely to the UVA (320–400 nm) region and sunburn (UVB, 290–320 nm) rays may be involved in the action spectrum. Sunscreens should be selected to include UVB absorbing action as well as protection against UVA.[254]

One can be confident that the FDA were also unaware of Kligman's refinement because after Mikulaschek had completed his presentation Powell asserted the view that Kligman's study "apparently identified the specific action spectrum of UVA band to which patients react."[255] Powell further advised the Committee:

> it seems to me it would be difficult to label this drug. It is impossible to put a sensible and accurate phototoxic reaction rate, because

it varies from nothing in Mexico to over 50 per cent with two or three investigators . . . It is probably true that most people are going to get out of the sunlight before they have any severe or dangerous sort of reaction because they are so uncomfortable. But it is also true that many people are going to not want to use factor 15 sun screens, many of which are greasy, heavy, coloured, some of which may discolour clothing . . . . Then lastly, what may be the most important question of all is how likely is it that repeated exposures to sunlight by these persons who are taking benoxaprofen over a period of years, is going to lead to increased incidence of accelerated ageing and carcinogenesis. But as I see it, that is a moot question. In the first place, *most of the damage to the skin is known to be due to the UVB spectrum, which is the shorter ultraviolet rays, and those are not in the action spectrum of this drug.* It is in the UVA range. On the other hand, damage is presumably being done to the skin and UVA radiation potentiates or adds to the damage done by the UVB and vice versa.[256] (Emphasis added)

It is clear from these comments that Powell had some reservations about approving benoxaprofen, but he appears to have been reassured that carcinogenesis consequent upon phototoxicity was unlikely on the grounds that benoxaprofen's action spectrum was confined to the UVA region. Since this was untrue, the carcinogenic risk associated with the drug was understated to the Committee.

The Committee agreed unanimously that benoxaprofen should be approved. On the question of labelling, Hepburn thought patients should be warned that the long-term effects (e.g. skin carcinogenicity) of long-term phototoxicity were not known. Hepburn and Pitts stated that they would only use benoxaprofen after other NSAIDs had not been effective, and voted for second line labelling. Citing the apparent low gastro-intestinal toxicity of benoxaprofen relative to aspirin, Wilske voted against labelling it for second line use. Gottlieb supported Wilske, stating that he thought the skin and nail adverse effects seemed to be transient and not very severe compared with the gastro-intestinal problems experienced with other NSAIDs.

The possible scientific justification for the reasoning behind the voting of Wilske and Gottlieb bears some questioning. During 1980 and 1981, in various contexts, Lilly had implied that clinical trials showed that benoxaprofen was of lower gastro-intestinal toxicity than other NSAIDs, and in August 1980 the CSM had approved an *Opren* data sheet which

149

stated that benoxaprofen caused less gastro-intestinal bleeding than other propionic acid derivatives.[257] Mikulaschek had claimed that there was a statistically significant difference in favour of benoxaprofen between "drug-related" gastro-intestinal adverse effects in rheumatoid arthritic patients taking benoxaprofen and those taking aspirin.[258] However, from the largest UK clinical trial, Tyson and Glynne reported in 1980 that the total incidence of adverse gastro-intestinal effects associated with benoxaprofen was greater than those with ibuprofen, and was considerably greater for patients over the age of sixty.[259] Indeed, in July 1981, when Gennery was informed by the CSM of reports of patients on benoxaprofen suffering gastro-intestinal haemorrhages he believed that "it was an attractive hypothesis" that they were related to the drug's prolonged half-life in some elderly people.[260] As for the FDA, agency scientists had accepted only the claim that in clinical trials the number of patients experiencing adverse gastro-intestinal effects while taking benoxaprofen was about half the number experiencing such effects on aspirin therapy.[261]

Furthermore, Wilske and Gottlieb made no mention of two articles published no more than a few weeks before the meeting; one by Stewart in the *British Medical Journal* and the other by Du Vivier in the *Lancet*. Stewart reported three serious cases of benoxaprofen-related gastro-intestinal haemorrhage, one culminating in death, and concluded:

> The assertion that benoxaprofen is less likely to cause serious gastro-intestinal disturbance than other non-steroidal anti-inflammatory agents requires further evaluation, especially in the elderly.[262]

And Du Vivier had reported a severe benoxaprofen-related photosensitivity reaction which lasted for at least two weeks, caused a severe skin reaction on the patient's face, V of her neck, arms, hands, legs and feet, and which required treatment at home because she was too unwell to attend a clinic.[263] Nevertheless, the Committee finally voted four to two in favour of benoxaprofen being labelled as a first line drug.

The supposition that benoxaprofen was of low gastro-intestinal toxicity relative to other NSAIDs was further challenged by Halsey & Cardoe, who, on 13 February 1982, published a summary of their survey of the adverse gastro-intestinal effects in 257 patients taking the drug in the UK. They reported an incidence of 31.9 per cent of such reactions in patients over 70 and concluded:

> Our results suggest that the manufacturer's recommended dose of 600mg benoxaprofen daily is associated with an unacceptable inci-

dence of gastric side effects in the elderly.[264]

Despite these comments by Halsey and Cardoe, and the FDA's own concerns about the reliability of Lilly's reporting of benoxaprofen-related onycholysis and photosensitivity,[265] on 19 April 1982 the FDA approved the marketing of *Oraflex*.[266] Unlike the *Opren* data sheets, the *Oraflex* package insert never described photosensitivity as "generally mild", but rather as a "sharp burning sensation", which might lead to the development of erythema and whealing. And it revealed that, in at least one patient, onycholysis had not subsided even after benoxaprofen had been withdrawn.[267] Nevertheless, the *Oraflex* package insert did not mention the involvement of UVB in the photosensitivity reactions, and failed to warn that the long-term effects of long-term photosensitivity were unknown, even though Hepburn had recommended that patients should be made aware of that fact. In particular, the possible link between long-term effects of skin photosensitivity and carcinogenicity continued to be ignored.[268]

Summarizing this section, the data on which Lilly marketed and the CSM and the DHSS approved benoxaprofen did not meet the standards demanded by the FDA. In fact, the British clinical trial data did not even meet the standards advocated by Lilly's own leading consultant clinical trialist. Significantly, the British regulatory authorities approved *Opren* without demanding its prior phototesting. In the context of the scientific knowledge of the time, and the declared opinions of other scientific experts, including Kligman, Lilly's own leading consultant, it may be concluded that that decision awarded a remarkable benefit of the scientific doubt in favour of the commercial interests of Lilly. By contrast, the FDA's insistence on phototesting experiments with benoxaprofen served a patient protective function.

As the clinical data began to show increasing incidence of photosensitivity and onycholysis, bias entered into some of Lilly's representation of the adverse reactions. For example, Barnett's self-contradictory argument that 20 per cent was not different from 10 per cent, and the inconsistencies between Lilly's proposed transformation of statements in Kligman's manuscript, on the one hand, and Kligman's knowledge, on the other.

The foregoing discussion illustrates how (more or less subtle) uses of language can function as bias in science. Discourse is extremely malleable; it can be manipulated so as to camouflage, or detract from, the truth without committing a falsehood. What is *not* said or written may be just as important as what is. The implications of this for social analysis is that scientific texts cannot necessarily be taken at face value. The going is tougher than that. It is often necessary to investigate the production of scientific discourse as well as its impact in order to assess its social significance. What this section demonstrates is that a path can be cut through the jungle of discourse in industrial and government science to reveal perhaps not the scientific truth, but at least the institutional biases and processes that inhibit it. Most notably the FDA decided to approve *Oraflex* in contradiction with the recommendations of the agency's dermatological reviewer, though that regulatory bias was less marked than in the case of the British regulatory authorities because of the FDA's more detailed and candid labelling of the drug's onycholysis and photosensitivity.

The risk of drug accumulation – when in doubt call for more data

From May 1982 a protracted controversy over benoxaprofen's potential to cause fatal liver toxicity manifest by a hepato-renal (liver and kidney) syndrome began to rage. It is often said that adverse drug reactions, including fatalities, are an inevitable consequence of modern drug therapy. But whatever the validity of that general claim it should not be used as an excuse for complacency about specific adverse drug reactions and investigations into how they could have been prevented. The picture is further complicated by the fact that such complacency can reflect an interest-based position that favours lax regulation on the grounds that since adverse drug reactions are to be expected there is nothing for regulatory authorities to be alarmed about when a particular drug exhibits toxicity. In that context there is much scope for bias. The role of bias in scientists' handling of benoxaprofen's hepato-renal toxicity is the focus of this and the next section. It is, however, a complex issue requiring an examination of events which significantly pre-date the public controversy itself.

Pharmacokinetics and the elderly

The story begins with some discoveries made about what is technically known as the *pharmacokinetics* of benoxaprofen, that is, how the drug is absorbed, distributed and eliminated (i.e. excreted) from the body. Pharmacokinetics can have important implications for the safety of medicines. Some particularly relevant parameters are: (a) *elimination half-life*, i.e. the time taken for concentration of a drug in the blood to drop to half its initial value; (b) *steady state*, i.e. the blood (plasma) level reached when additional doses cause no further accumulation; and (c) *renal functioning*, i.e.

the kidneys' ability to eliminate a drug from the body. If the latter is impaired then a possible consequence is toxic accumulation of the drug in the body.[269]

When initially marketed one of benoxaprofen's perceived therapeutic advantages was its long elimination half-life, enabling it to be taken only once a day. This was especially advantageous for elderly patients, whose compliance with taking tablets is known to decrease with the frequency with which they have to take them.[270] Benoxaprofen's long elimination half-life was known to Lilly and the regulatory authorities before marketing the drug in the UK, but until 1981, neither had investigated its pharmacokinetics specifically in the elderly.[271]

The Hamdy and Kamal studies

It was in this context that Ronald Hamdy, a specialist in geriatric medicine in St John's Hospital, London, approached Dista's medical department to arrange a pharmacokinetic study of benoxaprofen in the elderly, which was undertaken in March 1981.[272] Initially Hamdy had two groups of elderly patients. One group of six patients with average age 81.8 years and youngest 76 years received a single dose of 600 mg of benoxaprofen, while the other group of five patients with average age 86.2 years and youngest 72 received a single dose of 300 mg. For both groups plasma levels of benoxaprofen were measured for five days (120 hours). They found elimination half-lives of 111 hours and 86.4 hours in these two groups respectively.[273] This compared with an elimination half-life of 30–35 hours in "normal" subjects (i.e. a sample from a population including very few elderly patients).

These results were presented at a Paris Symposium in June 1981.[274] The possible relevance of Hamdy's findings to benoxaprofen therapy is illustrated by the following comment in the published version of his symposium presentation:

> The metabolism and excretion of compounds with a prolonged half-life, however, may be slower in old age as a result of impaired renal function commonly seen in this age group. The continuous administration of compounds [with long elimination half-lives] at the normally recommended doses to elderly patients, therefore, may result in unnecessarily elevated and potentially harmful plasma levels.[275]

Also presented at the Paris symposium was a paper by Kamal from St George's Hospital, Lincoln in England. He studied the blood profiles of benoxaprofen over a 17 days period in 10 elderly patients given a daily 600mg dose of the drug for the first 10 days. The mean age of these patients was 77 years; the youngest being 70. Kamal found an elimination half-life of 101 hours and drew the following conclusions:

The markedly extended plasma half-life could be attributed to an age-related reduction in benoxaprofen elimination. Since steady-state levels were not achieved within 11 days in these patients, a reduction in dosage may be necessary in elderly patients . . . The higher benoxaprofen concentrations and the long elimination half-life show evidence of accumulation in the elderly, probably due to several causes, including poor bowel motility, and decreased renal clearance common with increasing age. The recommended dose may require modification in geriatric patients.[276]

Thus Kamal's multiple dose study supported Hamdy's single dose analysis, and also showed stronger evidence of accumulation in the elderly since a steady-state was not reached even after ten days.

After the Paris symposium Lilly's pharmacokinetic group in Indianapolis, including Shedden, Mikulaschek and Karl Desante, reviewed Hamdy's data. They argued that blood samples should have been taken for as long as up to five times the half-life, and that the renal function of the elderly patients should have been determined before the study began.[277] Samples for up to five times the half-life had not been taken because neither Hamdy nor anybody at Lilly had anticipated that the half-life in the elderly would be so long.[278]

Significantly, Lilly's own pharmacokinetic research on benoxaprofen in Indianapolis did not meet the standards demanded of Hamdy. In early Spring 1982, Ridolfo, Senior Clinical Pharmacologist at Lilly in Indianapolis, and Desante, a Senior Pharmacokineticist at Lilly, co-authored a paper, which reported a single dose study of 20 patients, whose plasma levels were measured for up to seven days (168 hours). Yet the mean half-life for eight of these patients was just over 62 hours, and for another eight it was over 51.[279] For the former eight, five half-lives amounted to no less that 310 hours (12.9 days), and for the latter no less than 255 hours (10.6 days).[280] Clearly this research failed to study benoxaprofen's pharmacokinetics for as long as five half-lives for the majority of the patients in the study.

Nevertheless, Hamdy agreed to conduct a further single dose study with four other patients, measuring levels of benoxaprofen in the blood for as long as 21 days (504 hours).[281] These patients had a mean age of

79.5 years with the youngest being 71 years old. In this study, which was completed by the end of July 1981, Hamdy found a half-life of 147.9 hours. Based on Kamal's results and his own, Hamdy reached the conclusion that in elderly patients benoxaprofen tended to accumulate to a much greater extent than in younger patients, and that 600mg of the drug should be given to the elderly only once or twice per week, rather than on a daily basis because of the risk of adverse effects that could arise from its accumulation.[282]

Hamdy communicated this conclusion to Lilly in June 1981, whence he was referred to the company headquarters in Indianapolis. Hamdy wanted Lilly to set up a study "to look at the use of benoxaprofen using it once a week or twice a week in elderly patients with osteoarthritis"[283] because in his view there was no evidence that the drug would be effective at such infrequent doses. Instead, Lilly headquarters told Hamdy that they wanted more proof of his findings, even though he considered that his data, combined with that of Kamal's had:

> shown beyond doubt that giving 600mg daily to elderly patients leads to a considerable amount of accumulation.[284]

The parent company in Indianapolis was extremely reluctant to publish Hamdy's findings, or those of Kamal. Vaughan, one of Lilly's medical writers, who was responsible for preparing drafts for the publication of the Paris Symposium papers, has claimed that it was initially decided at Indianapolis not to do so. Any publication of either Hamdy's or Kamal's findings was to wait until after Ridolfo and Desante had carried out a further single dose pharmacokinetic study of benoxaprofen in five elderly patients,[285] because senior scientists at Lilly's headquarters demanded "further clarification" and found it "difficult to believe that benoxaprofen pharmacokinetics in the elderly are significantly different from those in young people in the absence of renal impairment.[286]

Yet a very significant body of medical literature was available which directly opposed the view taken by senior Lilly scientists on this matter. As early as 1950 Davies and Shock studied a sample of 70 men, aged between 24 and 89, none of whom had any history of renal or heart disease, and concluded that there was a decline in effective renal plasma flow amounting to 50 per cent between the ages of 20 and 90.[287] Even the authors of the Lilly-sponsored research into the effects on geriatrics of the Lilly NSAID, fenoprofen, commented in 1976:

> Elderly patients are characteristically susceptible to the toxic effects of drugs . . . Fenoprofen was well tolerated, although these

elderly patients would be expected to be highly susceptible to any drug toxicity.[288]

By the late 1970s concern about the accumulation of drugs in the elderly because of reduced drug elimination was *widespread* in the medical literature.[289] Indeed, in 1978 Castleden felt able to assert that it was "well-established" that drug elimination is "reduced with ageing even though there may be no clinical evidence of renal failure."[290]

Perhaps most significantly, in early 1981 the WHO's committee on "Use of Medicaments by the Elderly" concluded:

> The elderly differ from the young in the quantity of the drug delivered to the target organ, and possibly in the sensitivity of that organ to the drug. Although such knowledge has been present for a number of years, there are very few drugs for which a specific geriatric dosage is recommended, and dosage regimens for new drugs are still established on data obtained in younger individuals . . . The elderly are at risk from relative overdosage of drugs due to inefficient pathways for drug elimination and metabolism . . . In short, impaired elimination of drugs because of diminished renal function or hepatic metabolism is a major cause of the increased incidence of adverse drug reactions in the elderly.[291]

The Ridolfo study

Ridolfo's study, which was *single* dose, also featured prolonged half-lives (40–50 hours) in the five elderly patients involved, but less dramatically than the research of Hamdy or Kamal. Like other senior scientists at Lilly, Gennery took the view that Ridolfo's study was more scientifically rigorous than Hamdy's or Kamal's because it contained "good tests of renal function, and a good correlation between half-life and renal function".[292] It may be noted, however, that Lilly's decision to delay the publication of Kamal's multi-dose findings ostensibly to gain some corroboration from Ridolfo's single-dose study was inconsistent with the WHO's following advisory comments made in 1981:

> While most pharmacokinetic studies in the elderly have been conducted after single dose administration, for many drugs more clinically useful information will be obtained from studies carried out under continuous multiple dose conditions.[293]

Moreover, according to Gennery, the scientific justification for carrying out the Ridolfo study was not only to test the validity of the Hamdy and Kamal findings, but also to evaluate benoxaprofen's pharmacokinetics in the elderly aged 65–75, rather than the very elderly aged over 75, who were the primary focus of Hamdy and Kamal.[294] Such justification is, however, highly questionable. For if Ridolfo's study was designed to test the *validity* of the Hamdy and Kamal studies it should have attempted to compare patients of the same size and age group. Despite this, Gennery admitted that Ridolfo's patients were "substantially heavier and significantly younger".[295] If, on the other hand, Ridolfo's study was intended to explore the *reliability* of extrapolating the Hamdy and Kamal findings in the over 75 age group to the 65 to 75 age group, then there was an implicit assumption, on the part of Lilly, that age did indeed play an important role in defining benoxaprofen pharmacokinetics, as Hamdy and Kamal had claimed. Yet, on this assumption, there was no justification for Shedden's argument not to publish the Hamdy and Kamal findings on the grounds that they needed further confirmation from a study which measured the extent of renal function at the outset.

Lilly scientists seem to have been aware that there were safety implications of these pharmacokinetic studies in the elderly, because, on the basis of his findings, Ridolfo recommended, in an internal Lilly report on 25 September 1981, that the daily dose of benoxaprofen in elderly patients, with small body weight and reduced renal function, should be decreased by 50–75 per cent.[296] He suggested that this could be achieved by a dosage of 300 mg every 24 to 48 hours.[297] Desante, Ridolfo's co-researcher, concurred with these recommendations and believed them to have been made because of the study's "important implications for safety in those patients" and "important implications for the actual use of [benoxaprofen] in the marketplace".[298]

Similarly, Christensen, Vice President of Lilly's Research Laboratories in Indianapolis, has testified that the Hamdy, Kamal and Ridolfo studies were "a red flag in that you may want to use a reduced dosage in patients where it might accumulate" because "you're not sure what might come out of that sort of thing".[299] And Mikulaschek noted that the Hamdy, Kamal and Ridolfo studies implied that "you have to be careful because you have an accumulation of drug, and whenever you have accumulation of any drug there is increased risk".[300] Nevertheless, the Ridolfo study was never published.[301] This can be contrasted with the company's keen efforts to publicize the fact that benoxaprofen's long elimination half-life made possible the therapeutically convenient once-a-day dosage.

The publication of the Hamdy and Kamal studies

Despite his disagreements with the findings of Hamdy and Kamal, Gennery did not welcome the proposal from Lilly's headquarters not to publish their research. Fundamentally, he was concerned that the credibility and interests of the company might be damaged if Hamdy felt the need to submit his paper to a major journal such as the *British Medical Journal*:

Kellogg: And did you tell the people in Indianapolis that it would create a lot of attention to the subject if Dr Hamdy's paper were for some reason omitted from the European Journal and then he published it somewhere else?

Gennery: Well, yes. My approach to the publication was not based so much on the scientific finesse and nicety of the situation, but just the very pragmatic approach that we have had 85 rheumatologists at the meeting who have heard these papers presented, and we would find it difficult to explain to them why they weren't published.

Kellogg: Those 85 rheumatologists would in fact find it strange that these papers weren't in that journal.

Gennery: Absolutely.[302]

Gennery believed that the Hamdy and Kamal studies were technically satisfactory, but the dispute between Gennery and Lilly's senior scientists in Indianapolis was as much about where the best interests of the company lay on this matter as it was about the internal validity of the scientific arguments. By agreeing to publish the studies Lilly maintained greater editorial control over their fate because the company was sponsoring the journal edition in which the Paris Symposium proceedings were to appear. Ultimately Gennery's view prevailed within the company and the Hamdy and Kamal papers were published in early Spring 1982.

The regulatory inaction of the CSM

Throughout Lilly's deliberations about the pharmacokinetics of benoxaprofen in the elderly the company engaged in intermittent discussions with the CSM. The Committee decided that no regulatory action should be taken, but that Lilly should complete the Ridolfo study by 1 October 1981, when the situation would be reconsidered. The CSM made this recommendation even though, according to Sir Abraham Goldberg, then the Committee's chairman, they thought that Hamdy had conducted "a good study", and that the Hamdy and Kamal studies "warned there might be a problem with benoxaprofen in the elderly".[303]

Lilly complied with the CSM's suggestion, and on 7 October 1981 proposed to the Committee that the *Opren* data sheet should be changed to include a statement that elderly debilitated patients with evidence of renal impairment should be given only 300 mg benoxaprofen each day, and that debilitated elderly patients aged 75 or older should also receive the reduced daily dose of 300 mg. It is notable that of all the pharmacokinetic data being considered Lilly decided to adopt the Ridolfo study, which had the most conservative implications for dosage reduction, and to propose to the CSM the *smallest* dose reduction recommended by Ridolfo.[304] That approach may be contrasted sharply with advice in the *British Medical Journal* on 10 January 1981 to "always err on the side of *low doses* in the elderly.[305] (Emphasis in the original)

In any case, on 17 November 1981 the CSM did not accept Lilly's proposal for dosage reduction, and according to Gennery, had seen a conflict between the results of the Ridolfo study and those of Hamdy and Kamal. This seems to be confirmed by Goldberg in January 1983:

Mangold: Professor, you had two studies [Hamdy and Kamal studies] that warned you that benoxaprofen might be toxic to the elderly and it might indeed have a long half-life – there were your warnings. You already had two deaths, two unexplained liver deaths, benoxaprofen-related – what more information did you need before acting?

Goldberg: There were other pharmacokinetic studies, drug-handling studies, in relation to benoxaprofen which didn't fully confirm these initial studies.[306]

In particular, Gennery has testified that the CSM wanted Lilly "to repeat the Kamal protocol in patients aged 65 to 75,[307] when the situation would be reconsidered again.[308]

The *Opren* data sheet remained as approved in August 1980 until May 1982, making no reference to the elderly.[309] That decision by Lilly and the British regulatory authorities not to revise the data sheet was certainly controversial, especially since Michael Rawlins, chairman of the CSM in 1994 and a member of the Committee between 1979 and 1985,[310] stated under "Pharmacokinetics" in an article published in the *British Medical Journal* on 21 March 1981:

Patients with impaired renal function (including the elderly) are particularly liable to develop type A [quantitatively abnormal adverse pharmacological] reactions when given doses designed for healthy young adults.[311]

Moreover, in January 1983 Laurence Prescott, a toxicologist, who had sat on the CSM's Toxicology Subcommittee, argued that the Hamdy and Kamal studies implied that the dosage for the elderly needed to be reduced to a quarter of the dose given to a younger person.[312] In fact, on reviewing all the citations to the Hamdy and Kamal studies listed in the *Science Citation Index* from 1982 to 1990, I found many which treated the studies as authorities and none that challenged their findings.[313]

The approved safety warnings regarding the elderly

Lilly did carry out the further study requested by the CSM, but preliminary results were not available until the end of July 1982. Nevertheless, at the end of April 1982, following the deaths of several elderly patients from a hepato-renal syndrome while taking *Opren*, the CSM told Lilly that they were not prepared to wait for the additional study, and that they wanted the *Opren* data sheet changed urgently to stipulate that patients over 65 should receive no more than 300 mg per day because adverse effects were more common in the elderly.[314]

In fact, the new May 1982 *Opren* data sheet produced by Lilly and approved by the CSM stated merely:

A daily dosage of 300 mg may be advisable in patients with impaired renal function. This applies particularly to aged, frail patients.[315]

This was not an instruction to doctors not to prescribe more than a daily dose of 300mg benoxaprofen for elderly patients though it was advice not to do so for the elderly *and frail*. The findings of Hamdy and Kamal did not imply potential risks only to frail elderly patients, but to over 75 year olds in general. Though some very elderly patients may have extraordinarily healthy kidneys and livers, the view taken by Hamdy and Kamal was that such patients would, *in general*, have reduced renal and/or hepatic function, and so to err on the side of safety, doctors should have been warned about the drug's accumulation in this population group. However, the approach taken by Lilly and the CSM was to give a warning which minimized the elderly patient group at risk, disregarding the WHO's exhortations that ageing could alter drug metabolism in ways not reducible to renal function.

For Hamdy, the minimalist measures taken by Lilly and the CSM in May 1982 may have had severe consequences. He believed that his research, together with that of Kamal's, had anticipated the fatalities reported among elderly patients taking *Opren*.[316] Mikulaschek, however, denied that the

Hamdy or Kamal studies predicted deaths in the elderly, but he did consider that they implied the need for precautions, such as unusually frequent monitoring of kidney and liver functioning.[317] Yet Mikulaschek also acknowledged that the *Oraflex* package insert, approved by the FDA on 19 April 1982, stated no such precautions,[318] and nor did Dista's *Opren* data sheets.

He further admitted that none of Lilly's *Oraflex* package inserts or "Dear Doctor" letters told doctors in the US to be especially vigilant in monitoring liver and kidney functions in the elderly when prescribing the drug, with the possible exception of the very last "Dear Doctor" letter on 29 June 1982, more than 10 weeks after *Oraflex* had been approved in the US and no less than 10 months after Ridolfo had completed his single dose pharmacokinetic study.[319] These omissions are all the more remarkable in view of substantial evidence that doctors in general practice in the US prior to August 1982 did not usually monitor the liver functions of patients taking NSAIDs *at all*. For example, in a meeting about the hepatotoxicity of NSAIDs on 3 and 4 June 1982, the FDA's Arthritis Advisory Committee debated at length whether or not to instruct general practitioners to monitor monthly or quarterly the liver functions of patients being prescribed NSAIDs. The debate underlined the fact that general practitioners did not, as a matter of course, undertake such monitoring as illustrated by Bonnie Hepburn's remark:

> the fact is that these patients are not going to be monitored as well as you would like because those of us in rheumatology are used to monitoring carefully . . . but the general practitioner is not in a position to monitor this closely.[320]

Indeed, at least two of the six-member Arthritis Advisory Committee admitted that, even as rheumatology specialists, they did not administer tests to monitor the liver functions of patients taking NSAIDs.[321]

It was not until June 1982, following the publication of *Opren*-related deaths in the elderly in the *British Medical Journal*, that the CSM and Lilly issued a clear warning that the elderly should receive no more than a daily dose of 300 mg of *Opren*.[322] Moreover, the technical reason for the reduced dosage given in the June 1982 *Opren* data sheet confirmed the concerns expressed by Hamdy and Kamal in Paris one year previously:

> The elderly: In patients over the age of 65, a daily dose of 300 mg should not normally be exceeded, because the elimination rate of *Opren* is commonly reduced in such patients.[323]

I am not suggesting that Lilly scientists or members of the British regulatory authorities saw and ignored clear-cut risks to the elderly in the pharmacokinetic data. The toxicity of benoxaprofen to the elderly was a matter of some scientific uncertainty as is often the case in drug toxicology. Rather, the relevant issue is how the benefit of the scientific doubt was distributed.

Evidently Lilly scientists' technical objections to the Hamdy and Kamal studies were in contradiction with a massive body of scientific knowledge at that time, including the findings of some scientists who had conducted clinical trials on one of Lilly's other NSAIDs. This might be considered deviant behaviour were it not for the fact that those technical objections implied that Lilly scientists applied inconsistent criteria in judging the validity of the Hamdy and Kamal studies compared with those of their own scientists. Furthermore, Lilly's reasons for delaying publication of the Hamdy and Kamal studies until confirmed by Ridolfo's research were internally contradictory. These factors point to an institutional bias against the Hamdy and Kamal findings – a suggestion that is supported by Lilly's decision not to publish the first Ridolfo study even though it had important implications for the scientific profile of the drug and corroborated to some extent the safety concerns of Hamdy and Kamal about the prolonged half-life of benoxaprofen in the elderly.

It is also clear that when Lilly and the CSM did decide to recommend some dosage reduction in the prescribing of *Opren* it was initially minimalist in terms of defining the population at risk from taking the normal daily dose of 600 mg, and, therefore, also minimalist in terms of its negative commercial impact. When Dista and the CSM ultimately recommended a patient protective dosage reduction of benoxaprofen in the elderly the reason for the recommendation directly contradicted the earlier technical arguments by the Committee and senior Lilly scientists. At this stage the supposedly scientific and technical reasons for resisting major dosage reduction in the elderly evaporated and the CSM approved a warning in the labelling in agreement with Hamdy and Kamal – a warning that could have been approved six months earlier had the benefit of the scientific doubt been distributed more generously in favour of patients rather than the manufacturers.

Death – an inevitable risk?

On 24 April 1982 Goudie et al. reported in the *Lancet* three cases of jaundice associated with benoxaprofen in Scotland, including one death.[324] All three patients were elderly women and had been prescribed a daily dose of 600mg of the drug. In all three cases histological findings showed moderately severe canalicular and hepatocellular cholestasis (i.e. the diminution of the flow of bile due to obstruction of capillary passages and cell damage in the liver). The authors concluded:

> To the list of NSAIDs associated with occasional liver damage benoxaprofen can probably now be added. Although the association remains to be established we believe that caution should be exercised in prescribing this preparation in the elderly, particularly where there is evidence of hepatic or renal insufficiency.[325]

Two weeks later, on 8 May 1982, and independently of the Goudie et al. report,[326] Taggart reported five cases of fatal cholestatic jaundice (i.e. a type of jaundice in which the flow of bile is obstructed) in elderly patients taking 600mg benoxaprofen/day in Northern Ireland, [327] the details of which are shown in Table 8.

Taggart suspected benoxaprofen as the cause of death immediately in cases 3 and 5, and reported them promptly to the CSM. However, it was not until after the fifth case in January 1982 that the association of all five deaths with benoxaprofen occurred to Taggart. After subsequent re-examinations of the patients' records he reported the first death to the

Table 8 Taggart cases of fatal cholestatic jaundice.

Patient	Date began on *Opren*	Age	Date of death	Date death reported to CSM	Circumstances of death
1	15/12/80	81	13/7/81	10/2/82	Had developed jaundice
2	31/3/81	84	11/8/81	early April 1982	Died from jaundice and renal failure
3	May 1981	86	7/11/81	12/11/81	Died of jaundice and renal failure
4	24/8/81	88	14/11/81	early April 1982	Died from jaundice and renal failure
5	June 1981	82	26/1/82	late Jan. 1982	Died from jaundice and renal failure

Sources: H. McA. Taggart & J. M. Alderdice 1982. Fatal cholestatic jaundice in elderly patients taking benoxaprofen. *British Medical Journal* **284**, 8 May, 1372. US Court 1983 Deposition of *H. McA. Taggart & Clarence Borom* vs *Eli Lilly and Company*, 4 July, 151.

CSM on 10 February 1982, and the second and fourth in early April 1982. He had not reported the fourth death earlier because association in this case was much more difficult due to the absence of a postmortem.[328] In fact, only three of Taggart's five death cases had an autopsy.[329]

Following a chance meeting with a Dista sales representative in early February 1982, at the representative's suggestion, Taggart reported the deaths of patients 3 and 5 to Dista[330] no later than mid March,[331] but possibly as early as 9 February.[332] Meanwhile, on 10 February 1982 the CSM provided Gennery with a print-out of *Opren* adverse reactions up to January of that year. This listed a total of 25 deaths as well as 24 cases of serious liver disorders, including two fatal and three non-fatal cases of cholestatic jaundice.[333]

During a meeting on 22 February Gennery told Shedden about Taggart's two death cases, and mentioned that they were liver-related.[334] According to Gennery, he told Shedden that he did not have full details of the two Taggart cases, but that he was going to follow them up himself, and would keep Shedden "informed of anything that subsequently developed".[335] Shedden was also informed of 19 *Opren* deaths, about which Dista had detailed knowledge. Four of these resulted from kidney problems, and one from a liver problem.[336]

On 16 March Gennery met with Taggart in Belfast, where, Taggart has claimed, he told Gennery about all five death cases.[337] This has not been denied though, according to Gennery, Taggart "didn't have any great detail except for the information on two patients".[338] Taggart characterized Gennery's response as follows:

> there was incredulity in the conversation on his part that such a thing could possibly occur, and it was left that this [the liver toxicity] was probably due to something else on his part. He felt that this was likely to be due to some other reason.[339]

Taggart further claimed that no-one from Dista contacted him after the March meeting with Gennery until the publication of his article on 8 May, when "they suddenly took a lot of interest".[340]

In fact, Taggart's account of events is substantially supported by elements of Gennery's own account:

> Kellogg: Now, between March 16 and May 6, and apart from *The Lancet* article that you telecopied and that conversation [about the Goudie et al. article] did you personally have any other efforts to look into this liver disease question?
> Gennery: No, because until I received Dr Taggart's further re-

164

ports I couldn't be sure as to what actually I was dealing with. The first two cases: one I don't think there was any postmortem comment available; and the other was a rather complex case which involved pancreatitis as well as jaundice. The information I had at that time said that the patient was also taking another drug called *Ponstan*, and that drug has a well documented history of causing pancreatitis and hepatic failure. So until I got Dr Taggart's other case reports I couldn't really make any judgement as to how serious the problem might be.

Kellogg: And the one with the pathology report, was there mention of cholestasis?

Gennery: Yes.

Kellogg: Does *Ponstan* produce cholestasis?

Gennery: No, but if a patient had got pancreatitis they might well get cholestasis anyway.[341]

So Gennery's approach was to wait until there was compelling evidence that benoxaprofen was implicated in Taggart's cases and, in the meantime, to postulate alternative explanations. This approach was taken in the context of Dista having received about 10 inquiries in 1981 about benoxaprofen's possible association with jaundice, including at least one detailed case of cholestasis.[342]

Furthermore, despite the fact that Gennery told Shedden on 22 February that he would keep him informed of "anything that subsequently developed", Gennery did not contact Shedden after his mid March meeting with Taggart until around 24 April, when the Goudie et al. paper was published.[343] Yet at that meeting Taggart had given Gennery further details, including one pathology report, regarding the two death cases, of which Dista were already aware, and mentioned a further three deaths. This suggests that Gennery did not consider that additional information to be an especially important development.

By mid April 1982 Gennery had received Taggart's case reports of the three deaths, which Taggart had merely mentioned to Gennery during their mid March meeting. Some days later Gennery drafted a letter to Taggart stating that the reported pattern of jaundice was new. However, Gennery never sent this letter because on the same day he noticed the 24 April letter in the *Lancet* by Goudie et al. describing what he perceived to be the same pattern.[344] Thus, by the end of April 1982 Gennery had formed the opinion that the *same* pattern of jaundice, with fatal implications in some cases, had afflicted eight elderly patients taking benoxaprofen. That day Gennery telecopied the Goudie et al. article to Shedden in Indianapolis.

On 26 March 1982 the CSM asked Taggart for more details on the three death cases, of which they had been aware since mid February. He responded by sending more detailed pathology notes in early April 1982.[345] Nevertheless, the CSM did not insist that the *Opren* data sheet should warn of jaundice until May 1982, when cases of benoxaprofen-associated jaundice were published in the medical literature, and, as already noted, no clear warning to reduce the dose by half in the elderly was introduced into the data sheet until June 1982. Goldberg has provided the following justification for the Committee's approach:

Mangold: Taggart's first two deaths . . . were a confirmation of everything that Hamdy and Kamal were warning about.

Goldberg: They didn't warn about liver deaths, . . .

Mangold: They warned that there might be a problem with benoxaprofen in the elderly.

Goldberg: Yes, indeed, but . . . when one looks at comparative safety . . . up till that time, benoxaprofen, was no . . . there was no difference from a group of about three or four other drugs. If we had to sound warnings on benoxaprofen, we would have had to do the same for these other drugs as well.

Mangold: What made you finally reduce the dosage as late as June 1982? What had happened between February and June that made you change your mind?

Goldberg: Well, it was the accumulation of this data and substantiation of these other studies that made it quite clear that this should be done . . . and the dose was halved for the elderly.[346]

Evidently, like senior scientists at Dista and Lilly, the CSM, as a matter of policy, required compelling evidence of benoxaprofen's hepato-renal toxicity in the elderly before taking action. Goldberg acknowledged that the Hamdy and Kamal studies were a warning that benoxaprofen was problematically toxic in the elderly, but this, together with the first two Taggart deaths, was not sufficient to move the Committee to issue a warning to doctors. Rather, the CSM waited until there was such an accumulation of deaths and adverse reactions associated with the drug that it was, in their view, clearly substantially more toxic than other NSAIDs.

Approval in the US

The FDA had approved benoxaprofen for use in the US on 19 April 1982, but did so under conditions of considerable ignorance because Shedden had not reported any of the 29 benoxaprofen-associated deaths, of which he was aware, to the agency. Moreover, the package insert approved by the FDA on 19 April failed to list liver and kidney failures in the adverse reations section, despite purporting to include not only clinical trial experience, but also "reports since marketing outside the United States".[347]

It was not unreasonable for the FDA to expect to have been provided with such reports since, under the NDA regulations, which applied to approved drugs, companies were required to report to the agency "*any* unexpected side effect, injury, toxicity or sensitivity reaction as soon as possible and in any event within 15 working days of the [company's] receipt of notice of the event".[348] The regulations further defined "unexpected" as "not previously submitted as part of an NDA or not encountered during clinical trials of the drug or conditions or developments occurring at a rate higher than shown by information previously submitted as part of an NDA".[349] However, prior to 19 April, IND, rather than NDA, regulations applied to benoxaprofen because it was not then an approved drug in the US. Nevertheless, the agency issued the following statement in the *Federal Register* in April 1979:

All persons are encouraged to alert FDA as soon as possible after receiving the information regarding *any* serious adverse drug experience, death, or life-threatening problem that may reasonably be regarded as caused by or associated with a drug.[350] (Emphasis added)

Though not explicitly defined, it is reasonable to assume that the phrase "any serious adverse drug experience, death, or life-threatening problem" was intended to include deaths outside the US. Moreover, the IND regulations stated that serious adverse drug reactions should be reported "promptly" so the agency could have expected Shedden to report his knowledge of death cases in late February well before 19 April.

Notwithstanding the FDA's lack of information regarding some serious adverse reactions to benoxaprofen outside the US, the package insert did not satisfactorily reflect the data available to the agency. By early 1982, before *Oraflex* was approved by the FDA, at least four cases of jaundice, which occurred during US clinical trials, had been reported to the agency by Lilly.[351] Temple testified on 3 August 1982 that these jaundice cases were "reasonably important" to the agency, and worthy of mention on the package insert, rather than omission.[352]

As regards renal (kidney) toxicity the approved package insert stated:
There has been no evidence of renal toxicity in clinical trials.[353]

However, this claim is irreconcilable with the fact that a case of interstitial nephritis (inflammation of the kidneys) and a case of nephrotic syndrome (kidney disorder) had occurred during the US clinical trials – the latter certainly having been reported to the FDA by Lilly prior to *Oraflex* approval. Furthermore, interstitial nephritis was listed on the approved package insert as an adverse reaction, whose "causal relationship" to benoxaprofen was "unknown". Yet for the case of interstitial nephritis that occurred during US clinical trials, the clinical investigator and the patient's doctor both concluded that the condition was benoxaprofe-induced.[354] No other drug was even suspected.[355]

When asked to justify how such findings could be legitimately referred to as "no evidence", Alan Lisook of the FDA's Clinical Investigation Branch argued:

not only is there an internal inconsistency in the benoxaprofen label, but the statement concerning lack of evidence of renal toxicity is not consistent with the fact as known to Lilly at the time the statement was approved.[356]

Thus, Lilly marketed and the FDA approved *Oraflex* with labelling which considerably understated the toxicity of the drug. The FDA's approval of that labelling was partly due to ignorance, but *inconsistencies* contained within the labelling suggest that the agency did, in any event, award the company a substantial benefit of the doubt regarding the drug's renal toxicity.

Lilly's decision to market *Oraflex*

Benoxaprofen-associated deaths, whether published or unreported, did not deter Lilly's resolve to market the drug in the US. According to Wood, the company acted reasonably in so doing because:

The information concerning the liver–kidney reactions available to the company at the time the drug was introduced to the US market was not sufficient to assess the significance of the reports. Moreover, the reports were inconsistent with experience from the clinical trials of *Oraflex*, with the extensive marketing in Britain, and with a major post-marketing study in Britain that did not disclose unusual liver or kidney problems.[357]

However, these technical explanations are not very persuasive. First,

Dista had detailed reports on two of Taggart's five death cases, including one pathology report, and Gennery had come to the preliminary conclusion that the eight cases of cholestatic jaundice published by Goudie et al. and Taggart were of the same pattern. Secondly, according to Mikulaschek, during the US clinical trial programme some patients exhibited cholestatic jaundice.[358] Thirdly, by January 1982 the CSM's printout of benoxaprofen-related adverse reactions listed 24 cases of hepatic disorders including two fatalities, nine cases of jaundice and two cases of cholestatic jaundice, and these reports excluded most, if not all, of Taggart's cases.[359] And fourthly, one major post-marketing study in Britain, possibly the one to which Wood referred, was a "prescription event monitoring" (PEM) epidemiological study of benoxaprofen adverse reactions in England undertaken by Bill Inman, Director of the Drug Surveillance Research Unit, at the University of Southampton, who has proclaimed:

> I would like to dispel a misapprehension that PEM failed to identify the jaundice problem. In fact a small but quite clear signal of trouble did arise in the pilot study. Jaundice was reported as an event in 8 patients taking *Opren*. [360]

Surveillance in the US

The shortcomings of Lilly's scientific basis for marketing *Oraflex* reappeared in some of the company's post-marketing claims. On 14 May Christensen, Vice President of Lilly Research Laboratories, telephoned Temple, of the FDA, to discuss the recent reports of possible benoxaprofen hepato-renal toxicity in the British medical literature.[361] According to Temple, Christensen claimed that there were no cases of jaundice in the IND file.[362] Just over two weeks later on 29 May 1982 Shedden wrote a letter to the *British Medical Journal* entitled "Side effects of benoxaprofen" in which he claimed:

> No jaundice and no deaths due to hepatic failure were reported in approximately 2200 carefully followed patients who participated in clinical trials in the USA.[363]

As regards jaundice, the claims of both Christensen and Shedden were false, as is clear from the foregoing discussion. Indeed, Mikulaschek has acknowledged that "it would be wholly incorrect to say . . . that there were no patients who had jaundice in the US Phase III clinical trials".[364] Shedden has admitted that his statement to the *British Medical Journal* was incorrect, but has pleaded that he only became aware of this in June

169

1982.[365] Nevertheless, he never sent a further letter to the journal to correct his previous error, and by 17 June 1982 Lilly was still producing marketing letters for its sales staff claiming that no jaundice had been reported in US clinical trials.[366]

Subsequently, at a meeting on 23 June 1982 between senior Lilly staff, including Barnett, Christensen and Shedden, and senior FDA staff, including Meyer, Temple and Harter, Lilly told the FDA that there had been five cases of non-fatal jaundice from US clinical trials before *Oraflex* approval, only two of which had been reported in the IND file. The other three, Lilly claimed, had been discovered as the company surveyed its unprocessed IND data.[367]

At that meeting the FDA expressed surprise that Lilly had not submitted cases of jaundice "*prominently* to the NDA prior to its approval"[368] (emphasis added). Nevertheless, the agency was prepared to give the company the benefit of the doubt on this matter, as indicated by Temple's view that Lilly's overlooking of jaundice cases was due to "failures of perception", and to the problem that "there are too many events to cope with in an application".[369]

By 16 July 1982 the FDA had not attempted to verify the claim made by Lilly's officials at the 23 June meeting, that two cases of jaundice had been submitted to the IND in January and February 1982. Verification was still pending on 3 August 1982 despite the FDA Commissioner's stance that such claims should be verified before regulatory decisions were taken.[370] In fact, Harter stated that his Division had such a backlog that no IND submissions had been logged into the FDA system since 2 December 1981, and so there were was "no way to verify this claim".[371] Thus, Harter's Division had such a backlog that the agency was unable to monitor benoxaprofen's adverse reactions as reflected in the drug's IND file for over four months prior to approval. Moreover, senior FDA officials were aware that such a backlog existed and was problematic. Temple, for example, described it as "plainly unacceptable".[372]

The escalation of adverse hepato-renal reactions

While Lilly and the FDA debated the history of benoxaprofen-related jaundice more cases of cholestatic jaundice (many fatal) were reported in the British medical literature on 12 June 1982. In all these reports the doctors believed that benoxaprofen was the probable cause of the reaction, and they urged extreme caution in prescribing the drug.[373] In particular, Firth, Wilcock and Esiri reported a fatal case of jaundice accompanied by "gross intrahepatic cholestasis", whose progression was not halted *despite withdrawal of the drug* from the patient.[374]

Not untypically, Lilly's response to these developments was to argue that the evidence linking benoxaprofen to liver toxicity was not compelling. As late as 2 July 1982 Lilly contended that "a direct causal relationship has not been clearly established",[375] and further argued that, if such a relationship did exist, the incidence of adverse liver effects must have been low because of the small number of cases of jaundice during clinical trials.[376]

By June 1982 the CSM believed that benoxaprofen had "pulled away" from other NSAIDs in terms of comparative toxicity.[377] The Committee's response, however, was not to ban the drug, but rather to warn doctors to prescribe no more than 300 mg/day for patients over age 65, and to discontinue the drug if hepatic dysfunction were to occur.[378] As already noted, Firth et al. reported that in one case withdrawal of the drug after the onset of hepatic dysfunction was not in itself sufficient to prevent death.

The FDA's approach was not dissimilar. On 24 June the agency advocated revised labelling, which advised that in elderly patients benoxaprofen therapy should be initiated at 300–400 mg per day. The agency adopted this approach after the meeting with Lilly on 23 June 1982, in which 16 cases of benoxaprofen-associated jaundice, most fatal, were discussed. During that discussion the FDA and Lilly agreed that these cases seemed to be benoxaprofen-related and possibly related to the length of time on the drug.[379] Specifically, agency officials noted:

> The initial cases suggest a time relation. If this is true, the flurry of cases in the UK may be a harbinger of a great number of cases.[380]

Yet, like the CSM, the FDA were willing to have this prospective hypothesis verified by more cases of hepato-renal toxicity, rather than remove the drug from the market. Verification was forthcoming: before the drug was withdrawn from the market in August 1982 some 86 cases of jaundice were associated with benoxaprofen therapy, including at least 30 fatalities.[381]

In April and May 1982 Gennery took the reasonable step of asking two leading liver specialists, MacSween and Davis, to examine the tissue sample and clinical details regarding twelve people who had allegedly suffered severe liver toxicity due to taking benoxaprofen.[382] They presented their findings on 3 September 1982,[383] and, according to Gennery, concluded:

> that there was a distinctive histological pattern in the liver. That the type of jaundice and the associated renal failure was an unu-

sual combination and that there probably was a causal relationship [between benoxaprofen and the hepato-renal syndrome].[384]

Further examination of reporting of fatalities to the FDA

After prompting by a Congressional Committee the FDA undertook an inspection of Lilly's ADR reporting. The FDA's inspectors, David Duncan and Lawrence Lanvermeyer, alleged that Lilly had violated regulations by failing to: (a) promptly report 96 deaths associated with benoxaprofen marketing outside the US, 26 of which were known to the company's US headquarters and/or its affiliates prior to US approval; and (b) maintain records necessary to enable the FDA to determine whether or not approval should have been suspended.[385] For example, Duncan and Lanvermeyer claimed to have found one case in which a Dista form indicated the date of death as 5 January 1982 yet Lilly had reported this to the FDA on 8 October 1982 as a death occurring on 5 September 1982.[386]

Lilly's defence of their actions had regulatory and scientific elements. With respect to the former the official company position was that, though IND regulations required prompt reports of any finding during clinical trials suggestive of significant hazards associated with the drug, those regulations did not require sponsors to report adverse drug reactions associated with *foreign marketing* prior to US approval.[387] Thus, Lilly defended their actions by claiming that they had abided by the regulations. Yet, even if Lilly's interpretation of the regulations were correct, this would not necessarily be sufficient justification according to the company's own standards because Wood has stated:

> [FDA regulations are] a minimum set of standards. They are in written form, but beyond that you have an ethical code of conduct that scientists recognize as doing the right thing, and being completely honest, open and above board at all times.[388]

This, then, raises the question of what other possible justification the company's scientists had for failing to report death cases outside the US to the FDA. Regarding the Taggart cases, the official argument of the company was that the information regarding hepato-renal toxicity, which Dista had, was so sketchy that it "did not warrant special medical concern and . . . was not reported to the Indianapolis headquarters".[389]

Further justifications have been elaborated by senior Lilly scientists and officials. According to Peck, Lilly had a policy of reporting alarming *or* life-threatening adverse reactions to the FDA promptly (i.e. within 15 days).[390] He also believed that reports of the kind made by Taggart should be reported to the agency.[391] However, he considered that a well known adverse reaction, even if fatal, might not need to be reported within 15 days.[392] On the other hand, Mikulaschek argued unequivocally that serious and "certainly life-threatening" reactions should have been reported to the FDA, "even if they were not unusual".[393]

Christensen agreed with Mikulaschek that a 15 day report applied to "something serious, [and/or] alarming".[394] and described the Taggart cases as "a cluster of unusual and alarming events".[395] Initially Christensen attempted to justify Lilly's lack of reporting of deaths on the grounds of inadequate information, but under cross-examination he admitted that there were reports that provided adequate information to submit to the FDA:

> Kellogg: . . . but if you identified a patient, and if you identified that the patient was taking benoxaprofen, and if you identified that the patient died while taking benoxaprofen, is that enough to make out a 1639 [FDA adverse drug experience form]?
>
> Christensen: . . . that's about enough information . . .
>
> Kellogg: Okay, and the 1639 . . . if somebody dies one of these has got to go in within 15 days?
>
> Christensen: I think all deaths are reported in 15 days.
>
> Kellogg: Dr Christensen, isn't it true that information came to Indianapolis from sources outside the US where there was something to identify the patient, and something to say the patient died while taking benoxaprofen, that [was] not written up in 1639s and sent to the FDA within 15 days?
>
> Christensen: The only thing I can think of . . . would be those Spiers' reports and we just did not have a policy of filling out 1639s on those kinds of tabulations.[396]

In contrast to Christensen, Shedden, who had become aware of 24 benoxaprofen-associated deaths outside the US by February 1982, in one instance argued that they did not need to be reported promptly to the FDA because they were to be expected with the use of any NSAID.[397] It was for this reason, he attested, that the *Oraflex* package insert and "Dear Doctor" letters failed to advise doctors that, in rare instances, the death of a patient taking the drug was to be an expected result.[398]

It may be noted that, were Shedden's rationale for reporting fatal adverse drug reactions to be adopted, it would be impossible for regulatory authorities to conduct timely assessments of the incidences and relative incidences of deaths associated with NSAIDs. Yet this was precisely the kind of data on which the CSM purportedly depended to make its regulatory decision about whether or not to suspend the marketing of *Opren*. Shedden's explanation on this issue does not sit easily with his own previous statements that serious adverse reactions ought to be reported within 15 days[399] and that "clearly, an adverse effect resulting in death would generally be regarded as serious".[400]

One version of Wood's justification was directly opposed to Shedden's, expounding the view that before reporting a death to the FDA as associated with benoxaprofen therapy, a scientific determination that the drug was the cause of death must have been made.[401] Yet regarding the Taggart cases, he testified that "we'll never know" whether Taggart was correct in attributing benoxaprofen as the cause of death. The combined assertions of Wood, therefore, imply that some deaths associated with marketing benoxaprofen, including alarming and unexpected ones, should not have been reported until such time, no matter how long, as a determination of cause of death could be made by Lilly scientists, and that some might never be reported to the regulatory authorities because the precise cause of death might never be determined. Such a policy would have given benoxaprofen an extraordinary benefit of the scientific doubt. However, Wood's testimony is completely inconsistent with Lilly's actual practice because the company reported to the FDA several deaths occurring during the North American clinical trials with benoxaprofen, even though Lilly scientists did not think they were drug-related[402] and Mikulaschek reported a fatal case of Lyell's syndrome (an extremely toxic skin reaction) during the marketing of the drug in West Germany, even though he believed that the relationship of the death to benoxaprofen "could not be determined with any certainty".[403]

Furthermore, in a letter to Lilly shareholders on 5 December 1983 Wood adopted a justification for not reporting some benoxaprofen-related deaths similar to Shedden's:

> Serious [benoxaprofen] adverse reactions known to the company that occurred abroad consisted primarily of reactions that were known to be associated with NSAIDs as a class. Some of those reactions were fatal. Except in a few instances, none were reportable under Lilly policy because they were typical of reactions common to the drugs of the class to which *Oraflex* belongs and were consistent with the adverse reactions profile developed for *Oraflex* during the clinical trials.[404]

Yet this totally abandons his argument that the company had not reported those deaths because the precise cause of death had not been determined. For if deaths were not reported because they were an expected outcome of NSAID treatment, then there must have been an assumption, on Lilly's part, that the drug *did* play a key role in the cause of death.

Following the Duncan and Lanvermeyer report, the FDA referred Lilly's failure to report benoxaprofen-related adverse reactions to the US Department of Justice. By 21 August 1985 the Justice Department had filed 25 charges against Lilly and 15 against Shedden for breaking the regulations regarding adverse drug reaction reporting and for mislabelling *Oraflex*.[405] The Department concluded that Lilly "made no attempt" to incorporate into the *Oraflex* labelling information known to the company prior to US approval about fatal and non-fatal cases of benoxaprofen-associated hepato-renal failure and jaundice.[406] That the adverse reactions occurred outside the US was not deemed to be a legitimate reason for failing to report them to the FDA because, according to the Justice Department, there had been close contact between Lilly's US headquarters and its British affiliates.[407] Lilly pleaded guilty to all 25 charges and Shedden pleaded *nolo contendere* (i.e. no contest) to all charges brought against him.[408]

Regarding deaths associated with benoxaprofen therapy, the approaches of Dista and the CSM were remarkably similar. Both sought to exonerate the drug from blame for severe toxicity until the evidence implicating its involvement was irresistible. Moreover, the CSM delayed taking regulatory action against benoxaprofen until the drug's toxicity was overriding compared with other NSAIDs. Under this regime many deaths of patients while taking a non-lifesaving drug, such as benoxaprofen, may have to occur before the regulatory authorities decide that even a major warning about the drug's toxicity should be provided to doctors. Furthermore, tremendous trust is invested in senior scientists in pharmaceutical companies to determine how frequently and how publicly to report life-threatening and fatal ADRs. Yet it is clear from this case study of benoxaprofen that scientists and regulators could have acted differently; perhaps within different institutional contexts and imperatives. The CSM could have been more prudent and insisted on a reduced dosage earlier. Had Lilly scientists been organized so as to give patients' interests top priority they could have supported Taggart's reports in the British medical press by publicizing details about the jaundice cases during US clinical trials instead of there being a denial by Shedden that such cases existed. The FDA could also have been furnished with full details of all the deaths that had occurred during marketing outside the US prior to the agency's approval date. As a consequence the FDA might have denied approval altogether.

Such alternative scenarios may sound naïve to the hardened sceptic of corporate industry and Government regulators. But the point of highlighting these alternatives is to show that all the fatal and non-fatal risks associated with medicines are not an inevitable result of modern drug technology. Specifically, it is highly implausible that all the deaths associated with benoxaprofen were inevitable consequences that arthritic patients in search of therapy simply have to bear because such is the state of technology. Rather, it is more accurate to say that such is the state of the political and economic forces that frame technological risk and regulation.

Conclusion

The benoxaprofen case reveals many different aspects of corporate bias in science and regulation. There is bias in the generation of scientific papers which strikes at the very heart of the production of scientific knowledge. This is evident from Lilly's enthusiastic reception for the rather dubious claims of Bluhm et al. in favour of benoxaprofen as an exceptionally effective drug, compared with the company's extremely critical response to Hamdy's research which, though supported by a very substantial weight of medical thinking at that time, implied that the usual dose of benoxaprofen might need to be reduced in the elderly for safety reasons. However, bias is not necessarily uniform within a company as shown by the disagreement between Gennery and senior Lilly scientists about the publication of Hamdy's paper.

Furthermore, the exchange between Gennery and Lilly's headquarters suggests that the involvement of the wider medical profession can act as a check against crude forms of bias such as suppression of publication. The origins of that involvement also appear to be significant. For example, unlike Kligman, who was selected by the company as an expert consultant, Hamdy approached the company in order to further his independent research programme. The history of the benoxaprofen controversy indicates that Hamdy was willing to be much more critical of Lilly than Kligman.

Perhaps the most blatant aspects of corporate bias that emerge from the discussions in this chapter are the inconsistencies in interpretive extrapolations of animal and other non-human data to the human therapeutic situation. As just one example of this, Lilly scientists eagerly extrapolated positive efficacy studies involving experimental non-human data to the therapeutic effectiveness of benoxaprofen in the clinical setting, but emphasized the limited relevance of the positive carcinogenicity findings in mice to the carcinogenic risk posed to humans. Thus, scientific uncertainty was highlighted or downplayed in congruence with the commercial interests of the company.

The evidence adduced in this chapter suggests that corporate bias is also reflected in how the benefit of the scientific doubt is distributed in regulatory decisions. We can see this most clearly by comparing the permissive approach of the regulatory authorities towards approving benoxaprofen with the extremely cautious approach towards removing it from the market. The CSM approved *Opren* without requiring experimental phototesting on human subjects and after the completion of only one problematic carcinogenicity test in animals. By contrast, after approval the CSM was reluctant to act on incomplete scientific information and initially refused to support warning doctors to reduce the daily dosage of benoxaprofen in the elderly because, until May 1982, the Committee considered that the clinical evidence was not sufficiently compelling to do so. Here we see that the CSM awarded the benefit of the scientific doubt to the commercial interests of the company at both the pre- and post-approval stages. Furthermore, the CSM's handling of the Hamdy, Kamal and Taggart research shows that scientific uncertainty may not only be understated by regulatory authorities to maintain credibility, but also emphasized to defend inaction.

Similarly, the FDA approved *Oraflex* despite the unsatisfactory nature of the drug's carcinogenicity testing by reference to the agency's own standards, and despite the drug's lack of exceptional efficacy to outweigh its phototoxicity. Indeed, agency officials allowed the drug to remain on the market even though they were aware of the death cases reported by Taggart in the medical press and Lilly's failure to report jaundice cases to the agency during clinical trials, and despite having concluded that more benoxaprofen-associated deaths were imminent.

The adverse effects of benoxaprofen on patients gave rise to a major public controversy, especially in the UK. In concluding this discussion of corporate bias on the testing and regulation of benoxaprofen, therefore, it is fitting to consider how the foregoing analysis can shed some light on the official accounts provided by the British Government about the *Opren* experience. In his 1982 *Annual Report on the State of Public Health* the Chief

Medical Officer of the DHSS wrote:

The story of "Opren" illustrates one of the main difficulties in drug regulation. Even when a drug has been carefully tested over a period of years in animals . . . rare adverse reactions may only be detected when the drug is in wide use.[409]

and in January 1983 Kenneth Clarke, then Minister of Health, told Parliament:

The key point is that the [Hamdy and Kamal] studies did not contain specific evidence that the drug was harmful. Dr Hamdy was referring to the prospects of giving elderly patients smaller doses and still getting the beneficial effects.[410]

We may confidently conclude that, though the Chief Medical Officer may be correct in supposing that rare adverse reactions can only be detected after widespread prescription, it is highly questionable that benoxaprofen was *carefully* tested in animals for carcinogenicity according to many of drug toxicology's own scientific standards. Moreover, it is clear from the discussion in this chapter that Kenneth Clarke's account of Hamdy's research was potentially misleading, albeit unintentionally, because Hamdy and indeed some Lilly scientists believed that the accumulation of benoxaprofen in the elderly had implications for the drug's toxicity. That Hamdy explicitly mentioned his concern about benoxaprofen's potential for inflicting harm on elderly patients in his published paper suggests that he was not merely "referring to the prospects of giving elderly patients smaller doses and still getting the beneficial effects". By elevating this latter aspect of Hamdy's clinical work to "the key point" at the expense of drawing attention to concern about benoxaprofen's potential for toxic accumulation, Kenneth Clarke presented a biased account to Parliament.

Chapter Five

Feldene – the closure of technical dispute

A compound known generically as piroxicam was synthesized by Pfizer in 1967 in Connecticut in the US. By 1977 scientists at Pfizer felt that they had sufficient data to approach regulatory authorities for approval of the NSAID. Switzerland was the first to approve it in September 1979 with the UK soon following in January 1980. However, the FDA did not approve the marketing of piroxicam until April 1982. In both the UK and the US piroxicam was marketed under the tradename *Feldene*.

The *Feldene* product data sheet approved by the British regulatory authorities in 1980 stated that the drug was indicated for conditions such as osteoarthritis and rheumatoid arthritis. Doctors were advised that the normally recommended daily dose was 20 mg, though it was noted that some patients might be maintained effectively on just 10 mg/day while others might require up to 30 mg/day. However, the data sheet cautioned that long-term administration of daily doses of 30 mg or higher carried an increased risk of gastro-intestinal adverse effects.[1]

As discussed in Chapter 2, the 1962 Kefauver–Harris Amendment to American drug regulation demands substantial evidence of a drug's effectiveness before it can be approved for marketing in the US. The FDA's policy interpretation of this law has been, and remains, to require sponsors of NSAIDs to submit two well controlled (pivotal) clinical studies demonstrating efficacy for each of the two main arthritic conditions for which the drug is indicated; osteoarthritis and rheumatoid arthritis in this case.[2] According to the FDA that policy is based on the established scientific principle that experimental data usually need to be replicated in order to be credible.[3]

Efficacy – rules are made to be broken

When FDA scientists came to review Pfizer's clinical trials with piroxicam they experienced difficulty in finding what they regarded as satisfactory evidence of the drug's efficacy. The agency selected two trials by Ward et al. and Steigerwald & Messner as pivotal for rheumatoid arthritis and two trials by Stevens et al. and Abruzzo et al. as pivotal for osteoarthritis.[4] The Ward et al. and Abruzzo et al. studies were double-blind comparisons of piroxicam with aspirin, the Steigerwald study, also double-blind, compared piroxicam with indomethacin, and the Stevens et al. study compared the efficacy of daily doses of 10 mg, 20 mg and 30 mg.

On 22 March 1979 Leszek Ochota completed the first Medical Officer's Review of piroxicam for the FDA. At this time Ochota concluded that Pfizer's data were unsatisfactory to document effectiveness of piroxicam in osteoarthritis or rheumatoid arthritis[5] and recommended that the piroxicam NDA was "not approvable because of paucity (quantitative only) of data for effectiveness".[6] However, following the submission of the Ward et al. and Abruzzo et al. studies, Ochota undertook a second review in which he recommended approval of the piroxicam NDA on the basis of those additional studies *pending confirmation by FDA statisticians*.[7]

When on 26 August 1980 FDA statisticians Hoi Leung and Jerome Senturia examined the clinical studies supposed to serve as pivotal to the evidence of piroxicam's efficacy, they perceived several problems. They found that in the Ward et al. study, which was intended to compare piroxicam with aspirin for treatment of rheumatoid arthritis, there was the possibility of mixed-up or contaminated drug samples because the data showed significant levels of piroxicam in the bloodstream of patients purportedly receiving aspirin only.[8] Furthermore, they reported that piroxicam patients seemed to have been taking aspirin contrary to the study protocol:

> Patients who took concomitant anti-arthritic drug therapy or concomitant therapy with another investigational drug were supposed to be excluded from the study. This would imply that aspirin should not be allowed as a concomitant therapy for piroxicam patients since it is an investigational drug (to be compared with piroxicam in this study) as well as an anti-arthritic drug. The sponsor also stated in the protocol that aspirin therapy was stopped for one week (baseline period) before active therapy began. However, upon examining the data on the aspirin plasma level of patients, it

is obvious that many patients in the piroxicam group took concomitant aspirin therapy both during the baseline period and during the course of the study in violation of the protocol.[9]

Leung and Senturia found that the Abruzzo et al. study was afflicted with the same problems as the Ward et al. study.[10]

Hence the very clinical studies on which Ochota had based his recommendation for approval pending confirmation by FDA statisticians vis-à-vis efficacy were found to be unsound by those statisticians. Indeed, previously on 2 June 1978 William Gyarfus, the Director of the FDA Division responsible for NSAIDs, had written to Pfizer about some of its piroxicam clinical studies commenting:

> The concomitant use of aspirin is a flaw in the design of both studies, since it complicates the assessment of efficacy of piroxicam and its adverse effects. The data reported and summarised in this submission suffer from some serious deficiencies as do the analyses of that data.[11]

However, according to Robert Temple, the FDA's Acting Director for New Drug Evaluation, Pfizer thought their clinical studies were adequate and did not conduct any new efficacy studies prior to approval.[12]

On 16 January 1981, following a meeting with Pfizer, Leung and Senturia strongly reaffirmed their criticisms of the Abruzzo et al. study. They concluded that the data were "at best of questionable value", and that since there were "so many deficiencies in the design, conduct and analysis" even a re-analysis could at best render the study only "supportive rather than pivotal".[13] Later that month John Harter, the Group Leader for the reviewing of NSAIDs, concurred with Leung and Senturia about the Abruzzo et al. study of osteoarthritis, but felt that there was adequate evidence of efficacy in the treatment of rheumatoid arthritis.[14] Harter also stressed that though drug products effective in rheumatoid arthritis are generally also effective in osteoarthritis that was not a regulatory basis for approval if only because the effective dosage for osteoarthritis is usually different to that for rheumatoid arthritis.[15] Consequently, the dosage for osteoarthritis needs to be determined by separate adequate studies.[16] These considerations led Harter to recommend that piroxicam should be approved for rheumatoid arthritis but not osteoarthritis because "the firm ha[d] not met our requirements for 2 adequate and well controlled trials establishing efficacy" in the latter condition.[17]

Nevertheless, on 4 February 1981 Gyarfus, Harter's superior, decided to endorse Ochota's recommendation that the drug should be approved as effective in the treatment of both osteoarthritis and rheumatoid arthritis.[18] Yet Gyarfus's own previous doubts about the adequacy of Pfizer's clinical studies do not seem to have been entirely laid to rest even at this stage. In particular his justification for recommending approval for treatment of osteoarthritis seems to acknowledge that the clinical studies intended to establish efficacy in that condition were unsatisfactory:

> Both Dr Harter and the statistician point out that the sponsor did no placebo-controlled studies in osteoarthritis, but it is believed that with the information derived from the rheumatoid studies plus information from other clinical studies in osteoarthritis are adequate to show effectiveness of the drug in osteoarthritis. . . . Even though studies in osteoarthritis are not outstandingly well done and may have some procedural errors as pointed out by reviewers, there still is adequate information that the drug is effective in osteoarthritis. The studies in osteoarthritis may not stand alone to establish efficacy of the NSAID, piroxicam, but when coupled with the information from rheumatoid studies, it is felt that there is adequate data for approval for use in rheumatoid arthritis and osteoarthritis.[19]

Thus, certainly three FDA scientists, two statisticians and the Group Leader for NSAID evaluation, and arguably four, if one includes Gyarfus, believed that piroxicam had not been adequately studied to demonstrate clinical effectiveness in osteoarthritis by agency standards. Only Ochota, the Medical Officer, was convinced by the efficacy studies of piroxicam in osteoarthritis.

Despite Gyarfus's positive evaluation of piroxicam, the problems associated with the drug's efficacy review at the FDA multiplied. On 14 April 1981 Harter reviewed the Steigerwald et al. study which compared the effectiveness on rheumatoid arthritis of piroxicam with indomethacin. He observed that piroxicam and indomethacin patients took aspirin throughout the study and commented that controlled clinical trials with NSAIDs were, and remain, predicated on the assumption that:

> generally no other NSAID [e.g. aspirin] be given concomitantly with the study drug [piroxicam] and that all other concomitant anti-arthritic medicines be stabilized before the trial and kept constant during the trial.[20]

Moreover, according to Harter some of the patients in this study were not maintained on *stable* doses of aspirin. Harter concluded that the study design was "not suitable for establishing the basic efficacy of the test drug" and recommended that Pfizer should be told that the FDA required "another adequate and well controlled demonstration of efficacy in rheumatoid arthritis for approval for treatment of rheumatoid arthritis".[21]

On 28 July 1981 Harter reiterated his view that the Abruzzo et al. study was inadequate as a pivotal study to support efficacy of piroxicam in osteoarthritis, and referred to the Abruzzo clinical trial as a "methodological failure".[22] By this time Harter was recommending that Pfizer needed to provide the agency with "one well controlled trial in rheumatoid arthritis and one in osteoarthritis".[23] Several weeks later Leung and Senturia reaffirmed their conviction that the Abruzzo et al. study should at best be regarded as a supportive study and was too deficient to be pivotal for efficacy assessment.[24]

It was in this context that Marion Finkel, Associate Director for New Drug Evaluation and Gyarfus's superior at the FDA, reviewed the efficacy of piroxicam on 17 September 1981. She considered the Ward et al. study to be the "best" in support of efficacy and made no mention of the problems raised by Leung and Senturia that some of the piroxicam patients seemed to have taken aspirin and vice versa. Regarding the Steigerwald study Finkel did acknowledge that "there was, again, the problem of determining the effectiveness of an NSAID added to aspirin", but nevertheless argued that the study was sufficient to support the efficacy of piroxicam.[25] According to Temple, the Acting Director of New Drug Evaluation, she did not share Gyarfus's reservations about the *independent* validity of the efficacy studies of piroxicam in osteoarthritis.[26] Rather she not only concurred with Gyarfus that parts of the Abruzzo et al. study were supportive of efficacy in osteoarthritis, but believed that there were two adequate and well controlled studies in both conditions and concluded:

> Although the data for efficacy evaluation are scantier than we are accustomed to seeing in NDAs for new NSAIDs, I feel that the NDA can be approved. Dr Harter has suggested that additional studies be performed for both types of arthritis using placebo control. I see little to be gained by such studies since the drug is an effective NSAID.[27]

In a summary of the FDA's review of piroxicam efficacy on 9 March 1982, Harter referred to the decision to approve piroxicam as institutionally difficult because the opinions of the scientific reviewers had split 3–3 in their evaluation of whether Pfizer's clinical studies satisfied the agency's requirements for substantial evidence of effectiveness.[28] He further commented:

the concomitant use of aspirin in so many pivotal studies has made it difficult to demonstrate any other drug effect. . . . By the analyses we usually depend on the pivotal studies do not demonstrate statistically significant proof of effectiveness.[29]

Moreover, FDA scientists never managed to resolve the question of how piroxicam came to be in the blood of the aspirin-treated patients.[30] Consequently, the possibility that this finding was due to a mix-up in patient dosing was not entirely eliminated, though thought unlikely by Harter[31] – a mix-up, which, if it occurred, Temple testified "would have been a fatal lesion for the study".[32] Despite these and the many other problems identified by FDA scientists and discussed in this section, on 6 April the FDA approved piroxicam under the tradename *Feldene* as safe and effective for the treatment of osteoarthritis and rheumatoid arthritis.[33] When called upon to defend this decision on behalf of the FDA in front of Congress, Temple described the total data base on piroxicam efficacy as "marginal". He elaborated:

marginal means it can go either way depending on how you look at it.[34]

In particular, concerning the Steigerwald et al. pivotal study, Temple testified:

I do not think there were well-designed studies. It would not be my favourite choice of design, but a person could review them and conclude that the results are satisfactory anyway.[35]

The FDA's approval of piroxicam's "marginal" efficacy could not be justified on the grounds of the drug's greater safety than other drugs in its therapeutic class because FDA scientists had not found it to be significantly safer than other NSAIDs. In fact, just prior to approval Harter expressed concerns about the validity of its safety evaluation as well as its efficacy:

The evaluation of the adverse effects ("safety") is also confounded by the two problems. One is that the concomitant use of aspirin in most of their controlled trials makes it difficult to dissect our piroxicam contributions to the Treatment Emergent Signs and Symptoms (TESS). The other . . . is in their [Pfizer's] computerized adverse reaction file.[36]

Yet neither the FDA's official *Feldene Summary Basis of Approval* nor the package insert approved by the FDA for the labelling of *Feldene* in the US said anything of the above uncertainties or weaknesses in the clinical studies of the drug's efficacy. American doctors were not told that the FDA

184

believed that the evidence to support the effectiveness of the drug in treating osteoarthritis was "marginal". On the contrary the package insert stated merely:

In controlled clinical trials the effectiveness of *Feldene* has been established for both acute exacerbations and long-term management of rheumatoid arthritis and ostoearthritis.[37]

Prescribing doctors were to be kept in the dark about the "scantier" than usual basis for considering the drug to be effective.

Pfizer, however, exhibited no such reticence. Following approval the company felt able to claim in a *Feldene* Press Kit that the Abruzzo et al. study showed *Feldene* to be "statistically superior to aspirin".[38] It was not until 13 July 1982, over two months after the drug had been approved, that the FDA told Pfizer that this and some other statements in the Press Kit were "misleading".[39]

Carcinogenicity – approve and hope for the best

The FDA's approval of piroxicam is all the more remarkable if one considers the agency's assessment of Pfizer's carcinogenicity testing of the drug. Pfizer conducted two 18-month chronic toxicity studies for the purpose of determining the carcinogenicity of piroxicam – one in mice and the other in rats. When Manfred Hein of the FDA came to review these studies on 21 February 1980 he expressed reservations about their adequacy as tests for carcinogenicity.

According to Hein neither study indicated that piroxicam had carcinogenic potential. However, he also concluded that the rat study also failed "to suggest that piroxicam is not carcinogenic because of its limitations in duration and quality of data collection".[40] Specifically, he commented:

The validity of a study lasting only 18 months in the rat for the prime purpose of demonstrating carcinogenic potential is presently an open question. We have recommended that rat studies for this purpose be for at least 2 years and corresponding mouse studies to be designed to last up to 2 years. . . . It is questionable if the present rat (or mouse) study would meet the objectives spelt out in the now operative Good Laboratory Practice (GLP) regulations.[41]

Consequently Hein recommended "another adequate long-term administration trial in conformity with GLP regulations *as a precondition to any approval of the NDA*" (emphasis added).[42] Hein also noted the importance of taking into account the statistician's review before making a final recommendation.

The statistician, Leung, tended to confirm Hein's reservations. Leung described the rat study as being "plagued with problems of high variability of data, missing and/or unreported data".[43] As to the carcinogenic potential of piroxicam he concluded that:

the studies were inconclusive although there was no statistically significant difference in tumour occurrences between treatment and control groups. This could be attributed to the relatively short period (18 months) of study time together with problems of missing tissues.[44]

The *Feldene Summary Basis of Approval* made no mention of the fact that FDA scientists believed that the carcinogenicity testing prior to approval was "inconclusive". It did, however, state that Pfizer had agreed to undertake a 24-month carcinogenicity study in rats during the marketing of the drug, thus indicating that FDA management had decided to ignore Hein's recommendation that such a study should be a precondition for approval.[45] That study did eventually show that piroxicam was non-carcinogenic in rats and was acceptable to FDA scientists, but it was not completed until April 1985, three years after the drug was released on to the US market.

As for the initial *Feldene* package insert, it stated nothing whatsoever about carcinogenicity under the section headed "Carcinogenesis, chronic animal toxicity and impairment of fertility".[46] The 1980 *Feldene* data sheet approved by the CSM also said nothing about the drug's carcinogenic potential or the adequacy of the animal tests conducted in order to assess it, even though the ABPI Guidelines on carcinogenicity testing recommended that studies in rats should be of 24 months' duration.[47]

Gastro-intestinal toxicity – real or imaginary?

As with other NSAIDs piroxicam was found to be associated with some gastro-intestinal (GI) toxicity during clinical trials in the treatment of arthritis. Such toxicity was dose-related and GI ulcers in particular rose sharply when a 30 mg/day or 40 mg/day dosage was administered instead of a 20 mg daily dosage[48] as shown in Table 9.

The British *Feldene* product data sheet recommended a normal daily dose of 20 mg though acknowledged that:

A relatively small group of patients may be maintained on as little

Table 9 Gastro-intestinal toxicity of piroxicam.

Dose	N	GI ADRs (%)	Ulceration (%)	Discontinued (%)
10 mg/day	438	9.6	0.5	1.6
20 mg/day	2544	18.4	0.9	3.4
30 mg/day	717	22.3	2.6	4.3
40 mg/day	288	29.9	6.9	5.5

N = Number of patients treated.
Source: N. E. Pitts 1979. Review of clinical trial experience with piroxicam. *Piroxicam: a new non-steroidal anti-inflammatory agent,* 61. New York: Academy Professional Information Services.

as 10 mg daily. . . . Long term administration of doses 30 mg or higher carries an increased risk of gastro-intestinal side effects.[49]

It also stated that GI adverse effects were the most commonly encountered, including peptic ulceration and GI bleeding, but in most cases did not interfere with therapy. Unlike other NSAIDs on the market at that time (except benoxaprofen) conveniently *Feldene* could be taken only once a day because of its relatively long elimination half-life of 38 to 50 hours.[50]

The first *Feldene* package insert approved by the FDA in the US in April 1982 also recommended a daily dose of 20 mg, but did not entertain the option of maintaining some patients on 10 mg/day. Though the package insert warned of peptic ulcerations during clinical trials, GI bleeding was merely listed under adverse reactions with an incidence of less than one per cent. Indeed, Pfizer marketed *Feldene* as having "a generally lower rate of GI side effects" compared with many other NSAIDs.[51] Sales exceeded $386 million in the US during 1983.[52]

Complacency gives way to controversy

The assertion that piroxicam's GI toxicity was relatively low was first directly challenged by Ward & Weir who suggested that "the incidence of serious bleeding with piroxicam had been underestimated".[53] They reported that in a Dublin hospital during 1981, 6 out of 20 cases of peptic ulcer disease in which a NSAID was implicated involved piroxicam. In total these authors discussed eight cases of serious GI toxicity associated with piroxicam therapy, all of whom were over the age of 65 and two of whom died. The publication of these findings coincided with concern among the Irish drug regulatory authority, the National Drugs Advisory Board (NDAB), about the risks of GI toxicity in the elderly associated with piroxicam therapy. Consequently, by 1982 the NDAB had altered the Irish product data sheet to emphasize the long half-life of piroxicam and the increased risk of GI bleeding in the elderly with NSAIDs. The NDAB believed that in the elderly the lowest dose compatible with adequate and safe clinical control should be employed and, like the CSM, noted that some patients could be maintained on 10mg/day.[54]

In June 1982 Emery and Grahame voiced similar concerns in *The Lancet*. They reported five cases of "severe blood loss" (one fatal) associated with piroxicam treatment and suggested that the contra-indications for the British data sheet might require review because of the possibility of serious adverse effects in the elderly.[55] Simultaneously, the propensity of NSAIDs to cause ulceration in the elderly was studied by Gleeson in Jersey where he concluded that ulcers were more prevalent and more serious among patients, especially elderly women, taking NSAIDs than other patients not on NSAID therapy.[56]

In October 1981 British regulators ranked piroxicam as the worst NSAID regarding GI bleeding and perforations and expressed concern about this to Pfizer.[57] As a result the product data sheet was changed to warn that the drug should not be used in patients with active peptic ulceration or a history of recurrent ulceration, and that the drug should be withdrawn in the event of peptic ulceration or gastro-intestinal bleeding.[58] However, there was no mention of fatalities. The American package insert also changed in August 1982 to include a warning that peptic ulceration and severe cases of GI bleeding had been reported with piroxicam therapy with "a fatal outcome in rare instances".[59] The greatest concern about the drug's severe GI toxicity was shown at this time by the Federal German Health Authorities who were moved to hold a special hearing on the subject in Berlin in September 1983. The German authorities had received 45 reports of deaths possibly related to piroxicam, many of them due to GI toxicity.[60]

Meanwhile, the problem of whether elderly patients were particularly susceptible to serious adverse effects from taking piroxicam persisted. In February 1983 in the US, *The Medical Letter* expressed concern that "piroxicam, the newest NSAID and one with the longest half-life, might accumulate in elderly patients and cause more GI bleeding than other drugs in this class".[61] However, later that year Woolf et al. found no evidence that the pharmacokinetics of piroxicam was "grossly different" in elderly arthritic patients and so challenged the claim that the predisposition of such patients to piroxicam-related adverse effects was caused by an extended half-life of the drug in the elderly.[62]

Nevertheless, serious GI toxicity in the elderly continued to be associated with piroxicam. For example, in October 1983 the Ontario Medical Association's Committee on Drugs and Pharmacotherapy reported 82 cases of serious adverse reactions to NSAIDs, 29 of which were piroxicam-related and mostly GI problems in the elderly. Thirteen of those 29 were either fatal or unresolved.[63] And on reviewing the adverse effects associated with piroxicam during its first year of marketing in Norway, Laake et al. noted that the drug accounted for 103 out of a total of 711 suspected reactions submitted to the Norwegian drug regulatory authorities. Of these 103, 66 were GI reactions, including 2 deaths, 55 reactions which the authorities classified as "severe" and 8 classified as "life-threatening".[64] Many of these cases were elderly patients. Furthermore, in March 1984 in response to a parliamentary question in the House of Commons Kenneth Clarke, the British Health Minister, listed in descending order the total number of adverse reactions and deaths associated with each of the NSAIDs reported to the CSM during 1982. This revealed that piroxicam was prescribed less than ibuprofen, indomethacin or naproxen but was associated with more adverse reactions than all three combined and with more deaths than naproxen and ibuprofen combined, though with fewer deaths than indomethacin.[65]

In April 1984 a number of significant changes were made to the piroxicam package insert in the US. It now warned that peptic ulceration, perforation and GI bleeding were sometimes severe and fatal in *some*, rather than rare, instances. The attention of doctors was drawn to the precaution that

> patients with impaired renal function . . . as well as elderly patients who have decreased renal function are more at risk. Because of the extensive renal excretion of piroxicam and its biotransformation products, lower doses of piroxicam should be anticipated in patients with impaired renal function.[66]

Six months later John Harter at the FDA prepared a ranking of the 11 NSAIDs marketed in the US according to number of fatal and non-fatal adverse reactions per million prescriptions associated with each drug in reports to the agency. The ranking was prepared as a basis for discussion at the 26 October Arthritis Advisory Committee meeting where some FDA officials proposed the possibility of designating some NSAIDs as "not for initial use".[67] The Committee rejected that proposal, but the ranking revealed that piroxicam had the most fatal and non-fatal adverse reactions in total and the most fatal and non-fatal GI adverse reactions in particular.[68]

By January 1985 Richardson et al. had published a pharmacokinetic study of 12 young and 13 elderly healthy subjects claiming that "piroxicam body clearance in elderly women was approximately 33 per cent lower than in young women"[69] and Fok et al. had reported "a high incidence of ulceration induced by piroxicam" in their patients.[70] Two months later Beerman argued that the concerns of Fok et al. were supported by reports to the Swedish Committee on Adverse Drug Effects and that "the frequency of complications from the upper GI tract seem[ed] to be very high for piroxicam in relation to its sales".[71] Simultaneously representatives of the Belgian Ministry of Health suggested that reports to their Centre for Drug Postmarketing Surveillance suggested that piroxicam was not associated with a low incidence of GI ulcers.[72] On the other hand, other commentators, such as Inman and Rawson of the Drug Surveillance Research Unit at Southampton cautioned against using anecdotal reporting to estimate the incidences of adverse drug reactions because of variation in reporting rates between different drugs and of unknown patient exposure.[73]

Pfizer enters the controversy

On 29 April, Roger Sachs, Medical Director of Pfizer Laboratories, echoed Inman's sentiments at an FDA Arthritis Advisory Committee meeting. Sachs directed his attention to Harter's rankings of NSAIDs according to adverse reaction per million prescriptions. He argued that Harter's data needed to be adjusted for *product life-cycle characteristics* (i.e. the evidence that historically the peak of reporting of adverse reactions to other NSAIDs had tended to be in the early years of marketing) and corrected for the degree of patient exposure (i.e. the "length" of prescription on different drugs). Sachs emphasized that piroxicam was then still only coming to the end of its third year on the US market compared with say indomethacin which had been on the market for 20 years. Indomethacin, therefore, would be expected to have a low reporting rate relative to piroxicam. And regarding length of prescription he argued that a typical prescription for piroxicam was four weeks, but only two weeks for ibuprofen. Hence, a patient developing an adverse GI reaction after four weeks might do so on one piroxicam prescription but two ibuprofen prescriptions – making piroxicam responsible for twice as many adverse reactions per number of prescriptions as ibuprofen because of length of prescription rather than toxicity of the drug.[74]

Harter, however, had prepared a modified ranking of the NSAIDs according to number of cases of non-fatal upper GI perforations, bleeding and ulcers per million prescriptions and also per million daily doses. By this method, which is not open to Sachs' criticisms about length of prescriptions, piroxicam also ranked the highest (though tied with diflunisal).[75] (See Tables 10 and 11.)

In both Tables 10 and 11 the NSAIDs have been ranked by Harter according to the number of *cases in the US* of fatal or non-fatal GI adverse reactions per million prescriptions in the US (i.e. by the figures appearing in the last column) and not according to number of adverse drug reactions (ADRs) either in the US or outside the US. Table 10 shows that in 1984 piroxicam ranked as having the highest number of non-fatal cases of GI adverse reactions in the US per million prescriptions in the US. Column

Table 10 Ordering by United States (US) non-fatal (N-F) non-hepatic GI ADR cases (C)/ million prescription 1984 (MRx).

Rank	NSAID	MRx	N-F	N-F/MRx	US C	US C/MRx
1	piroxicam	7.53	534	70.96	145	19.27
2	diflunisal	2.50	138	55.27	40	16.02
3	phenylbutazone	2.81	56	19.95	24	8.55
4	sulindac	5.47	131	23.94	35	6.40
5	meclofenamate	1.80	25	13.87	8	4.44
5	indomethacin	9.02	157	17.41	40	4.44
7	fenoprofen	3.26	58	17.80	12	3.68
8	naproxen	11.86	175	14.76	33	2.78
9	tolmetin	2.57	59	22.92	5	1.94
10	ibuprofen	20.45	129	6.31	26	1.27

Table 11 Ordering by United States (US) fatal (F) non-hepatic GI ADR cases (C)/million prescription 1984 (MRx).

Rank	NSAID	MRx	F ADR	F ADR/ MRx	Foreign F C	F US C	F US C/ MRx
1	diflunisal	2.50	9	3.60	0	3	1.20
1	meclofenamate	1.80	5	2.77	0	2	1.11
3	piroxicam	7.53	85	11.30	52	8	1.06
4	indomethacin	9.02	25	2.77	4	7	0.78
4	sulindac	5.47	21	3.84	3	4	0.73
4	phenylbutazone	2.81	8	2.85	0	2	0.71
7	tolmetin	2.57	10	3.89	0	1	0.39
8	fenprofen	3.26	6	1.84	0	1	0.31
9	naproxen	11.86	12	1.01	0	3	0.25
10	ibuprofen	20.45	10	0.49	2	2	0.10

two of that table shows that the FDA received substantially more reports (inside and outside the US) of non-fatal adverse reactions associated with piroxicam than any of the other NSAIDs listed and column three shows that piroxicam also ranked as having the highest number of associated non-fatal GI adverse reactions (inside and outside the US) per million prescriptions in the US. Table 11 ranks piroxicam as third for number of cases of fatal GI adverse reactions in the US per million prescriptions in the US associated with its use. However, it also reveals that piroxicam ranks by far the highest for number of associated fatal GI adverse reactions (inside and outside the US) per million prescription in the US. Moreover, the FDA received reports of 52 fatal cases of GI adverse reactions associated with piroxicam outside the US, but only 9 such foreign fatal cases associated with all the other NSAIDs combined during 1984.

The question of GI toxicity in the elderly in view of piroxicam's long half-life was also raised during Sachs' presentation at the Arthritis Advisory Committee. Specifically, the following transpired:

Weisman: An alternative explanation for this [Harter's] data could be that there are some groups that are at particular risk to develop GI toxicity from piroxicam. A possibility exists that the medication, that was marketed at a schedule with a very long half-life of over 24 hours, that perhaps certain patients would be put at particular risk to have difficulty with the long half-life and effective dose level of piroxicam. Those patients might be elderly patients, patients with diminshed renal function. . . . Do you think that is a reasonable hypothesis?

Sachs: Well, I think all hypotheses are reasonable until disproven. I don't think there is enough data to prove or disprove that.[76]

In the same year further evidence was provided by Collier & Pain that the elderly, and especially elderly women, were particularly susceptible to NSAID-related peptic ulcer perforation.[77] On the other hand, as regards patients under 65, Jick et al. concluded that "the risk of hospitalization for upper GI bleeding from the stomach attributable to the NSAIDs used [including piroxicam] is very low".[78] The safety of piroxicam came under even closer scrutiny when on 7 December O'Brien & Burnham published an article claiming that the drug was associated with over twice as many ulcer cases in the Romford area of England as would be expected from regional data. The mean age of the patients was over 68 and the vast majority were over 60.[79]

A few weeks later debate was further fuelled by press coverage of the

CSM's investigation into the safety of NSAIDs. This revealed that during the five years on the British market piroxicam was associated with 77 fatalities, most due to GI perforation and/or bleeding, and over 2,000 serious adverse effects.[80] The O'Brien & Burnham article prompted three letters to the *British Medical Journal* expressing concern about GI toxicity associated with NSAIDs and piroxicam in particular, and a fourth letter by Inman in which he reiterated his criticisms that anecdotal data, even when related to regional prescribing rates, cannot be used as a basis for comparing different NSAIDs because of different reporting rates between different drugs and the non-uniform nature of prescriptions.[81] Later O'Brien & Burnham provided a rejoinder to Inman's second point by asserting:

> We know of no evidence that the size of the prescriptions of any individual non-steroidal anti-inflammatory drug should be greater than that of the rest, and this seems an unlikely occurrence with so many prescriptions.[82]

The public citizen campaign

It was in this context that on 8 January 1986 the Public Citizens' Health Research Group (HRG) petitioned the Secretary of the US Department of Health and Human Services (DHHS) and the FDA to "immediately ban, as an imminent hazard to public health, the use of Pfizer's widely sold anti-arthritic medication *Feldene* (piroxicam) in people aged 60 and older".[83] Citing Harter's aforementioned ranking of NSAIDs, the Swedish adverse reaction data reported by Beerman, reports from Belgium and Norway, and the O'Brien & Burnham study in Romford, HRG claimed that GI toxicity was more common and more severe with piroxicam than other NSAIDs, especially in the elderly.

The Public Citizen Group further argued that piroxicam was particularly dangerous to elderly patients for three reasons: (1) the elderly tended to have a decreased capacity to eliminate the drug; (2) it exhibited a long elimination half-life increasing the possibility of accumulation in the bloodstream, reminiscent of the benoxaprofen controversy; and (3) it had a low margin of safety with respect to ulcerogenicity (i.e. at doses above the normal recommended 20mg/day the risk of ulceration increased markedly).[84] According to HRG, for reasons (1) and (2) above, the elderly were likely to be exposed to what was, in effect, a dosage greater than 20mg/day, and consequently to a very toxic medication.[85] To support their contention that the drug was particularly dangerous to the elderly

HRG cited the study by Richardson et al. suggesting that elderly women excreted the drug at 33 per cent of the rate of young women, and the fact that Pfizer's communications with the Irish regulatory authorities had indicated concerns about the relatively large number of reports of serious GI toxicity in the elderly culminating in a labelling change on the Irish product data sheet.

On the basis of internal Pfizer memoranda, HRG also claimed that "at least one Pfizer official believed that proper studies had never been performed by the company to determine whether elderly patients are at risk of adverse reactions to the drug".[86] However, those memoranda were dated no later than August 1983. Moreover, HRG omitted to mention that Pitts, the Pfizer official in question, stated in October 1982 that he believed that "the local effect of an NSAID at the mucosal level is more important than blood level in producing GI toxicity".[87] That belief directly opposed HRG's contention that piroxicam-related GI toxicity was aggravated by drug accumulation in the blood due to a long half-life and/or inefficient elimination. Nevertheless, these memoranda did reveal some important observations by Pitts regarding the relationship between piroxicam kinetics and therapy in the elderly (especially elderly women) and reports of adverse reactions to the drug. For example, regarding piroxicam clinical trials Pitts reflected:

> Phase II kinetic data, albeit from an uncontrolled setting, indicated the possibility that blood levels were higher dose for dose in women. . . . However, we have *never* generated controlled data on this point. I would contend that, in its absence the possibility remains. . . . I suggested that future controlled kinetic studies should separate groups of males and females.[88] (Emphasis in original)

And regarding "suggestions from post-marketing experience" he commented:

> When the initial adverse GI experience was reported in Ireland it was noteworthy that the patients were (a) very old, (b) female. The latter fact could be kinetics related but it could be equally due to other factors. The female predominance appears to have held true for the UK and Scandinavian adverse GI experience. Impaired renal function becomes increasingly common with advanced age. After the initial Irish experience I suggested that further controlled kinetic work be done in the elderly and in patients with renal impairment, with particular attention to male and female subgroups.[89]

In August 1983 Pitts reiterated his view that evidence concerning

NSAID-related GI ulceration "used at therapeutic doses" is "overwhelmingly against" the toxicity being "a function of systemic blood levels" and "favours a predominant local effect".[90] However, he elaborated and concluded as follows:

> I myself am still not convinced that, with piroxicam, there is not a sex related difference in kinetics. The kinetic data from the clinical research program, casual and uncontrolled though it was, certainly seemed to suggest this. . . . If one is really concerned to demonstrate the safety of a long half-life drug then one should thoroughly adequately document the kinetic profile in the elderly patient (at least >65 years and preferably >70 years). This should address age related differences in drug handling completely separate and distinct from considerations of impaired hepatic and/or renal function. It should also address possible sex related (male v female) and disease (rheumatoid arthritis v osteoarthritis) differences. *I have not seen any data which reassures me that the 70 year old plus female osteoarthritic, for instance, is not at special risk because of different kinetics.* I seem to recall that the severe "bleeds" reported some time ago in Ireland were all female and in the over 70 years age group. Whilst GI irritation is predominantly a local effect at therapeutic doses *this does not preclude a systemic component if doses and/or blood levels are high enough.*[91] (Emphasis added)

In response to the HRG's petition the FDA announced that there would be a public hearing on 28 February 1986 in which HRG and Pfizer would be given an opportunity to put forward their views on the safety of piroxicam.[92] In the interim Adams et al. published a major article on NSAIDs in which they reiterated a claim made by O'Brien in 1983 that "NSAIDs with long half-lives are more likely to cause gastric side effects than those with short half-lives".[93] They further advised:

> Clearly, caution should be exercised when these drugs are used in the elderly and a compound with a short half-life favoured.[94]

Furthermore, Moebius published results, derived from spontaneous reports of adverse drug reactions to the CSM over the period 1979–84, which showed that piroxicam was associated with far more fatal and non-fatal cases of peptic ulceration per million prescriptions in the UK than any other NSAID except for benoxaprofen.[95] Based on these data Moebius questioned the safety of piroxicam, although his analysis did not take account of the possibility that product market life-cycles could exaggerate the comparative ulcerogenicity of the newer NSAIDs such as piroxicam.

The controversy goes public

The FDA public hearing opened with an overview by John Ward, a Professor of Medicine and Rheumatologist at Utah University. He argued for caution in reaching conclusions from anecdotal and spontaneous reporting of ADRs on the grounds that the reporting rate of ADRs is highest during its first two years on the market and then subsides. Ward believed that that phenomenon was supported by the data regarding piroxicam-related ADRs. For this reason any comparison of toxicity between NSAIDs based on spontaneous ADR reporting had to take account of product life-cycles on the market.[96] He did acknowledge, however, that if an analysis did take this into account together with relative uses of the NSAIDs via prescription data, then a "statistically significant difference" in serious toxicity between one NSAID and another would be sufficient for him to consider using other drugs in favour of the more toxic one.[97]

Later the HRG cited internal Pfizer memoranda and the fact that the recommended dosage for the drug was 20 mg/day regardless of patients age or size to support their claim that piroxicam had a "low margin of safety".[98] In support of HRG's contention that blood levels of piroxicam were elevated in elderly patients Richardson presented her published Canadian study which suggested that the elimination half-life was significantly longer in older than younger women and a second study suggesting that half-life tended to increase with increasing age for men and women.[99]

HRG had petitioned for a ban on the use of the drug in the elderly rather than merely a reduction in dosage because, they argued, the variability in the drug's half-life in the elderly and the difficulty in determining which elderly patients took a long time to eliminate the drug meant that a reduced dosage would be ineffective for some patients.[100] This point seems particularly pertinent in view of the marginal nature of the clinical trial evidence submitted in support of the drug's efficacy prior to approval. According to HRG the high blood levels in elderly patients were especially significant because piroxicam-related GI toxicity was partly, if not mostly, systemic rather than local. In support of this concern they cited the fact that the Australian labelling of the drug recommended a starting dose of 10mg/day due to reservations about the drug's long half-life.[101] HRG also revealed that Pfizer officials had attempted to dissuade the editors of the *British Medical Journal* from publishing an article which concluded that "piroxicam produced an unnecessarily high incidence of severe ulcer disease".[102] The paper was rejected by the *British Medical Jour-*

nal. Pfizer's attempt to suppress publication shows the length to which the company was willing to go in order to influence the medical press received by piroxicam. However, the evidence suggests that Pfizer's intervention did not actually influence the final editorial decision of the *British Medical Journal.*[103]

That unpublished paper was one of six sources which HRG cited to argue that piroxicam was associated with markedly greater serious GI toxicity than other NSAIDs. They did this by calculating for each of the seven NSAIDs common to the studies the ratio of the observed number of serious GI adverse effects to the number that would be expected from NSAID treatment given the particular drug's prescription share. That ratio was consistently high for piroxicam – always the highest except in the comparison with ketoprofen, which had a higher ratio than piroxicam in two of the studies.

Pfizer's defence of piroxicam therapy was in three parts. First, they reviewed 11 pharmacokinetic studies with piroxicam, including two Richardson studies and some studies conducted by Pfizer investigators as shown in Table 12.

The Norwegian research by Rugstad, comparing piroxicam with Naproxen, was by far the largest of the pharmacokinetic studies reviewed by Pfizer. According to the company that study revealed a "statistically significant trend for plasma [blood] concentrations of both drugs to in-

Table 12 Pfizer's summary of studies examining effect of age on piroxicam kinetics.

Study type	Investigator	N	Age	Influence of age
Single dose	Richardson #1	25	20–75	Clearance signif. lower in elderly women
	Campbell	24	19–86	NSE
	Darragh	44	20–80	NSE
Multiple dose	Richardson #2	23	27–79	SE
	Darragh	44	20–80	NSE
	Woolf	19	27–94	NSE
Kinetic monitoring	Hobbs	264	21–83	NSE
	Bollet	93	17–88	NSE
	Lochead	68	20–71	NSE
	Kraag	54	31–79	NSE
	Rugstad	635	24–90	Mean blood levels signif. higher in elderly women only; small effect.

Key: N = number of patients; NSE = no significant effect; SE = significant effect.
Source: FDA Public Hearing Transcript.

crease with age".[104] Thus, Pfizer concluded from all the data in Table 12 that "while there may be a tendency toward increased serum [blood] concentrations of piroxicam in elderly females, these changes are relatively small and similar to those seen in other NSAIDs, such as naproxen".[105]

Secondly, Pfizer argued that the hypothesis that increased blood levels of piroxicam in the elderly caused greater toxicity was not supported by clinical evidence. Pfizer acknowledged that there was an increased risk of GI toxicity in the elderly associated with all NSAIDs, but disputed both that there was any clear relationship between such toxicity and the half-life of piroxicam, and that piroxicam was any more GI toxic to the elderly than other NSAIDs. Specifically, company representatives asserted:

> This elegant Norwegian study [Rugstad] clearly refutes the HRG assertion. There is no difference in GI adverse reactions in piroxicam versus naproxen-treated patients. There is no correlation of blood concentration with either GI adverse reactions in general or serious GI adverse reactions. And the difference in half-lives between piroxicam and naproxen has not been shown to be clinically significant with regard to GI toxicity.[106]

At the hearing Pfizer explained these findings by reiterating Pitts's view that although higher doses of piroxicam were associated with more GI toxicity, and although higher concentrations were found in the blood levels of the elderly, these two findings did not result clinically in greater GI toxicity because such toxicity was "at least in large part due to a local effect rather than a systemic effect".[107]

Thirdly, Pfizer reviewed several epidemiological studies, including the O'Brien & Burnham research in Romford. Data from a Norwegian study by Giercksky was cited as showing that all the NSAIDs "have almost the same potential to induce GI bleeding".[108] Similarly a study by Somerville, argued Pfizer, supported the view that there was no difference between the NSAIDs in GI bleeding and peptic ulceration in the elderly, although the study could only detect a greater than twofold difference.[109] As regards the O'Brien & Burnham study Pfizer scientists disputed its methodology and claimed that the authors should have reached the conclusion that there was no statistically significant difference between piroxicam and other NSAIDs with respect to the risk of GI bleeding.[110]

In concluding, Pfizer reiterated their critique of using anecdotal and spontaneous ADR reporting without correcting for prescription share, product cycle factors and background changes in reporting rates. Background changes, it was argued, relate to the fact that overall reporting rates change over time (e.g. Pfizer maintained that overall reporting rates had increased in the US since 1980 and in the UK since 1976) and that the mass media can influence reporting rates about particular drugs.[111] According to Pfizer if the NSAIDs are compared for spontaneous GI ADR reports for their first two years of marketing then piroxicam is not the most toxic – it is about average relative to the other NSAIDs.[112]

Spiers, a lecturer in clinical toxicology in the UK, who worked for the CSM between 1979 and 1984, presented evidence at the hearing in support of Pfizer's critique of spontaneous reporting ADR data. He argued that regulatory action could not be based on such data and that the latter "does not produce data which aid comparisons of the risks of drugs within the same therapeutic group".[113] Although, somewhat in contradiction with this he stated:

> We can't look for small differences, but I think we can look for, say, 20-fold differences, 16-fold differences [between corrected ADR reports data for different NSAIDs].[114]

He also noted that prescriptions for NSAIDs in the UK are generally for the same length of time and so the correcting for length of prescription advocated by Pfizer was not necessary when using British prescription data for NSAIDs.[115]

Finally, Jick, Director of the Boston Collaborative Drug Surveillance Programme, presented the results of an epidemiological study funded by Pfizer to examine trends of serious GI bleeding in patients over 65 taking NSAIDs. Among his population Jick found that the rate of GI bleeding for all the NSAIDs was similar except for piroxicam which was associated with double the rate of the others, though based on just two piroxicam patients. Regarding the question of whether piroxicam therapy had a greater incidence of serious GI toxicity than the other NSAIDs, he concluded:

> Our conclusion here is not that there is no effect. Our conclusion is that there is no obvious strong effect.[116]

The regulatory authorities decide

The CSM also published their latest views on NSAIDs. The Committee had reached the conclusion that use of NSAIDs was likely to be one of the factors predisposing the elderly to ulcer perforation and advised that those drugs should be given to the elderly only after other forms of treatment had been carefully considered. However, the CSM also took the view that:

it is not yet possible to conclude with confidence that any one member of the class is more toxic than another.[117]

A few months later the CSM published an analysis of the number of fatal and non-fatal serious GI adverse reactions to NSAIDs. The crude numbers of reactions from 1964–85 showed that piroxicam was associated with far more non-fatal serious GI ADRs than any other NSAID and more fatal GI ADRs than any other NSAID, except indomethacin which had been marketed in the UK since 1964. However, figures for the number of such fatal and non-fatal ADRs per million prescription during the first five years of marketing of each NSAID featured piroxicam lower than some other NSAIDs, though higher than most NSAIDs.[118] The British regulatory authorities took no specific action against piroxicam based on such ADR data.

On 28 April 1986 Harter, the FDA's Group Leader for NSAIDs, reviewed Pfizer's submission of evidence to deny HRG's petition. He was deeply critical of Pfizer's submission, describing the company's statements about ascertainment of GI bleeding and ulceration as "meaningless and not thoughtful".[119] He further elaborated:

> They are completely silent on the critical questions of the effect of how often patients were seen, what questions they were asked and what tests are performed, when and on what basis. Most of the studies they give in any detail, including the Norwegian study which is the largest comparative trial they submitted, are silent on these issues.[120]

Regarding the controlled clinical trial data submitted by Pfizer, Harter found that they did not provide "substantial evidence" that a twofold difference in GI ADRs did not exist between piroxicam and other NSAIDs.[121] Overall Harter concluded:

> The clinical trial data submitted . . . is so poorly presented and analyzed that it is virtually worthless to assist us in dealing with the HRG petition. . . . My opinion is that HRG has declared an imminent hazard on the basis of a major misunderstanding of FDA's Voluntary Reporting System plus very weak other evidence. I believe we should concentrate our attention on deciding whether or not HRG have made their case. . . . I am disappointed that Pfizer after a year and a half of working on these studies has come up with such a pitiful effort. . . . I still am of the opinion that piroxicam is high dose NSAID prescription, that many doctors don't realize this (based on personally talking with physicians), partially

because of the way Pfizer initially promoted the drug, and that the suggestion that I made for the labelling last July to warn physicians not to treat patients, who can be maintained on lower dose therapy of some other NSAID, with piroxicam for convenience alone is sensible, good medical advice and a conservative statement that is in the patient's and physician's best interests. . . . I recognize that I am in an analogous position to HRG's, in that I am making a proposal based on 6–8 conversations with physicians to change piroxicam's label.[122]

On 14 May 1986 the FDA made its recommendation to deny HRG's petition. The agency rejected HRG's analysis of FDA spontaneous ADR report data and accepted the arguments put forward by Pfizer that such data must be adjusted to take account of: (1) "secular" changes in reporting rates (e.g. it was argued that the reporting for all NSAIDs had increased since 1982, which the FDA believed was due to greater reporting rather than more risks associated with drugs); (2) the difference in reporting for newly marketed drugs relative to old; and (3) differential age and use patterns between NSAIDs.[123] The FDA also asserted that any use of the agency's spontaneous ADR reporting database needed to exclude foreign reports because such reports could not be reliably related to the number of prescriptions dispensed for the drug in the US.[124]

There are a number of key regulatory principles that were developed in the agency's attempt to close this controversy. These principles take the pseudo-scientific form of epidemiological rationality. For instance, it is assumed that increases in the reporting of adverse effects associated with NSAIDs is merely due to increases in reporting rates rather than a *real* increase in adverse reactions. That assumption builds into regulators' appraisals a bias which implies that *new drugs*, such as piroxicam, only *appear* to be more toxic than their predecessors because of increased reporting rates. The product cycle argument has similar ramifications; it is assumed that because in the past reporting on drugs decreased over time then this must follow for any new drug in the future. That assumption permits regulators to claim that if a new drug exhibits a much higher rate of ADR reports than other drugs in its therapeutic class then that phenomenon is because of the drug's newness rather than its exceptional toxicity. Such assumptions award the new drug manufacturers a substantial benefit of the scientific doubt and help to ensure a respite period from regulatory action during a drug's most vulnerable period on the market. Conversely, patients and consumers may be exposed to a real increased risk from a new drug – a real risk that could be mistaken for more vigilant reporting.

Yet even by making all these adjustments favourable to Pfizer the FDA still found that the number of upper GI adverse effects per million prescriptions reported with piroxicam was 1.65 times that which would be expected for an NSAID as new and as heavily used (especially in the elderly) as piroxicam. According to the FDA this finding was significant, but the agency felt able to conclude:

Although a reporting rate 1.65 larger than expected is statistically significant, it is not alarmingly large.[125]

The agency found no evidence that the rate of fatal upper GI adverse effects per million prescriptions was higher for piroxicam than other NSAIDs, though that conclusion depended on excluding a considerable number of foreign fatal cases associated with piroxicam.[126] The agency considered the small retrospective case studies, such as the O'Brien & Burnham study, to be statistically insufficient to allow a conclusion that a real difference in GI toxicity between piroxicam and the other NSAIDs was being observed.[127] Regarding the epidemiological studies presented at the hearing, such as Jick's study, the FDA interpreted them as showing no evidence of an increased risk of serious GI toxicity with piroxicam compared with other NSAIDs, though the agency acknowledged that all these studies had limitations and were somewhat inconclusive.[128]

The FDA argued that because there was no sound epidemiological or clinical trial evidence that piroxicam posed a greater risk of GI adverse effects than other NSAIDs the pharmacokinetic characteristics of the drug became irrelevant to the question of imminent hazard. However, the agency accepted that its pharmacokinetics were:

potentially pertinent to the labelling of piroxicam: evidence of delayed excretion in a particular population would be reason to urge a lower dose in such persons on theoretical grounds alone, even in the absence of documented risk.[129]

Concerning the pharmacokinetic studies, such as Richardson's, the FDA concluded:

While the data are not consistent they suggest some tendency for plasma concentrations to increase modestly with age. . . . and not a need for major dosing adjustments. It is probably prudent to start a very small person on a lower dose of piroxicam.[130]

Piroxicam remained on the US market without being contra-indicated in the elderly and also without a warning that piroxicam was high-dose therapy as Harter had recommended. The drug survived on many other markets as well, but in Ireland and West Germany there remained severe labelling restrictions about using the drug in the elderly.[131] The Australian regulatory authorities continued to recommend a low starting dose and from July 1986 the Canadian regulatory authorities required Pfizer to state on their Canadian label that:

> The usual maintenance dose is 10–20 mg daily. . . . As elderly patients appear to be at a higher risk from a variety of adverse reactions from NSAIDs and as elderly, frail or debilitated patients tolerate GI side effects less well, consideration should be given to a starting dose that is lower than usual and to an increase of the dose only if symptoms remain uncontrolled.[132]

Moreover, by April 1986 the labelling for Novopirocam, the generic version of *Feldene* in Canada, manufactured by Novopharm Ltd rather than Pfizer, advised:

> *Use in Elderly, Frail or Debilitated Patients*:
>
> Since GI side effects and ulceration from piroxicam are dose related, persons with a decreased ability to eliminate the drug may be more susceptible to adverse effects. Treatment in the elderly, frail or debilitated patients, especially those aged 65 and over should be started with 10 mg a day and increased to 20 mg a day, if necessary.[133]

By the end of 1986 the British Pfizer product data sheet was more liberal than its Australian, Canadian, Irish or German counterparts. Nevertheless, it recommended:

> *Use in the elderly*: Elderly, frail or debilitated patients may tolerate side-effects less well and such patients should be carefully supervised. As with other NSAIDs caution should be used in the treatment of elderly patients who are more likely to be suffering from impaired renal, hepatic or cardiac function.[134]

Conclusion

The piroxicam case shows how regulatory authorities can establish closure of scientific disputes about drug safety and efficacy. These disputes illustrate closure because there is no sense in which the efficacy or GI toxicity of piroxicam were *technically* resolved. The scientific controversies were dissipated by socio-institutional and political means.

The achievement of closure in the UK is different from that in the US.

In the former minimal information is deposited in the public domain; just enough to enable the regulators to help bolster their authority and regulatory decisions based on privileged access to data. Indeed some British medical scientists involved in the dispute about the GI toxicity of piroxicam specifically noted that they had had difficulty in locating official data on prescribing frequency of individual NSAIDs because of a secrecy agreement between the pharmaceutical industry and the DHSS for commercial reasons. By contrast, the FDA's methods of closure are fairly transparent. Internally senior agency officials may override the majority assessment of their scientists irrespective of the technical subtleties of the scientific dispute. In the public context the agency sets protagonists against each other and pronounces its own verdict having listened to the various arguments put forward.

Such actions reveal that scientificity is something that may be mobilized or discarded by regulators in the face of corporatist objectives. In this sense scientific standards can be both a help and a hindrance to regulatory authorities. They are a help when they can be used to give credibility to political decisions, but a hindrance when there is political motivation to reach certain decisions in spite of scientific developments.

The dispute over the efficacy of piroxicam shows how the socio-institutional imperative for closure within regulatory authorities can mitigate technical standards of clinical drug testing. The FDA finally decided to approve piroxicam as effective even though the agency's own rules concerning controlled clinical trials had not been adhered to strictly while the drug was tested for efficacy.

If the debate about the efficacy of piroxicam within the FDA shows the transgression of certain established standards, then the assessment of the drug's GI toxicity reveals the negotiation of standards within the regulatory science of drug epidemiology. There is clearly extensive interpretive flexibility in the evaluation of non-controlled ADR data. The degree of risk attached to a drug relative to others in its therapeutic class can be affected dramatically by how the data are constructed. Are secular changes in reporting patterns over time taken into account or not? Are product life-cycle factors used to modify the comparative raw data? While Public Citizen believed that the relatively large number of piroxicam ADR reports of GI toxicity relative to other NSAIDs reflected a *real* and exceptionally high risk to patients, Pfizer, the CSM and eventually the FDA argued that there was no exceptionally high risk if secular reporting and product life-cycle factors were introduced into the comparison. In taking that approach the regulatory authorities set up an interpretive principle that erected a high threshold of significant risk for new drugs. No science dictated the logical superiority of that approach. Thus, what might appear to be a purely technical regulatory tool was, in fact, a social judgement about acceptable risk.

As regards bias, what is most striking about the closure of the technical disputes about piroxicam is how the benefit of the scientific doubt was *consistently* awarded to the interests of the manufacturers by the regulatory authorities. In particular the FDA closed the dispute about carcinogenicity and efficacy by neglecting its own preferred regulatory standards so that piroxicam could be marketed, yet went to great lengths to establish new and rigorous standards of epidemiological evidence to justify maintaining the drug on the market. And even according to those new standards the FDA found piroxicam to be statistically significantly more GI toxic than other NSAIDs. Regulatory inaction against the manufacturers was justified by reference to the arguably arbitrary and emotive standard that the statisitical significance was not "alarming".

Finally, the controversy over the GI toxicity of piroxicam raises further questions about the adequacy of the British regulatory authorities' handling of *Opren* risks. For example, the FDA believed that pharmacokinetic data could be sufficient to urge a reduction in piroxicam dosage in the elderly in the absence of demonstrated harm. That principle directly conflicts with the argument developed by Kenneth Clarke in Parliament to justify the British regulatory authorities' delay in warning that the daily dosage of *Opren* in the elderly should be reduced.

Chapter Six

Zomax – the persistence of data

Analgesics play the important role in medicine of relieving and/or treating pain. For many years one goal of analgesic drug research has been to find an analgesic more effective than aspirin, but without the adverse effects of narcotics. Such adverse effects include the development of tolerance (which induces patients to increase continually their medication to obtain its positive effects), a feeling of cloudiness and the inability to perform/work satisfactorily. The pharmaceutical company called McNeil Laboratories claimed that they had developed such a non-narcotic analgesic NSAID during the 1970s. It was known generically as zomepirac with the tradename *Zomax*.

Acceptable carcinogenic risk

McNeil Laboratories, a fully owned subsidiary of the Johnson & Johnson company, synthesized zomepirac in 1969, began clinical studies with the drug in the US during 1974 and on 18 December 1978 sought to market it there by submitting a NDA to the FDA.[1] The company submitted two 24 month studies in rats and two 18 month studies in mice as tests for the carcinogenicity of the drug.[2]

FDA evaluation and approval

On 25 October 1979 Manfred Hein, an FDA pharmacologist, found that the incidence of tumours in the soft internal part of the adrenal glands (adrenal medullary tumours) in the male animals in the first rat study increased with the dose.[3] Hein concluded that the NDA was not approvable at that time. A few weeks later FDA statisticians determined that this increase in adrenal medullary tumours with increasing dose was statistically significant.[4]

FDA scientists further determined that the second carcinogenicity study in rats was "confirmatory of the first one".[5] On this basis they concluded that zomepirac should be considered a "tumourigen".[6] McNeil scientists did not dispute the incidence of the tumours, but did challenge the FDA's interpretation of their significance by suggesting three possible ways in which the tumours might have developed even if zomepirac were not a "tumourigen": (a) rats metabolize many compounds differently to humans; (b) the rats may have developed lesions because they were so debilitated by the large experimental doses of zomepirac, which McNeil scientists described as "near lethal levels for the species";[7] and (c) other variables, such as the diet or the environment could have caused the tumours.[8] In addition, McNeil scientists consistently characterized those adrenal medullary tumours as "benign",[9] and concluded that "an increased frequency of benign adrenal medullary lesions is specific to male rats and did not indicate an increased tumourigenic potential".[10]

Thus McNeil scientists attempted to invalidate their own work as a test for carcinogenicity in order to undermine the positive result. Specifically, the experimental design of carcinogenicity tests in animals is supposed to eliminate the possibility that diet, environment and factors other than the presence of the test drug could have a significant impact on the differences detected between tumour occurrences in the test animals and the control animals. That the increase in adrenal medullary tumours with increasing drug dose was statistically significant suggests that it is unlikely that other variables caused the tumours, unless one rejects the fundamental principles of drug toxicology. Moreover, if the rats developed tumours because they received excessively large doses of zomepirac, then this only serves to show that McNeil conducted an inappropriate experiment. As regards differences between humans and rats in metabolizing zomepirac, this possibility does not alter the tumourigenicity of the drug in rats – a finding which implies some carcinogenic risk to humans that needs to be taken into account.

When Hein again came to review zomepirac carcinogenicity on 20 May 1980, he recommended:

> If zomepirac is to be approvable on other grounds a box warning in the labelling as a minimum is indicated alerting to the carcinogenic potential based on 2 yr rat study.[11]

Moreover, on 16 October 1980 William Mulloy, the only FDA pathologist to examine the tumours in the first rat study, concluded that they were malignant.[12] This was clearly a significant conclusion because just over a week earlier Marion Finkel, the agency's Associate Director for New Drug Evaluation, recommended that whether the tumours were benign or malignant should be stated on the *Zomax* package insert.[13] Yet on 28 October 1980 the FDA approved a daily dose of 400–600 mg zomepirac for marketing with labelling that included no box warning and merely read under "Carcinogenesis, mutagenesis and impairment of fertility":

> In two 2-year studies in rats at doses up to 7.5 mg/kg/day (approximately the human dose in mg/kg), the incidence of adrenal tumours was increased. In two 18-month studies in mice at doses up to 10 mg/kg/day zomepirac sodium did not show evidence of tumourigenicity.[14]

Furthermore, in connection with a proposal from the manufacturers that the labelling should refer to the dose in the first rat study as twice the human dose, on 21 September 1981 the FDA pharmacologist, Sydney Stolzenberg, argued that the drug's labelling was misleading:

> The first paragraph under the heading of "Carcinogenesis, Mutagenesis and Impairment of Fertility" is misleading. The first sentence indicates that "doses up to 7.5 mg/kg/day (approximately the human dose in mg/kg)" were used. Actually, this dose was reduced to 7 mg/kg on week 18 and to 6 mg/kg on week 35. Therefore, the dosage during 69 weeks of this two year study was 50–75% human dose of 400–600 mg/day.[15]

However, Temple, Acting Director of the Office of New Drug Evaluation, believed that stating "approximately the human dose" was a sufficient indication of the kind of dosage that had produced the tumours and he noted that that statement was "meant to be scary" since positive carcinogenicity findings usually result from doses in the test animals that are several times the expected human dosage.[16]

McNeil believed that the ratio of the dose in the first rat study to the human dose should be based on the blood levels of the drug in the body, thus taking account of the different pharmacokinetics of the drug in rats and humans, rather than simply the amount ingested. Stolzenberg recommended that McNeil's proposed changes to the labelling should be rejected. However, on 7 March 1983, three days after McNeil had withdrawn the drug from the market worldwide, the FDA approved a request by the manufacturers to replace the above carcinogenicity labelling with the following:

In a 2-year rat study at dosage levels approximately twice the human dose (based on blood level determinations) the incidence of benign adrenal medullary tumours was increased in males. In another 2-year rat study at doses approximately the human dose there was an increase in adrenal medullary hyperplasia, but no increase of tumours in males. There was no increase in adrenal lesions in two 18-month studies in mice at doses approximating the human dose or in the 12-month study in monkeys at three times the human dose.[17]

Thus, the agency accepted a representation of the dosage of the first carcinogenicity test in rats, which the FDA's own pharmacologist regarded as misleading, and removed the supposedly "scary" aspect of the warning. It was also willing to characterize the significant tumours of the study as benign, contrary to the evaluation of the only FDA scientist who undertook the appropriate histopathological examination, and contrary to the following position later taken by Temple on 19 August 1983:

> I don't think we would be prepared to say they [the adrenal medullary tumours] are unequivocally benign.[18]

UK approval – saying nothing

As for the British regulatory authorities, they approved zomepirac for marketing in March 1981 "for the treatment of pain in . . . osteoarthritis and rheumatoid arthritis" as well as other conditions such as "post-traumatic pain related to musculoskeletal injury", "post-operative pain", "pain secondary to oral surgery" and "pain secondary to malignancy".[19] In the UK the drug was marketed by another Johnson & Johnson subsidiary known as Ortho-Cilag. It is clear from the initial *Zomax* data sheet produced by Ortho-Cilag and approved by the British regulatory authorities, that the drug was expected to be used chronically as well as in other ways since doctors were advised to monitor patients "on long-term therapy" because of concerns about possible adverse effects on kidney or liver functioning.[20] Moreover, the indication for treatment of pain in osteoarthritis and rheumatoid arthritis implied an indication for chronic use. There certainly was no warning against chronic use. Prescribing doctors were also informed that "no teratogenic effects [fetal toxicities] have been found in animals", and that:

> Animal studies have indicated that bicarbonate alkalinization significantly enhances zomepirac elimination from the plasma and suggest that this measure would have benefit in a clinical overdosage situation.[21]

Thus, Ortho-Cilag and the British regulatory authorities did think that it was worth mentioning the negative teratogenicity findings in animals and the possible extrapolation of how the drug was eliminated in animals to certain human situations. Yet in all the *Zomax* data sheets they omitted to make any mention whatsoever of the carcinogenicity studies with the drug, including the positive "tumourigenicity" finding in rats, much less explicitly suggest that positive findings might be extrapolated to the human risk situation.

Substituting non-approval with warnings

Regarding the malignant character of the adrenal medullory tumours, Finkel has claimed that Mulloy told her in an FDA internal discussion that he concluded that they were benign. According to Finkel she was able to remember this discussion because it was about "a very important issue".[22] Yet agency files contained no written record of this discussion. Furthermore, in response to Finkel's claims Mulloy has stated:

> I diagnosed the adrenal rat tumours as malignant. . . . Communication with Dr Marion Finkel was by memo which would become a permanent record of the Department, not in personal meeting with her.[23]

> At no time did I represent to Dr Marion Finkel of the FDA that these tumours were of no consequence in consideration of the drug which had been administered to the rodent population. The potential for malignancy was raised by me, in view of the frequency of the tumours and the appearance of the cells which composed them. . . . Malignancy in this type of tumour is reported as high as 10 per cent.[24]

It is impossible to say with certainty who – Finkel or Mulloy – is correct in their recollection. What is clear is that the written record implies that Mulloy believed the tumours were malignant, and that this was his final judgement on the matter. While the *Zomax* product data sheet approved by the CSM recommended chronic use of the drug, the labelling approved by the FDA warned doctors:

> Because of animal tumourigenicity findings . . . caution should be exercised in considering *Zomax* for chronic use.[25]

Regarding communications with the medical profession, FDA Commissioner Hayes maintained that it was important to point to what was known and important.[26] Nevertheless, Harter acknowledged that the above zomepirac labelling was somewhat less than explicit:

The labelling essentially attempted to make the drug not of choice for chronic use. *It didn't say specifically that you should try other drugs first,* but it really suggested all these reasons why chronic use was not its preferred use. The labelling in a sense was *trying* to send a message to physicians to use it only after other means had not been successful.[27](Emphases added)

The agency was aware that zomepirac would almost certainly be used chronically by many patients. For example, on 9 February 1979 John Harter wrote to several of his senior colleagues asserting:

It is my opinion that all drugs with anti-inflammatory properties should meet the same chronic toxicity and carcinogenicity require-ments no matter whether they are submitted for one or all of the indications which members of this class of drugs have been ap-proved for. This is because the likelihood is quite high that they will . . . be used chronically.[28]

In fact, agency officials have estimated that in the US 20 per cent of the patients on zomepirac (i.e. 100,000 people per month) were chronic users who, therefore, took 55 per cent of the tablets.[29] Moreover, McNeil adver-tised zomepirac stressing its usefulness in treating chronic pain and claim-ing that it represented "a logical first choice in both chronic and convalescent pain".[30] Evidently, although the agency wished to warn against the chronic use of zomepirac, it was willing to permit extensive chronic use of the drug. This occurred in the context of an FDA regulatory policy that a drug found to be carcinogenic in animal tests should not be approved unless there were no therapeutic alternatives of at least equal efficacy.[31] That policy seems to have been reaffirmed by Temple regard-ing zomepirac in April 1983:

If all one were able to say is that the drug [zomepirac] is another NSAID with no advantage over other similar agents, it is obvious that making it available for chronic use would not be consistent with the attitude toward the tumourigenicity findings in the first place.[32]

Gross's analysis

In connection with Congressional hearings concerning the FDA's regula-tion of zomepirac held on 26 and 27 April 1983 and at the request of the Congressional House Committee on Government Operations, Adrian Gross, a senior scientific advisor at the Environmental Protection Agency (EPA) and former FDA pathologist, reviewed the animal carcinogenicity tests of the drug in rats and mice. He supported Hein's overall recommendation that zomepirac was not approvable because it had not been satisfactorily tested for carcinogenicity and his conclusion that increased dose of the drug was associated with increased incidence of medullary tumours of the adrenal gland in male rats. Gross was not able to determine himself whether those tumours were malignant, but he accepted Mulloy's evaluation that they were malignant.

Gross's analysis, however, was much more critical than any emanating from the FDA. The first rat study, the centrepiece of the zomepirac carcinogenicity controversy, had the dosage regime in body weight terms shown in Table 13.

Hence, on a body weight basis only the high-dosed rats received approximately the human dose. Moreover, Gross argued that, because pharmacokinetic and metabolic processes in general are more directly related to surfaces than to weight, it is more appropriate to conduct a "species-translation" of dosage based on body surface area instead of body weight. This makes a considerable difference because on a body-surface basis a 60 kg human is no longer "equivalent" to about 141 rats weighing 425 g each, but only $141^{2/3} = 27$ (approx). Applying the appropriate calculations Gross estimated the dosages shown in Table 14.

According to Gross, the dosages given to the rats in this carcinogenicity study should have been regarded as a small fraction of the recommended human dose for the drug. He described the statement in the package insert claiming that zomepirac had been given to the rats at approximately

Table 13 Dosage of first zomepirac carcinogenicity study in rats.

Dosage group	Average doses in rats (mg/kg/day)	Average daily doses given to rats (mg/day)	Equivalent total human dose (mg/day)	Percentage of recommended human daily dose
low	2.2	0.9	129.8	21.6–32.5
mid	4.3	1.8	259.6	43.3–64.9
high	6.1	2.6	368.6	61.4–92.2

Table 14 Dose in rats as a percentage of human dosage.

Dosage group	Average doses in rats mg/kg/day	Percentage of recommended human daily dose on body-surface basis (%)
low	2.2	4.2–6.2
mid	4.3	8.3–12.5
high	6.1	11.8–17.7

the human dose as "vastly misleading".[33] Notably, the FDA's official response to Gross's analysis accepted that his use of body-surface species translation was more appropriate than the body weight approach if the drug was metabolized identically in both species.[34] But, argued the FDA, pharmacokinetic data suggested that zomepirac was absorbed differently in rats and humans and so blood level interspecies comparisons were more appropriate.[35] More generally the FDA commented:

> Regarding the preferable use of surface area over body weight, it is well recognized, certainly among toxicologists and clinical pharmacologists, that any attempt to extrapolate doses between species is inevitably arbitrary, regardless of the exact method chosen as a basis for the extrapolation. As a matter of practice, if not for any scientifically persuasive reason, mg/kg is accepted as a common and convenient means of comparing doses in animals and humans in acute and chronic toxicity studies, and there is no overriding reason to assume that extrapolation based on surface area is any more reliable or precise for most drugs.[36]

Assuming that the FDA is correct in asserting the arbitrariness of interspecies extrapolations (and this is questionable since at least one major toxicology text, published in 1980, considers the surface area method superior to the body weight method[37]) it is significant that the agency consistently selected methods of extrapolation (first body weight instead of body surface and then blood levels instead of body weight) which represented the dosage in the rat studies as being higher, rather than lower, relative to the recommended human dose. In each case the manufacturers received the benefit of the scientific doubt.

Like the FDA statisticians who reviewed this study, Gross found that the dose-related increased incidence in medullary tumours of the adrenal gland of the male rats was statistically significant. He further found that there was an "acceleration" in the appearance of such tumours, that is, the time to "death with tumour" was shortened in a dose-dependent manner. According to Gross "this, by itself, is a sufficient criterion for carcinogenicity".[38] He concluded:

> In view of the highly significant trend of the incidence of these malignant tumours with dose, one can conclude without much doubt that this study had *not* established that any dose of the agent on test, *Zomax*, can be viewed as *not* being associable with carcinogenic activity; in other words, this particular drug product ought to be viewed as a carcinogen.[39] (Emphasis in original)

For these reasons Gross believed that it was misleading for the package insert to state merely that "the incidence of adrenal tumours was increased". He recommended that it should have said:

> Malignant tumours primary in the medulla of the adrenal gland were increased in incidence in a highly significant dose-dependent fashion in male rats at dosage considerably below those recommended for human use.[40]

As regards the other carcinogenicity tests in rats and mice, Gross agreed with FDA scientists that the second rat study tended to confirm the first – particularly important, in his view, because the doses given to the rats in the second study were even smaller than in the first.[41] He considered the quality of two mice studies as insufficient to draw any reliable conclusions and was not convinced by McNeil's data that the statement on the package insert claiming that the two mice studies "did not show evidence of tumourigenicity" was justified.[42]

Tumourigen or carcinogen?

Another difference between Gross's characterization of zomepirac and that of the FDA is that Gross concluded that the drug ought to be regarded as a potential carcinogen in humans, whereas the agency labelled the drug as a "tumourigen". Scientists agree that a particular tumour can be benign or malignant, and that a malignant tumour is defined as cancerous. Often, though not always, whether or not a tumour is benign or malignant can be ascertained from histopathological analysis. A carcinogen is a cancer inducing substance and, therefore, the term "tumourigen" implies a substance that induces tumours, which may or may not be malignant. However, Gross considered the term "tumourigen" as a misnomer because, of those substances which produce tumours there is none known to induce solely benign tumours.[43] (That is, all "tumourigens" produce some malignant tumours hence all "tumourigens" are actually carcinogens).

Temple seems to have agreed that no tumour-producing substance induces solely benign tumours for he testified:

> it is a general dogma – *and I basically believe it* – that any drug that causes tumours in an animal should be considered as having some potential to cause malignant tumours in that animal in a different dose or in a different animal or conceivably in man. Therefore, I more or less agree with what Dr Gross said about that question.[44] (Emphasis added)

Temple further acknowledged that the FDA "accepted the idea that the findings in the rats could represent some degree of carcinogenic risk for man", and explained that it was for this reason that the package insert included "a warning against chronic use".[45]

What's a few tumours between friends?

Temple defended the agency's decision to label zomepirac as a tumourigen and asserted that the data from the animal studies showed that the drug should be called a tumourigen rather than a carcinogen, even though the only FDA pathologist to examine the medullary adrenal tumours characterized them as malignant.[46] According to Temple, scientists have reported extreme difficulty in defining adrenal medullory tumour as either benign or malignant[47] – a view supported by Gross. Nevertheless, speaking on behalf of the FDA, Finkel testified:

we felt that the tumours did not behave in a malignant manner.[48]

Moreover, Temple emphasized that "the tumourigenic finding was not perceived as a particularly scary one" because there was not "clear cut malignancy",[49] and whatever malignancy there was was of a "very low" order.[50] Finkel also took the view that the carcinogenic risk of zomepirac was minimal, arguing that "prudence dictates that one consider, unless it can be ruled out, that the drug does, in fact, have some *mild tumourigenic effect*".[51] (emphasis added). These judgements partly account for the FDA's conclusion in its official Summary Basis of Approval (SBA) for *Zomax* that:

The adrenal tumourigencity findings in rats are not sufficiently conclusive to prevent approval of this drug. However, because of these findings *Zomax* is not recommended for use in children and caution is recommended in using it chronically in adults.[52]

Indeed on the 5 February 1982 the FDA agreed to McNeil's request to omit the word "tumourigenicity" from the warning section of the package insert because senior officials at the agency agreed with the firm that "the label had perhaps just too much emphasis on the word 'tumourigenicity'".[53]

In addition to the above comments by Finkel and Temple, Commissioner Hayes justified the evaluation of the adrenal medullory tumours provided in the SBA by arguing that (a) mutagenicity studies were negative; (b) such tumours were not found in the two mice studies nor were they increased above controls in female rats in the two rat studies; (c) such tumours are common in untreated rats; (d) no other tumour type was increased in any of the rodent studies; and (e) a 12 month monkey study did not show any precursor lesion to such tumours.

These justifications illustrate the relentless way in which senior FDA scientists sought to underplay the positive carcinogenicity finding in one rat study and its partial confirmation in a second. For it was well known within the field of carcinogenic toxicology that a substance can be carcinogenic despite negative mutagenicity findings; that failure to find a significant association between a certain type of tumour in one species or one sex does not negate a positive tumour finding in another species or sex; that failure to find a plethora of drug-related tumour types in the species in question or other species does not undermine the carcinogenic risk associated with such a positive drug-related finding for one type of tumour in that particular species; that the common appearance of a tumour type in untreated animals does not undermine a statistically significant drug dose-related increased incidence of those tumours compared with control animals in an experimental setting; and that a 12-month study in monkeys is far too short a period to provide any reliable reassurance that a drug is not carcinogenic. As for the 18 month mouse studies FDA pharmacologists believed that they should have been run for two years and that one of them was started at doses that were too high.[54]

FDA's risk–benefit assessment

In October 1979 Finkel provided the FDA's policy rationale for recommending the non-approval of a drug intended to treat gout called benzbromarone, as follows:

> We concur with your scientists that while not appearing to be a potent carcinogen there can be no question but that benzbromarone is a definite carcinogen in the rat. Although this does not prove it is a carcinogen in man, it is well accepted that it indicates a potential risk of carcinogenicity to humans. We feel that this potential carcinogenic risk must be judged against the benefit which the drug may provide to those individuals for which it would be prescribed. Currently there are available marketed therapeutic alternatives for the treatment of hyperuricaemia [gout] which have not been shown to have a similar carcinogenic potential and which are equally efficacious. Therefore, in our judgement the potential risk outweighs the potential benefit which the drug may provide, and

under section 505(b)(1) of the [Food, Drug and Cosmetic] Act, approval of this application must be denied.[55]

In keeping with this policy on 20 May 1980 Hein recommended that zomepirac should not be approved for marketing "pending resolution of whether adrenal medullory tumourigenicity can or cannot be tolerated in a drug for which there are alternative therapeutic agents available".[56] FDA Commissioner Hayes has explained how the agency resolved to approve the drug as follows:

> There has been a long quest for a non-narcotic analgesic with greater effectiveness than aspirin. The data showed that zomepirac represented such a drug. The analgesic specialists in FDA . . . believed that it had been shown to be as effective as 8–12mg of morphine and all reviewers found it equivalent to 2 acetaminophen plus 60mg codeine. These factors were considered sufficient to support approval for predominantly short-term use as an analgesic, despite the tumourigenicity in male rats.[57]

However, FDA scientists had not determined that zomepirac was of superior efficacy to alternative drug therapies that were not carcinogenic in animal studies. Indeed, in a meeting between the agency and McNeil on 4 March 1983 Temple "questioned the need for another analgesic equal to aspirin with codeine or acetominophen with codeine"[58] and Harter proposed:

> labelling *Zomax* not for initial therapy and for use only when all other NSAIDs have been unsuccessful. Patient information should include a warning about . . . using it only as last resort.[59]

Temple testified that when he made the above comment on 4 March 1983 he was not aware that the analgesic group in the FDA considered zomepirac equivalent to and a potential replacement for modest doses of morphine. For Temple, if that were true, it would make zomepirac a drug of considerable value.[60] Thus, it was zomepirac's potential for replacing morphine therapy which crucially defined the drug's unique effectiveness according to the agency.

Yet on 24 September 1980, just one month before approval, Harter, the leader of the group in the FDA responsible for regulating NSAIDs, described the studies submitted to the agency by McNeil, which compared the efficacy of zomepirac with morphine, as "confusing".[61] Previously FDA statistician Jerome Senturia had raised a number of problems concerning those studies[62] and as late as 22 September 1980 he concluded that McNeil had "not responded adequately" to the problems raised.[63]

On 26 April 1983 Harter reiterated his view when he testified that he was not convinced of zomepirac's equivalence to morphine:[64]

> I recognized that we didn't know whether it was equivalent to morphine. I couldn't say it wasn't equivalent to morphine. I just felt the tests that were performed didn't establish it and I thought it was still an open question and feel that way today.[65]

In fact, the FDA did not approve zomepirac as equivalent to morphine; deciding instead to wait for the results of further ongoing studies.[66] However, Harter also found these studies inconclusive and the agency never approved such claims of equivalence to morphine as part of the *Zomax* labelling.[67]

Despite his questioning of the need for another analgesic equal to aspirin with codeine or acetaminophen with codeine on 4 March 1983, Temple, on 26 April 1983, testified that zomepirac was "uniquely effective compared to other NSAIDs that had been approved for lesser degrees of pain".[68] However, Finkel took the view that other NSAIDs might be found to be just as effective for treatment of such pain had they been so tested.[69] In justifying the approval of the drug, despite its carcinogenic potential, she stressed that "it was not intended to treat arthritis a disease of many years duration", but rather "was largely intended for short term use".[70] Yet this is entirely inconsistent with the agency's policy of requiring analgesic NSAIDs to meet the carcinogenicity standards as anti-arthritic NSAIDs because of the FDA's knowledge that a substantial proportion of patients would, in fact, use such analgesics chronically. It may also be noted that Finkel's justification contradicts considerably the recommendation by Ortho-Cilag and the British regulatory authorities that zomepirac could be used for the long-term treatment of pain in arthritis.

Anaphylactoid reactions – predictable shocks?

Anaphylaxis is a hypersensitive state of the body to a foreign agent (usually protein) such that the injection of a second dose of the agent brings about an acute shock-like reaction which may be fatal. Anaphylactoid reactions are those that resemble anaphylaxis.

On 16 April 1981 the first published report concerning an association of an anaphylactoid reaction to zomepirac appeared. The author noted that in a personal communication McNeil had told him that "anaphylactoid reactions to zomepirac had not previously been reported".[71] According to the FDA Commissioner, the agency received its first report of a serious hypersensitivity (anaphylactoid) reaction associated with zomepirac on 5 May 1981, approximately six months after the drug's approval for marketing in the US. This report was incorporated into an FDA *ADR Highlight* published on 26 May 1981 which focused attention on anaphylactoid reactions to NSAIDs.[72] That publication had been preceded by another *ADR Highlight* published on 20 June 1979 describing anaphylactoid reactions to tolmetin – another NSAID, with a chemical structure very similar to that of zomepirac, which was associated with a disproportionately high number (27 per cent) of such reactions compared with other NSAIDs relative to its market share (2 per cent).[73] Many of the tolmetin-associated anaphylactoid reactions had been published in the medical literature prior to zomepirac's approval.[74]

By 4 March 1983, when the drug was withdrawn from the market, the FDA had recorded 923 acute hypersensitivity reactions associated with its use, including five fatalities. McNeil, however, had recorded 1,026 such reactions, of which they classified approximately 58 as life-threatening, 160 very serious (i.e. requiring hospitalization), 300 reasonably serious, 300 mild reactions, such as rashes, and 300 unclassified.[75] In the first seven weeks subsequent to withdrawal of zomepirac the FDA received a further 400 reports of anaphylactoid reactions, including between five and ten fatalities, and McNeil also classified more reactions – 18 life-threatening, 54 serious, 113 reasonably serious and 229 as mild.[76] Moreover, the senior FDA staff were in no doubt that these data reflected the causal fact that there had been fatal and very serious reactions to zomepirac.[77]

When zomepirac was approved for marketing in the US in October 1980 its labelling did not mention anaphylactoid reactions.[78] Indeed Harry Meyer of the FDA has testified that the clinical trials involving several thousand people did not indicate that the drug was associated with anaphylactoid hypersensitivity reactions.[79] McNeil scientists also claimed that "no anaphylactoid reactions had occurred in [zomepirac] clinical trials, so anaphylactoid reactions were not mentioned in the original prescribing information".[80] When post-marketing cases of anaphylactoid reactions to zomepirac began to be reported it was against a background of extensive use and so the supposed absence of such reactions during clinical trials tended to reinforce the FDA's view that those reactions were "rare".[81]

It was not until 21 July 1981 that McNeil revised the zomepirac package insert to include anaphylactoid reactions,[82] even though Robert Gussin,

Vice President for Scientific Affairs at McNeil has testified that "during the period November 1980 to June 1981 anaphylactoid reactions were first noted",[83] with the company receiving its first report of a post-marketing anaphylactoid reaction in the US on 28 January 1981 over a month before approval in the UK.[84] Despite this, Ortho-Cilag's product data sheet for *Zomax* approved by the British regulatory authorities in March 1981 made no mention of anaphylactoid reactions to the drug. The data sheet merely warned against giving zomepirac to patients who had manifested hypersensitivity to other NSAIDs.[85] However, by 1982 the British data sheet did specifically acknowledge anaphylactoid reactions, stating:

As with other NSAIDs anaphylactoid reactions have been reported. Because of the possibility of cross-sensitivity due to structural relationships which exist among NSAIDs anaphylactoid reactions may be more likely to occur in patients who have exhibited allergic reactions to these compounds, particularly tolmetin sodium.[86]

This echoed precisely some of the general precautions stated in the US package insert of April 1982. Notably neither the British data sheets nor the American package inserts mentioned the fact that by April 1982 at least one anaphylactoid reaction had been *fatal*.

Furthermore, a Congressional Committee discovered adverse reactions, occurring in three patients taking zomepirac during US clinical trials, which a consultant expert allergist characterized as anaphylactoid reactions.[87] He considered one of those reactions, involving a patient "with respiratory impairment requiring intensive treatment in a hospital emergency room", to be "life-threatening".[88] Though FDA officials challenged the assessment of the other two adverse reactions as zomepirac-induced anaphylactoid,[89] they did accept that the latter case was likely to be zomepirac-related and was a "serious anaphylactoid reaction".[90] In retrospect the FDA acknowledged that it could have provided more explicit warning about such reactions.[91] The agency's failure to do so in the light of zomepirac's close chemical relationship with tolmetin, a known anaphylactoid-inducer, suggests a rather permissive approach to pre-marketing clinical risk assessment.

More specifically, according to a McNeil memorandum dated 19 February 1985, in the course of an FDA retrospective review of *pre-approval* zomepirac clinical trial case report forms Harter found "approximately 23 instances of *Zomax*-related allergy-anaphylaxis" with an incidence "roughly between 3 and 7 times that which obtained with aspirin usage in these trends".[92] This implies that there may have been very good reason to include a warning about anaphylactoid reactions to zomepirac therapy in both the initial US package insert and the British product data sheet.

Defying reason

Following the first post-marketing report of a fatal anaphylactoid reaction to zomepirac the FDA met with McNeil on 22 and 29 March to discuss labelling revisions and a "Dear Doctor" letter to be sent to physicians regarding anaphylactoid reactions.[93] As previously noted zomepirac was approved in the US with a warning about chronic use, and although a substantial number of patients used it chronically, many patients took it intermittently. At the March 1982 meetings McNeil informed the FDA that the intermittent use of zomepirac posed a particularly problematic risk and proposed that the "Dear Doctor" letter should warn about patients who might be at greater risk:

> . . . anaphylactoid reactions have been reported, and patients with the following characteristics are at a higher risk of developing anaphylactoid reactions: . . . Patients with prior history of uneventful exposure to *Zomax* or other NSAIDs – most patients have taken *Zomax* uneventfully. However, the development of hypersensitivity with intermittent re-exposure cannot be ruled out.[94]

According to Temple this information from McNeil was no surprise and the agency had already formed such an impression about zomepirac and indeed tolmetin.[95] However, the actual "Dear Doctor" letter which was finally sent to physicians on 9 April 1982 omitted the reference to a greater risk in "patients with prior history of uneventful exposure to *Zomax*".[96] Harter has testified that he decided to delete such reference in order to stress the higher risk to patients who had experienced a mild reaction to the drug previously. He justified this action as follows:

> I felt that of all the people who had developed anaphylaxis it was not those people who showed nothing on previous exposure. It is true that they had some risk, but more importantly the high risk people were the people who had any evidence of allergic reaction on previous exposure. In fact, as we have gone through the reports coming in, it is not uncommon for a person to have a mild reaction, not recognize it as such, not take it for a while. Then when they take it again those are the people who have the highest risk. A person who took it before and didn't have any problem at all is at a lower risk.[97]

Yet, the data contained in the FDA's May 1981 *ADR Highlight* suggested that only two out of seven (28.6 per cent) of the individuals having an anaphylactoid reaction to *Zomax*, who had earlier taken that drug, previously reacted to it. Only 6 out of 42 (14.3 per cent) of patients having an anaphylactoid reaction to zomepirac or tolmetin, who had earlier taken the same drug, previously reacted to it. By comparison, 17 out of 43 (39.5 per cent) of patients having anaphylactoid reactions to NSAIDs (including aspirin) other than zomepirac or tolmetin, who had earlier taken the same drug, previously reacted to it.[98] Thus the FDA's own data implied that only a minority of zomepirac-related anaphylactoid reactions were characterized by a previous reaction to the drug.

Moreover, this suggests that it was significantly more difficult to predict serious hypersensitivity reactions to zomepirac and tolmetin, based on prior allergic history, than to other NSAIDs. In short, what follows from the agency's database is inconsistent with the FDA's justification for permitting McNeil to remove the warning about the risk of zomepirac associated with prior uneventful exposure and intermittent use. Furthermore, according to a McNeil memo, by 31 March 1982 the company had received reports of allergic/anaphylactoid reactions in 178 patients, of whom 7 had experienced the reaction on first dosage, 25 on continuous therapy and 68 on the first dose following a break in therapy (i.e. intermittent use) with the remaining 78 patients' records not containing dosing information.[99] Evidently by March 1982 substantial evidence was available to McNeil and FDA scientists that the greatest risk of anaphylactoid reactions to zomepirac was in patients taking the drug intermittently.

According to Harter, if he had decided that it was necessary to warn of an increased risk of anaphylactoid reaction associated with the intermittent use and a prior uneventful history of zomepirac therapy, then that would have suggested that "anybody is in danger" and he would have been inclined to require extensive relabelling of *Zomax* as a "second-line drug" (i.e. one which should only be used after all alternative therapies have been exhausted).[100] Nevertheless, the FDA elected to give the drug the benefit of the doubt and Commissioner Hayes even testified that it would have been misleading to warn physicians that, compared with other NSAIDs, zomepirac was especially anaphylactic to patients without a prior allergic reaction compared with other NSAIDs.[101]

By August 1982 some McNeil staff had become extremely disturbed by the large number of anaphylactoid reactions to zomepirac and urged an action plan of "top priority" to investigate "the cause, detection and prevention" of those reactions.[102] It was not until 11 February 1983 that the agency recommended that McNeil should consider changing the labelling of zomepirac to stress the greater risk of anaphylactoid reactions in patients using the drug intermittently, and not until 28 February 1983, less than a week before the manufacturers withdrew zomepirac from the market, that it recommended that *"Zomax* be labelled not for initial therapy but for those patients who do not get satisfactory relief from other NSAIDs".[103] In fact, the drug's labelling never was changed to warn of the increased risk of intermittent use or to recommend second-line usage only.

Expert advice and the repackaging of risks

On withdrawing zomepirac from the market McNeil told the FDA that 75 per cent of the anaphylactoid reactions to the drug were "with intermittent use or restarts".[104] Subsequent to the withdrawal of zomepirac, McNeil sought to *re-market* the drug specifically for chronic use, even though long-term administration of the drug was likely to increase its carcinogenic risk. The FDA referred the question of whether the drug should be re-marketed for chronic use to its Arthritis Advisory Committee on 19 August 1983.

By that time FDA scientists had acknowledged that anaphylactoid reactions were "much more numerous" with zomepirac than other NSAIDs.[105] One epidemiologist estimated that the risk of an allergic reaction for a patient exposed to zomepirac was 2.55 times greater than for other NSAIDs.[106] Moreover, Temple argued that this figure of increased risk relative to other NSAIDs should be taken as a minimum and for that reason was "pretty impressive".[107] Data produced by the CSM in the UK also indicated that zomepirac was associated with a greater frequency of reported anaphylactoid reactions than other NSAIDs.

At that Arthritis Advisory Committee meeting McNeil argued that the relatively high risk of anaphylactoid reactions to zomepirac resulted from the drug's intermittent use, but not its chronic use:

> Approximately 75 per cent of them [anaphylactoid reactions] occurred on the first dose after reinitiation of therapy . . . there is a subset of the general population for whom *Zomax* can be prescribed appropriately. Such patients are those suffering from intractable pain, such as cancer pain, that have not been responsive to other NSAIDs or analgesics. . . . The available data suggests that such patients are at a reduced risk of suffering an allergic [anaphylactoid] reaction *while they remain chronically on the drug.* For these patients in whom the benefits outweigh the risk of an allergic

reaction, the analgesic properties of *Zomax* make it the drug of choice. We believe, therefore, that with changes in labelling and a strong educational programme for physicians and patients that *Zomax* can be used with minimal risk by those patients who need it and for whom acceptable alternative therapy is unavailable.[108]

The significant changes in labelling proposed by McNeil included a prominent box-warning highlighting the higher incidence of anaphylactoid reactions to zomepirac, a warning about allergic reactions from intermittent use of the drug and an indication that because of the anaphylaxis zomepirac should not be given to patients unless alternative drugs had been tried unsuccessfully.[109]

In 1982 the FDA established a policy for new drugs which tolerated a "somewhat greater incidence of side effects" in a drug compared with other drugs in its class "if those side effects are sufficiently offset by greater benefits".[110] Moreover, with respect to zomepirac FDA Commissioner Hayes testified in April 1983 that "to allow the return of zomepirac to the marketplace [the agency] would have to conclude that there is a population of patients in whom the risks of its use would be outweighed by its benefits".[111] Even if such a population did exist one of Commissioner Hayes' "conditions for remarketing zomepirac" was that the drug should demonstrate its superiority to other NSAIDs:

> there might be a population in which a relatively high risk might be acceptable, e.g. patients who cannot tolerate narcotics and who do not respond to non-narcotic analgesics. In this case, however, studies would be needed to determine whether other NSAIDs could function as well as zomepirac against narcotics. To date these have not been done.[112]

At the Arthritis Advisory Committee meeting Temple reiterated the FDA's view that it was important to identify a "real population" for which zomepirac was uniquely effective.[113] During that meeting, however, William Beaver, one of McNeil's expert consultants implied that such a population could not be identified:

> The question, can we identify *a priori* the kinds of patients who would do better on this drug than, say, some other nonsteroidal? Well, no. That's the problem. We can identify patients that we *suspect* will do better on this drug than, perhaps, narcotic-containing combinations.[114] (Emphasis added)

The FDA acknowledged that since April 1983 when Commissioner Hayes had noted that no studies to identify such a population had been carried out, "no additional data from adequate and well controlled studies were provided to the [Arthritis Advisory] committee regarding patient population identification".[115] This problem was posed squarely by Saul Bloomfield, a member of the FDA's Arthritis Advisory Committee:

> in order to come to an informed decision as to whether or not this agent [zomepirac] should be re-introduced, we need to see studies performed in the exact, specific patient population that [it] is proposed that this drug be introduced for, namely patients with intractable chronic pain, and that these include a comparison with other non-steroidal anti-inflammatory agents to indeed determine whether zomepirac will be effective in those patients that are unresponsive . . . we need controlled studies giving us good data that will show substantiated evidence that zomepirac will indeed be a useful addition to the armamentarium for analgesics used for patients with chronic pain.[116]

Nevertheless, the Committee voted in favour of re-marketing zomepirac as a second-line drug, and indeed conditioned its recommendation on the manufacturer's undertaking to conduct studies *during* re-marketing in order to identify and define such a "real population".[117] That recommendation directly contradicted the FDA's position that those studies should be completed *prior* to re-marketing.

As regards the re-marketing of zomepirac for chronic use, it may be noted that FDA scientists were not necessarily convinced that the increased incidence of anaphylactoid reactions associated with zomepirac relative to other NSAIDs was a result of the drug's intermittent use. In this connection Temple stated in April 1983 that patients could suffer a serious anaphylactoid reaction "on the first time of use" and on using the drug chronically, as well as intermittently.[118] And Commissioner Hayes testified that the relatively high frequency of hypersensitivity reactions to the chemically similar tolmetin, which was not used intermittently, suggested that the increased frequency of anaphylactoid reactions to zomepirac might be "related to the drug itself" rather than to its intermittent use.[119] The Commissioner concluded that it would be difficult to prove in advance that re-marketing zomepirac for chronic use would significantly lower the risk of anaphylactoid reactions,[120] and Temple declared that before such re-marketing one would have to conclude that:

> the risk of anaphylaxis would not be so severe where the drug is given chronically. . . . it is not clear how you would reach that conclusion.[121]

Furthermore, at the Arthritis Advisory Committee meeting Judith Jones, an FDA epidemiologist, acknowledged that whether the increased risk of zomepirac-associated anaphylactoid reactions compared with other NSAIDs was due to chemical difference or type of usage remained unresolved, and that "critical" studies still needed to be done to ascertain "whether or not repeated intermittent exposure in fact increases the risk considerably".[122]

Evidently, even by the time of the Arthritis Advisory Committee meeting the FDA did not have the data it considered necessary to conclude that the risk of zomepirac-associated anaphylactoid reactions would be less severe when the drug was given chronically. Hence, according to the criteria of the agency's own senior officials, it did not have the data required to make a proposal to re-market zomepirac for chronic use. Furthermore, FDA scientists, including the Commissioner had determined that zomepirac "seems to have no advantage in chronic use over aspirin or other NSAIDs in arthritis",[123] and Temple testified that before even considering the re-marketing of zomepirac for chronic use there would have to be "substantial new information" that such use of the drug had some advantage over other NSAIDs.[124] Yet again McNeil's own expert consultant scientist, William Beaver, acknowledged the "lack of data" in this respect:

We just simply don't know what happens when you move into these other models [of chronic pain], and these other models are the ones that are relevant to the question being put today. . . . There is very little data that other NSAIDs compare in the way you have seen zomepirac comparing with morphine in, say, cancer pain or chronic pain. So we are suffering from a lack of data in this regard. . . . To my knowledge, there are no nose-to-nose comparisons of zomepirac with the other non-steroidals in, say, cancer pain or other chronic pain problems that are even ongoing or have been done.[125]

Beaver further noted that "from the limited data available in the treatment of rheumatoid arthritis, zomepirac doesn't look particularly impressive at all".[126]

That this lack of data persisted even until March 1985 was later confirmed by the FDA.[127] And yet again the Arthritis Advisory Committee recommended that such efficacy comparative studies in "chronic pain models" should be undertaken *during* the re-marketing of zomepirac to determine whether the drug did have advantages over other NSAIDs in that context of use.[128] This was completely contrary to the FDA's supposed criteria for re-marketing, which stipulated that such comparative advantage in efficacy should be demonstrated as a *precondition* of re-marketing.

In addition, Commissioner Hayes testified in April 1983 that before re-marketing zomepirac for chronic use "it would be necessary to reconsider the implications of the rat adrenal medullary tumour finding".[129] More specifically, Temple, elaborated:

> In deciding whether the drug should be available for long-term use as opposed to the short-term uses now stressed in the labelling . . . you would have to conclude something new and different about the risk of tumourigenicity. . . . If all one were able to say is that the drug is another NSAID with no advantage over other similar agents, it is obvious that making it available for chronic use would not be consistent with the attitude [of the FDA] toward the tumourigenicity findings in the first place.[130]

At the time of the Arthritis Advisory Committee the FDA had not received any new information about the tumourigenicity of zomepirac and had not reached a new or different conclusion to that stated in the initial labelling regarding the meaning or significance of the tumourigenicity findings in the rat.[131]

Given the situation described above there seems to have been little or no basis on which the FDA could properly seek the advice of the Arthritis Advisory Committee about whether to re-market zomepirac for chronic use because, according to the agency's own scientific and regulatory criteria, no such re-marketing could be justified. Moreover, during the Committee meeting the FDA provided the Committee with regulatory options which violated the agency's own established scientific criteria by asking the Committee whether additional studies to establish a population in which zomepirac was uniquely effective should be conducted as a condition of re-marketing, and if so, whether they should be carried out before or during re-marketing.[132] At one stage during the Committee meeting Harter even recommended to the Committee that those studies should be conducted after the drug had been permitted to return to the market.[133] Although later he recognized that such a proposal was problematic:

> I think part of the problem is, if you answer no, has a population been adequately identified, and you have to do the study to identify it, how are you going to market it in the meantime, who are you going to market it for in the meantime?[134]

Evidently some senior FDA scientists gave serious consideration to re-marketing zomepirac *before* determining whether it was safe and effective in use, as defined by the agency's own scientific and regulatory standards.

The penny drops

Ultimately the FDA did not fully accept the Arthritis Advisory Committee's recommendations. By March 1985 Harter had reached the conclusion that "because the risk of an anaphylactoid reaction is substantially greater with *Zomax* than with other NSAIDs, about 10 fold based on spontaneous reporting, *Zomax* should only be used in patients with chronic moderately severe to severe pain, such as the pain of malignancy, who have not obtained adequate relief with several other NSAIDs and who cannot be managed satisfactorily with other analgesics".[135]

The agency concluded that either: (a) McNeil would have to conduct studies which demonstrated unique effectiveness in chronic pain models in patients who had not responded to other NSAIDs *before* re-marketing; or (b) the company could re-market the drug without such prior testing but the labelling would indicate the drug's use "primarily for chronic pain of malignancy, but also for carefully selected patients with other chronic pain, in patients unresponsive to other NSAIDs or intolerant of analgesic narcotics, and only in a setting where safe use can be assured, such as an in-patient or medically controlled setting".[136]

Even this latter option, which reduces the risk from anaphylactoid reactions ignores the potential carcinogenic risk with chronic use of zomepirac in patients other than those already suffering from malignant cancer pain or perhaps pain from other fatal diseases, and fails to provide evidence that zomepirac is any more likely to be effective in such patients than alternative NSAIDs. The FDA's reasoning here seems to be based on a sort of desperate trial and error approach. Although the situation of chronic pain sufferers unresponsive to NSAIDs and/or narcotic analgesic may well be desperate, as Congress has noted, the agency has a legal responsibility to conclude that a drug is safe and effective *before* it approves it for marketing.[137] Notably, McNeil decided not to re-market zomepirac under the above conditions set out by the FDA and the drug never returned to the market, presumably for commercial reasons.[138]

Finally, on 27 April 1984 the British Medicines Commission held a hearing to consider whether zomepirac should be re-marketed in the UK. The Commission rejected the proposal for re-marketing because it was concerned about anaphylactoid reactions and was not convinced of any unique benefit to outweigh that risk. In addition, and most significantly, the Commission found that the results of the carcinogenicity studies were a cause for concern.

This is important because the Commission did not review any *additional* animal carcinogenicity tests. If those tests were cause for concern in 1984 shouldn't they also have been a cause for concern in March 1981 when zomepirac was approved in the UK? If that concern was a reason for with-holding re-marketing in 1984 should it not also have been a reason for withholding approval in 1981 or at least sufficient reason for some mention of the drug's carcinogenic potential on the approved *Zomax* data sheet? Unfortunately, because of the secrecy surrounding the British regulatory authorities' activities it is impossible to obtain conclusive answers to these questions. Nevertheless, the stark inconsistency between the position of the Medicines Commission in 1984 and the British Licensing Authority in 1981 remains.

Conclusion

This chapter confirms many of the insights about corporate bias developed in the previous chapters. The manufacturers of *Zomax* attempted to undermine their own positive carcinogenicity findings in order to persuade the regulators that the drug should be approved. They were also willing to market the drug in the US with a caution against chronic use, while simultaneously recommending its chronic use in the UK. Moreover, having previously marketed *Zomax* in the US with a caution against chronic use McNeil later advocated re-marketing the drug specifically for chronic use without any new evidence to suggest that the carcinogenic risk was reduced. This shows how the industrial imperative of marketing a drug can give rise to a corporate bias that is characterized by discarding the troublesome results of industrial science itself.

The zomepirac case study provides further detailed evidence of how the regulatory authorities in the UK and the US are consistently willing to award the benefit of the scientific doubt to manufacturers rather than patients. The depth of that bias in the US was probably greater in this case than any previously considered in this book because it filtered through to the very basics of toxicological science, such as the definition of a carcinogen and the conventions of dosage extrapolations from animals to humans.

Yet such bias cannot make tumour findings or anaphylactoid ADRs disappear. That persistence of data creates major problems for industrial and government scientists who do not want to undermine the corporate interests of pharmaceutical companies, but also feel the need to defend the credibility of science for reasons of public legitimation or otherwise. This produces a tension and helps to generate inconsistencies in argumentation. Once again the technical inconsistencies contained in the accounts and actions of the regulators are in congruence with a steady trend prioritizing industrial interests over patient safety. Many more technical inconsistencies can be identified in the American than in the British regulatory context. However, that does not imply that the British regulatory decisions are less biased, merely that they are more protected from public scrutiny. That secrecy could suggest that, were the British regulatory decision-making processes to be exposed to rigorous public examination, as many inconsistencies might be found as currently obtain in the relatively open US situation.

In the case of the FDA these inconsistencies can be seen in the form of senior scientists' self-contradictory stances as well as in their decisions to overrule the recommendations of their own expert staff without credible reasons. For example, FDA management ignored the recommendation of their own scientists that the *Zomax* package insert should contain a box warning highlighting the carcinogenic risk of the drug. And rather than alert doctors to the possibility that all patients might be in special danger of anaphylactoid reactions from zomepirac, the FDA decided not to warn of the increased risk even with a prior uneventful history of treatment with the drug.

Furthermore, the zomepirac case confirms the proposition that serious ADRs are not an inevitable consequence of drug therapy. The hazards of zomepirac could have been markedly reduced by taking into account all clinical trial results, and even avoided entirely if the drug had not been marketed in the first place. The zomepirac case, however, did break new ground at the FDA in the sense that it heralded a policy in which carcinogenic drugs, which had no significantly greater efficacy than existing therapies, could be put on the market. The crucial shift in thinking that was emerging within the FDA management was that risks, rather than being grounds for non-approval, should as far as possible be tolerated and put on the label. That approach is clearly visible also in the way that the FDA handled the anaphylactoid risks of zomepirac. The broadening of the expert advice sought does not necessarily offer much comfort to patients as the performance of the Arthritis Advisory Committee who recommended the re-marketing of *Zomax* has shown. The fact that the British and American regulatory authorities decided against such re-marketing is a measure of the extremely high risk–benefit ratio associated with the drug.

Chapter Seven

Suprol –
anything goes?

Suprofen was manufactured by Ortho Pharmaceuticals, a wholly owned subsidiary of Johnson & Johnson. Ortho Pharmaceuticals first filed an NDA for suprofen with the FDA in October 1978. That was withdrawn because of alleged irregularities and possible falsification of data by some clinical investigators of the drug (independently of the company), and then re-filed in August 1981.[1] In 1982 the British regulatory authorities approved the marketing of suprofen for the treatment of pain, including pain in osteoarthritis and rheumatoid arthritis. Use of the drug was indicated for long-term therapy on all the UK-approved data sheets.[2] Notably, according to Andrew Veitch, as late as October 1986 a spokesperson for the British regulatory authorities said that they were not aware of any false data submitted to the CSM.[3] However, official secrecy under the Medicines Act prevents us from knowing whether or not suprofen was approved partly on the basis of falsified data. Meanwhile, in the US suprofen was developed as a pain killer for arthritis.

Carcinogenicity – moving the goal posts

On 7 July 1980 Manfred Hein reviewed Ortho's first carcinogenicity study in Wistar rats for the FDA. He considered that the "high mortality alone" (60 per cent in control males after only 15–18 months) was "adequate to invalidate the study as a carcinogenicity trial". In support of his view he cited PMA guidelines which recommended that carcinogenicity studies should be terminated when mortality reduces the original number of control animals to 40 per cent, and that carcinogenicity tests of two years in rats were desirable. Hein concluded that this study was:

inadequate in meeting our standards for a well controlled test of carcinogenicity in rats.[4]

Consequently, the FDA recommended a repeat carcinogenicity study in rats.[5]

In December 1984 Ortho submitted a second carcinogenicity study in rats; this time Long Evans rats. On the 18 July the FDA pharmacologists, Conrad Chen and David Richman, reviewed both two-year carcinogenicity studies in rats and an 18-month carcinogenicity study in mice which had also been submitted by that time. For the Long Evans rats study there was a statistically significant positive finding regarding adrenal tumours (pheochromocytoma) in the test animals compared with controls. This prompted these FDA scientists to re-inspect the incidence of pheochromocytoma in the first Wistar rat study. They discovered that there was also a statistically significant drug-related increase in the incidence of pheochromocytoma in that study.[6] Chen considered this finding particularly significant because the high rate of mortality among the Wistar rats on test made it difficult to detect drug-related increases in tumour incidence since tumours are most likely to be induced over a long period and hence in the latter part of the animals' life-spans.[7] As for the 18-month mouse study, Chen & Richman reported a statistically significant drug-related finding of liver tumours (hepatomas). Consequently, Chen concluded:

> Suprofen causes pheochromocytoma in two strains of rats and causes hepatoma in one strain of female mice. It is felt that [the] NDA should be approved only if the clinical benefits would outweigh this possible risk.[8]

These views were fully endorsed by Richman who argued:

> It is concluded that we do have adequate evidence that suprofen produces an increase of pheochromocytoma in two strains of rats and of hepatomas in both sexes of mice and that these findings are not random. It is recommended to our medical reviewers that these findings be given adequate weight on the risk portion of the benefit/risk equation when making their decision to approve or not to approve this product.[9]

In the light of these findings John Palmer, Director of the FDA's Division of Oncology and Radiopharmaceuticals, recommended to Robert Temple, Director of Drug Research and Review, that suprofen should not be approved since it lacked "sufficient redeeming intrinsic features" in terms of safety or efficacy compared to other drugs in its class to compensate for its carcinogenicity, and because labelling it as a tumourigen would pass on the judgement regarding the drug's carcinogenic risk to prescribing doctors, who would be even less equipped than FDA scientists to make that judgement.[10] By contrast, John Harter, the FDA's Group Leader for NSAIDs, argued that there were as many negative tumourigenicity findings (i.e. where the incidence of tumour types in the control group is statistically significantly higher than in the test animals) as positive ones, and that positive findings involved types of tumours common in untreated mice and rats. He further commented:

> Although our statisticians feel that the statistical methodology is sound, I am not convinced that we are not studying random variation. Further, assuming that these findings are reproducible, I personally am not convinced that such findings have any meaning for man.[11]

Thus Harter sought to undermine the statistically significant positive findings of some tumour types by citing the existence of negative findings regarding other tumour types. On this basis he challenged the conclusions of the FDA's own statisticians. In any case he seems to dismiss the whole exercise of animal carcinogenicity testing by implying that even sound positive findings may not be worthy of much attention in assessing human risk.

Moreover, Harter was "not convinced that there are patients who have such a unique response to one NSAID that no other gives them the same quality of life" so he recommended approving suprofen as a drug which has caused "statistically significant increases in common animal tumours", and which should be "not for initial use".[12] Nevertheless, on 24 December 1985 Temple, on behalf of the FDA, approved suprofen as a *first-line drug* (i.e. for initial use) for the treatment of mild to moderate pain. Under "Carcinogenesis, mutagenesis, impairment of fertility" the labelling stated:

> Two 2-year studies in rats and an 18 month study in mice were performed to evaluate the carcinogenic potential of the drug. The initial rat study had inadequate survival. In mice, an increased incidence of benign liver tumours occurred in females at a dose of 40 mg/kg/day (approximately three times the human dose). Treated male mice also had an increased incidence of hepatomas (not dose related) when compared to control animals. No evidence of carcinogenicity was found in doses as high as 40 mg/kg/day in the rat and mouse.[13]

Temple defended this decision by claiming that there was extensive scientific debate about whether the liver tumours in mice were "unique to the mouse" with "uncertain if any significance for man".[14] He acknowledged, however, that "there is no absolutely clear way to answer the debate".[15] As a consequence, according to Temple, the labelling referred to the liver tumour findings because "some people would want to know that", but FDA's final regulatory decision seems to have been non-committal about suprofen's potential carcinogenic risk to humans, leaving that judgement to prescribing doctors.[16]

As for the positive findings of adrenal medullary tumours in the two rat studies, Temple maintained:

> They can arise when the animal is stressed in a variety of ways, it is not at all clear they correspond to what we think of as carcinogenesis. . . . the drug was clearly not gene active . . . So whether those [rat tumours] have any meaning I think it is impossible to say with absolute certainty.[17]

Despite the fact that the FDA's own pharmacologist and Director of the Division of Oncology and Radiopharmaceuticals had concluded that suprofen produced adrenal medullary tumours in two strains of rats and recommended that that finding be taken into account in the overall benefit–risk assessment of the drug, Temple felt able to omit such conclusions in approving the drug's labelling on the grounds that there was not absolutely certain evidence of carcinogenic risk to humans. Although he admitted that he could not assert that there was no carcinogenic risk to humans from suprofen.

As Director of the Office of Drug Research and Review, Temple's approach reflects the official regulatory position of the FDA's management. That position may be contrasted with the views expressed by Temple about zomepirac's carcinogenicity in 1983 when he had similar official status within the agency:

> It is widely stated by people who study tumourigenicity that a finding, even of benign tumours, could represent some carcinogenic risk for man. And that is a position that is really impossible to disagree with. I think that is true. If we did not believe that was true we would not have reflected the finding in labelling at all because there would be nothing to worry about. So we accepted the idea that the findings in rats could represent some degree of carcinogenic risk for man. That is true. I don't think anybody disagrees with it.[18]

Evidently, Temple's downplaying of the human carcinogenic risk of suprofen-related "benign" tumours in mice flatly contradicted his own views about carcinogenicity expressed four years earlier. That there is no chemical agent which elicits exclusively benign tumours remains the position of expert pathologists, such as those working at the US National Cancer Institute.

Furthermore, unlike the FDA's approval of zomepirac, suprofen's labelling did not warn against chronic use due to positive carcinogenicity findings. According to Temple, this was because in the suprofen case "we [senior FDA officials] felt the finding was often more uncertain".[19] Yet it is clear from the reviews of the FDA scientists who actually evaluated the carcinogenicity tests with suprofen and zomepirac (as discussed in Chapter 6) that those scientists' evaluations do not imply that the carcinogenicity of suprofen was more uncertain than zomepirac.

According to Gross, who was asked to review the FDA's carcinogenic risk assessment of suprofen by Congress, Temple not only believed that the drug's carcinogenicity was uncertain, but also wrote to the manufacturers on 9 October 1985 stating that "we [the FDA] believe the adrenal medullary tumours cannot be considered treatment [suprofen] related" because of "marginal statistical significance".[20] By contrast, Gross calculated that those tumours and the liver tumours in the mouse study were related to suprofen in a highly statistically significant way, including the animals given dosages at 40 mg/kg/day (three times the human dose), and concluded that "*Suprol* is much more of a tumourigen or carcinogen than was demonstrated for *Zomax*".[21]

As for the manufacturers, they remained adamant that suprofen did not pose a significant carcinogenic risk to patients. For example, according to Veitch, Medical Director of Ortho-Cilag, who marketed the drug in the UK argued that the tests had shown that suprofen might cause tumours in animals but provided no evidence that it could cause cancer in humans. Here again we see senior industrial scientists seeking to undermine the significance and fundamental purpose of their own carcinogenicity testing in animals when the results are positive. For a crucial principle of chemical toxicological testing (especially carcinogenicity testing) is that the tests are conducted in animals in order to inform an assessment of the cancer risk in humans. If a positive result in such animal tests can be considered as "no evidence" that the drug could cause cancer in humans, then there seems to be little point in undertaking the tests in the first place.

The FDA's approval and labelling of suprofen is even more remarkable because, according to Gross's report to Congress, in response to Temple's communication on 9 October 1985, Ortho Pharmaceuticals stated that: (a) for the mouse study benign *and malignant* liver tumours occurred in the females in a positive (i.e. suprofen-related) statistically significant way (p = 0.0021); (b) for the Wistar rat study benign adrenal medullary tumours occurred in males in a positive statistically significant way (p = 0.0423); (c) for the Long-Evans rat study benign *and malignant* tumours occurred in females in a positive statistically significant way (p = 0.0087).[22] This suggests that senior FDA officials not only overruled some of the views of their own scientists, but also rejected the manufacturer's scientific assessment that suprofen induced tumours, including malignant ones, in a statistically significant drug-related fashion in both mice and rats.

Gross also testified that in a memorandum concerning the carcinogenicity tests with suprofen, on 23 October 1985, Temple suggested a p = 0.01 rather than the usual p = 0.05 probability criterion for determining statistical significance.[23] Thus, according to Gross, the Director of Drug Research and Review was proposing to alter statistical analyses at the fundamental level of significance decisions. That is, an alteration which increases the probability of accepting the null hypothesis (that there is no quantititative difference between the tumour induction in the control animals and the test animals) when, in fact, it is not true – a "false negative". Consequently, a significance criterion of p = 0.01 is necessarily less patient protective than one of p = 0.05. Nevertheless, the former p value does make it easier to argue that the suprofen-related adrenal medullary tumours in the rats were only marginally significant, although the liver tumours in the mice are still clearly significant even on a p = 0.01 decision value, as shown by the p values given above.

Finally, by considering the relationship between the recommended human daily dose and the daily doses given to the test animals in terms of body-surface ratios instead of body-weight ratios, Gross determined that the doses given to the rats were approximately half the recommended human dose and the doses given to the mice about one-fifth of the human dose. The package insert asserted that the drug produced "benign" tumours in mice at doses "three times the human dose". Gross concluded that this statement was a "15-fold exaggeration".[24]

Not untypically the suprofen data sheets approved by the British regulatory authorities reported negative teratogenicity results from animal studies, but did not mention the positive carcinogenicity results in animals. Nevertheless, according to Veitch, the CSM had studied the data from carcinogenicity tests in animals that McNeil had submitted to the FDA. Indeed, Veitch has reported that, according to a spokesperson for the DHSS, "the CSM assessed it [the carcinogenicity data] carefully before deciding that a product licence should be granted".[25]

Efficacy and risk–benefit analysis

Suprofen was first developed in 1972 in Belgium and was introduced into Europe for treatment of pain and arthritis in 1982.[26] The efficacy of suprofen was not impressive according to FDA scientists. When Harter reviewed suprofen on 25 June 1985 he concluded that it "probably has the least favourable benefit to risk ratio of the NSAIDs we have approved recently".[27] Moreover, on 25 November 1985, just one month before the agency approved the drug, the FDA informed the drug's sponsors that "suprofen will be the first drug to be approved in about 10 years that has demonstrated no benefit, efficacy or safety, over aspirin".[28]

During November and December 1985 Cilag, another wholly owned susbsidiary of J & J in Switzerland, contracted the Institute for Clinical Pharmacology (IPHAR) in West Germany to conduct two studies to see how effectively the suprofen liquid formulations were broken down and used by the body (i.e. bioavailability) compared with the 200mg capsules that were finally marketed. Nine of the 24 healthy volunteers in these two studies (i.e. 37.5 per cent) developed mild to severe flank (lower back) pain after taking the liquid formulation and three of those nine experienced flank pain again upon re-challenge with suprofen in capsule form, while five showed signs of kidney damage. In addition to those nine, three volunteers showed signs of acute kidney toxicity, making a total of half the subjects on the two studies exhibiting signs and/or symptoms of acute kidney toxicity.[29]

According to an FDA inspection the results of the IPHAR studies became available to McNeil's International Division on 26 February 1986 and 29 April 1986,[30] and McNeil's medical personnel by 19 June and 30 June 1986.[31] It was not until 29 July 1986 that McNeil informed the FDA of the IPHAR studies.[32] No major findings of flank pain were uncovered in other pre-approval clinical trials. Consequently, when suprofen was first approved in the US its labelling did not mention the flank pain syndrome.[33] However, following post-marketing reports of 16 cases of flank pain

McNeil proposed, and FDA approved, revised labelling on 24 April 1986 and a "Dear Doctor" letter on 25 April 1986 warning of the adverse reaction and its association with signs of abnormal renal functioning.[34]

By June 1986 about 100 cases of flank pain had been reported to the FDA who required McNeil to send a second "Dear Doctor" letter issued on 10 July 1986, which updated physicians about the status of the reaction.[35] That letter informed doctors that the reporting rate from the flank pain reaction was 1 in 5000, but did not mention the IPHAR studies which suggested a much higher incidence, even though it was issued 10 days after McNeil medical personnel were found to have become aware of the IPHAR results.[36]

Both Temple and Harter acknowledged that if the FDA had known about the IPHAR results by 10 July 1986 then the agency might have required them to be mentioned in the "Dear Doctor" letter in addition to the statement about a 1 in 5000 reporting rate.[37] Indeed, an FDA memorandum dated 27 August 1986 recounted:

> Dr Harter stated that he thought suprofen should be relabelled as second line use only for its present indications and that FDA would have pushed for this relabelling sooner if FDA had known about the two foreign studies conducted by IPHAR. . . . These studies suggest that the incidence of mild flank pain with suprofen is more common than previously thought by FDA.[38]

Eileen Barker, a medical officer for the FDA's Division of Oncology and Radiopharmaceutical Products regarded the IPHAR results as "astonishing" because they were so inconsistent with other pre-marketing data, and because they pointed so clearly to the drug's acute kidney toxicity.[39] McNeil scientists, however, argued that the company was not required to report those results within 15 days under FDA regulations because the findings were neither "serious" nor "unexpected".

As a result of the IPHAR studies, according to Temple, during the summer of 1986 the FDA concluded that "the flank pain syndrome was potentially fairly frequent in some patient groups" and "although certainly painful and unpleasant . . . continued to be reversible in all cases followed".[40] On 10 September the agency, therefore, required McNeil to relabel suprofen explicitly as a second-line drug and to issue a third "Dear Doctor" letter drawing attention to that labelling change.[41] Thus, the FDA permitted the drug to remain on the market (albeit as a second-line drug) even though FDA scientists had concluded that "it provided no unique benefit".[42] Moreover, the agency scientists were not at that time able to rule out the possibility of "long-term kidney damage" for the patients who experienced adverse acute kidney reactions to suprofen.[43]

In permitting suprofen to remain on the market as a second-line drug the FDA decided to adopt, in effect, a policy of "trial and error" with respect to medication. Suprofen was to be used if other therapy failed despite the fact that no real population had been identified that would uniquely benefit from the drug.[44] FDA officials recognized that this was a "close decision" and so they referred it to the agency's Arthritis Advisory Committee on 2 December 1986.[45] In fact, at that meeting Temple argued:

> The idea of a last resort analgesic needs to be probed. We have temporized, pending a trip to this committee, with the idea that suprofen should be used for people who do not respond to or cannot tolerate other drugs. *But it is very important to try to figure out whether that is a real population, whether there is any such thing.*[46] (Emphasis added)

Yet, according to Temple, the FDA had no scientific evidence that identified a patient population who responded better to suprofen than any other drug in its class.[47] Moreover, Temple told the Arthritis Advisory Committee that suprofen "has no unique benefit".[48] Nevertheless, in apparent contradiction of the well established FDA policy that "a somewhat greater incidence of side effects may be tolerated in a drug . . . as compared [to its] class as a whole, if those side effects are sufficiently offset by greater benefits"[49] the FDA and its Arthritis Advisory Committee agreed that suprofen should remain on the market, although the Committee recommended that the flank pain reaction be cited in a black box warning on the label.[50]

On 11 March 1987 a fourth "Dear Doctor" letter was issued to explain the recommendation of the Arthritis Advisory Committee.[51] By this time there had occurred several hundred cases of suprofen-related flank pain in the US alone. On 12 May 1987 the European Community's expert committee on the safety of medicines declared that they would no longer permit suprofen to be marketed in the EEC. A few days later McNeil decided to withdraw the drug from the market worldwide.[52]

Conclusion

The suprofen case demonstrates that the political penetration of regulatory science by corporate bias can run so deep as to involve the "re-writing" of statistical rules. Such "re-writing" helped the FDA management to represent a clear-cut statistically significant result as a marginal one, thereby apparently increasing the scientific uncertainty regarding the carcinogenicity of suprofen in animal tests. The discussion in this chapter also provides further evidence of the FDA's reluctance to remove drugs from the market even if they provide no special benefit to patients, and are especially hazardous relative to others in the same therapeutic class.

The agency's preference for warning about hazards on the label instead of removal from the market, in effect, passes on regulatory decisions to prescribing doctors who receive much of their information about new drugs from pharmaceutical company representatives. It is, therefore, a regulatory approach in the interests of industry, but against the interests of patients, because it increases the risks of hazardous prescription.

Once again the trust that regulatory authorities invest in pharmaceutical companies proved problematic because significant risks from pre-approval human studies emerged only after approval in the US. Perhaps the most serious instance of corporate bias concerning suprofen was the way in which the FDA permitted the drug to remain on the market despite the possibility of long-term kidney damage from the flank pain reactions. However, that was just one instance in a consistent trend in which the agency awarded the benefit of the scientific doubt to the manufacturers rather than to patients.

This case study also suggests that the CSM did not insist that the positive carcinogenicity findings in animals should be reported to prescribing doctors on the product data sheet, even though they had reviewed the relevant animal tests. In the absence of comprehensive access to CSM files conclusions must be tentative, but it does seem that animal tests which showed the drug in a poor light were treated with intense secrecy.

Chapter Eight

Conclusions and policy implications

In this chapter I draw out the main conclusions from the discussions in the previous chapters. This will enable us to crystallize more clearly the key facets of corporate bias in drug development and regulation.

Too often research in science and technology studies provides rich accounts of the social processes of science and technology, but stops short of discussing the implications for political change. In my view that academic internalism is a mistake. Social science research should attempt to provide an intellectual basis for social and political intervention and should not, therefore, shy away from the policy implications of its findings. With these principles in mind I close this book by considering what kinds of political frameworks for drug testing and regulation should be developed in order to provide patients with a rational medical science which supplies safe medicines that are needed.

Industrial drug testing

The findings in this book provide further evidence that the Mertonian perspective on the norms of science, which holds some sway,[1] is of limited relevance to the conduct of science in industry. Merton supposed that bias in science was restricted to the abuse of scientists by politicians, and to anti-meritocratic distortions internal to the academic reward structure (e.g. the "Matthew Effect"). For Merton, the "ethos of science" demanded "logical consistency and consonance with the facts". However, investigation of drug toxicology and pharmacology suggests that people who are institutionally defined and recognized as scientists can be very much involved in bias in science.

Rather than evaluating the therapeutic value of new drugs in terms of "logical consistency and consonance with the facts" many of the industrial scientists featured in this book have put forward self-contradictory arguments or made claims that were logically inconsistent with the established scientific standards of drug testing and medication at the time. At the company level this can extend to recommending the chronic use of a drug in the UK while simultaneously cautioning against such use in the US, as occurred in the *Zomax* case. Moreover, those technical inconsistencies repeatedly coincided with the commercial interests of the pharmaceutical company involved, often by emphasizing drug efficacy or by downplaying drug toxicity.

Thus, the preceding analyses of technical controversies concerning the safety and effectiveness of NSAIDs has demonstrated that there is plenty of scope for a divergence and even conflict of interest between patients and pharmaceutical companies when the therapeutic value of a drug becomes controversial. The case studies in this book do not support the complacent industrial viewpoint that commercial interests can be relied upon to deliver the best marketing decisions for patients.

A likely explanation for these technical inconsistencies is that senior industrial scientists share the commercial perspectives of their company managers to some extent. It seems that these perspectives lead them to take an "instrumentalist" view of their science as a means primarily to produce data that will demonstrate product safety and efficacy in order to overcome regulatory hurdles. Similar instrumentalism among scientists was found by Ellis, who reported:

> Each interviewee [scientist] was asked whether the academic who was faced with a choice between publishing or selling the results of his [or her?] work had a moral obligation to make his knowledge public to his fellow scientists. Most industrial scientists felt that he should follow his immediate self-interest; e.g. do what was best for his future.[2]

Other research has suggested that even university undergraduates, who enter industry without an instrumentalist view of their science, soon develop such a view through enculturation or, as Barnes suggests, in response to the demands of success in their new situation.[3] Consequently, what Schwarz & Thompson refer to as "the moral commitment . . . to a particular institutional perspective" may become central to scientists' actions.[4] Furthermore, Lynn's research suggests that a common feature of the industrial institutional perspective is that technological risks in society are exaggerated.[5] When that commitment diverges from patients' interests and is subjected to critical scrutiny it is likely to generate technical contradictions and inconsistencies as industrial scientists attempt to serve the master of commercialism in a context where they are required to represent their actions as primarily beneficial to patients.

Evidently, economic and political goals structure the social practices of scientists. The commercial imperatives of the industry direct scientists to conduct studies of specific use to companies in clearing regulatory hurdles, rather than to engage in research strategies intended to advance scientific knowledge about the pharmaco-medical needs of patients *per se*. Perhaps the most pronounced feature of this is the fact that many scientists in the pharmaceutical sector involve themselves in the testing of "me-too" drugs, which offer no therapeutic advance. For example, in May 1979, even before the Reaganite deregulatory crusade of the 1980s, the FDA calculated that of the 1,816 pending INDs, 39 represented important therapeutic gains, 157 offered modest therapeutic gain, and the remainder were of little or no therapeutic importance.[6] This is not to suggest that the commercial goals of scientists in industry never converge with patients' medical needs. In particular, as noted in Chapter 2, many of the regulatory standards which the pharmaceutical industry has been required to meet have been in the interests of patients at the margins. Nevertheless, because neither the British nor American regulatory authorities are routinely permitted to refuse approval of a drug on grounds of comparative efficacy, it is commercially viable for companies to manufacture drugs which do not offer any therapeutic benefits over existing medicines.

Cozzens & Gieryn are right when they conjecture that "laboratories are political and economic forces".[7] The case studies of NSAIDs in this book provide some details about the nature of those forces in the pharmaceutical sector. Industrial scientists may expend considerable effort in an attempt to produce evidence that a drug is exceptionally effective, but only undertake important toxicity checks if required to do so by regulatory authorities. And in responding to the latter regulatory demands, a company is likely to mobilize scientists who are sympathetic to the company's commercial concerns.

At a more micro-social level, corporate bias may be involved in the production of scientific papers through various degrees of editorial control and intervention exercised by drug manufacturers. In some contexts where positive claims about the therapeutic effectiveness of the drug are put forward editorial intervention by the company will be minimal and directed towards strengthening the certainty of those claims. In other contexts where claims about adverse toxicity of the drug are being made then the editorial intervention of the manufacturers is likely to be substantial and concentrated on emphasizing the uncertain and tentative nature of the claims.

In noting the profound ways in which the commercial goals of industrial drug testing can, and have been shown to, bias the work of scientists, it is important to appreciate that such bias is neither all-pervasive nor uniform. This is particularly so at the interfaces between pharmaceutical companies, clinical investigators and prescribing doctors. When their product comes to be tested in clinical trials and in the marketplace, firms have to involve themselves in negotiations with scientists not in the full employment of the company. The nature of that involvement can vary from one of close sponsorship by the company, as in Lilly's relationship with Kligman, to one of virtual independence between the two parties, as in Lilly's interactions with Hamdy and Taggart.

Consultant scientists' vulnerability to corporate bias can be affected by the degree of their mutuality of institutional interests with the company. For example, institutionally Kligman was an "insider" *vis-à-vis* Lilly scientists. He had a close and long-standing relationship with the company, and was willing to co-operate very substantially with Lilly in pre-publication negotiations about how the problem of phototoxicity should be finally presented in the scientific journal. By contrast, Hamdy was an institutional "outsider" who approached Lilly to explore the pharmacokinetics of benoxaprofen as part of his own research agenda regarding geriatric medicine. Potentially this could have proven to be very damaging to the perceived value of benoxaprofen as a safe and effective NSAID for the elderly. Lilly responded by demanding confirmation of his results by the "insiders" Desante & Ridolfo. Consideration was even given to refusing to publish Hamdy's work.

Gieryn's concept of "boundary work"[8] has usually been invoked to describe how professional scientists exclude non-scientists from policy debates,[9] and how professional interests police the established methodologies of orthodox medicine.[10] The benoxaprofen controversy highlights "boundary work" to protect industrial *institutional* interests rather than professional interests. Key Lilly scientists sought to monopolize scientific authority by attempting to undermine the legitimacy of Hamdy's clinical methodologies even though, as a professional "insider", he and his methodologies had substantial credibility within the medical world.

Thus, within the medical–industrial complex corporate bias becomes entangled with some of the more traditional reward structures of science because a significant criterion of publishability can be conformity to industrial interests. Indeed, this affects the production of scientific knowledge at an early stage via grant awards for research. Since the career structure of academic medics rewards them for publications, there is an institutional incentive for such medics to work co-operatively with an industry that can provide the funding for publishable research.[11] Moreover, the authority structure of science can be used to amplify corporate bias. For example, Kligman seems to have been swayed in his perceptions of benoxaprofen's efficacy by the high status of the scientists supposedly endorsing the drug's exceptional efficacy. This is why drug companies consider it of such strategic importance to persuade high status medical scientists to value their pharmaceutical products.

Also of significance is the authority of the paper itself. Through citation there is the potential for a multiplier effect on corporate bias because readers rarely request the raw data on which claims in scientific papers are made. For example, Dawson positively cited the Bluhm et al. paper as an authority to support his arguments, and in so doing helped to advance the status of Bluhm's research on benoxaprofen.

In saying this, it is important to appreciate that commercial and institutional interests are dynamic. Even within a single pharmaceutical company individual scientists may respond differently to the commercial pressures upon them with significant consequences for the extent of corporate bias in the science they practice. This is illustrated by the disagreement between Gennery and Shedden about the publication of the papers by Hamdy and Kamal on *Opren* safety in the elderly, the discrepancy between Ridolfo's recommendations for the dosage reduction of *Oraflex* in the elderly compared with that finally recommended by Shedden, and the contrasting views of Pitts and senior scientists at Pfizer on the significance of *Feldene*'s GI toxicity in the elderly.

These different responses derive partly from the fact that scientists may construct their company's interests slightly differently to their colleagues. This is most evident in Gennery's argument that Lilly had vital interests in maintaining professional credibility among its medical public by being willing to publish at least some version of the Hamdy and Kamal studies. Clearly Gennery's intervention affected the bias of the medical literature about *Opren* by influencing the course of publication. An important conclusion from that episode is that agents' constructions of interests, including expectations about "social viability" and "public legitimacy" need to be incorporated into an understanding of corporate bias in science.[12]

Government scientists and regulatory bias

When scientists in Government reach conclusions about whether a drug should be marketed they are involved in an eminently trans-scientific activity because they are judging what constitutes an acceptable risk for the public, rather than merely attempting to produce quantitative estimates of risk. That technical procedures do not lead government scientists ineluctably to precise regulatory conclusions is clear from the contradictory institutional decisions taken by the CSM and the FDA, and the opposing judgements reached by individual scientists within the FDA. My research, therefore, supports Weinberg's concerns about the limitations of science and scientists' interpretations as the sole basis for regulatory decision-making.

Furthermore, the empirical research in the previous chapters refines Weinberg's distinction between science and trans-science by providing a political analysis of the institutional and commercial interests that can affect the regulatory judgements of government scientists in the US and the UK. Notwithstanding possible secret disagreements between scientists in the British regulatory authorities, the scientists at the FDA seem to have been more scrupulous towards industrial testing of NSAIDs than their British counterparts.

The close institutional relationship between the regulators and the pharmaceutical firms in the UK has been associated with a sympathetic view of scientific data from the pharmaceutical industry on the part of the Government scientists and scientific advisers. That regulators have been trained by, or hold consultancies with, industry does not mean that the individuals involved are necessarily biased in their regulatory assessments, but it may increase the likelihood of conflicts of interest that might generate bias, albeit unconsciously.

Often individuals on regulatory committees with direct interests in the particular manufacturer or product under consideration will not be permitted to vote on the regulation of that product. However, conflicts of interest can be much broader than is appreciated by such attempts to safeguard against regulatory bias. Regulators may be sensitive to their aspirations to provide consulting services in the future to pharmaceutical firms with whom they have no current financial links. Moreover, regulators may not only come from industry with a sympathetic view of industrial interests, but may also view their career prospects in terms of a return back into industry at a higher position. This "revolving door" situation creates conditions in which regulators might feel uncomfortable about treating the regulated industry too harshly. In addition, the official secrecy which surrounds British drug regulation results in there being very little scope for scrutiny of, or challenge to, regulators' assessments by the public, including the wider medical profession. As Eijndhoven & Groenewegan argue, such secrecy is likely to encourage flexibility and inconsistencies in experts' applications of scientific standards because there are no dissenting voices in a position to call the experts' credibility into question.[13]

In general, this has been less true of FDA scientists, who have maintained greater independence from the industry, and are required to be seen to be independent by Congress. In particular, American drug regulation functions within the legal framework of the 1966 Freedom of Information Act, and acknowledges explicitly the possibility of conflicts of interests between industry and patients. In 1978 the US Congress passed the Ethics in Government Act, which prohibited employees of any American federal agency, including the FDA, from joining the industry they were regulating for at least two years after leaving the agency.[14]

In the US there is far greater legislative and judicial review of regulatory decisions. The FDA can be required to answer for its actions in public by Congressional committees keen to probe into its affairs, and it may be frequently challenged in the courts by pharmaceutical companies or by influential consumer groups such as Public Citizen. By contrast, in the UK, provision for legislative oversight of the CSM and the DHSS has been minimal, judicial review infrequent and subordinated to legal concerns about official secrecy, and consumer organizations are relatively weak. There are, therefore, many good reasons why the FDA is likely to be less biased towards industrial interests than its British counterparts.

The discussion in Chapter 2 suggests that a further source of corporate bias in drug regulation can be the economic viability of the Government's position in terms of balance of payments. This has been particularly true in Britain since the Second World War when the Government has been a major sponsor of the pharmaceutical industry because of the latter's contribution to a positive trade balance and domestic employment via a prosperous export performance. Indeed, currently the British Department of Health (formerly the DHSS) is both sponsor and regulator of the pharmaceutical industry. Since the interests of the British Government and the pharmaceutical industry converge in this way, the former has been, and remains, reluctant to damage the commercial success of the latter through regulation. In the UK when the pharmaceutical industry *en masse* perceives that regulatory policies are detrimental to its commerical interests, it applies pressure on government to relax those policies – as occurred during the early 1950s regarding the categorization of brand name products according to the Cohen Committee's drug standards, and during the late 1970s regarding the scientific standards required to obtain a clinical trial certificate.

By contrast, in the US there exists no such institutionalized common interest between the FDA and the industry. Consequently, the American regulatory authorities are likely to be less vulnerable to industrial pressure than the British. However, pharmaceutical companies often have commercial links with the two major political parties in the US, as well as with individual members of Congress. As a result, the drug trade can muster substantial resistance to unwelcome regulatory activity by negotiating deals with the Executive and Congress – as illustrated by industrial opposition to the Tugwell Bill in 1933 and the implementation of the Drug Efficacy Study during the 1960s and 1970s. Moreover, the neutralization policy at the FDA suggests that key regulatory personnel at the FDA can assimilate some of the perspectives of the pharmaceutical industry. Under such conditions senior scientists in the agency may look for ways of approving drugs rapidly with minimal adversity towards industry. Yet this approach cannot always be made consistent with the FDA's declared scientific standards, which cannot anticipate the perceived shortcomings of companies' drug testing. Consequently, scientific standards and their conscientious application by some FDA scientists may be set aside so that industry instead of patients can be given the benefit of the scientific doubt.

In the review of risk studies in Chapter 1 I noted that contributors to that literature often complain that senior government officials and scientists try to give the impression that potential risks to the public are under control by downplaying scientific uncertainties or by framing them to appear "normal". However, taken as a whole, the evidence in this book implies that an indicator of regulatory bias which is more relevant to patients' exposure to risk is the consistent way that the British and American regulatory authorities awarded the benefit of the scientific doubt to industry. That this is the case is shown by the occasions on which the regulatory authorities in the UK and the US have *emphasized* scientific uncertainty as a justification for regulatory inaction, thereby prioritizing the commercial interests of manufacturers over patients' interests in drug safety. The evidence suggests that in regulating NSAIDs both the FDA and the British regulatory authorities have taken a permissive approach.

Perhaps what is most disconcerting is that the case studies discussed here reveal that the regulatory authorities may have become *more* permissive during the 1980s. For example, consider the FDA's carcinogenic risk assessment of NSAIDs. In March 1977 the Director of the Bureau of Drugs stated the agency's regulatory principle that prior to approval uncertainty about carcinogenicity resulted in non-approval. In October 1980 the FDA were willing to approve *Zomax* with a warning against chronic use after carcinogenicity tests had proved positive. Evidently in 1977 uncertainty about carcinogenicity was deemed sufficient to deny approval, but three years later even a positive carcinogenic risk was considered insufficient to refuse approval. In 1985 *Suprol* was approved without any caution against chronic use despite positive results from carcinogenicity tests. Meanwhile, the British regulatory authorities have provided doctors with no assessments of the carcinogenicity studies in question, but because they approved *Suprol* we can reasonably conclude that they too do not believe that a positive result in carcinogenicity tests is sufficient reason to caution against chronic use. As a second example, consider the CSM's approach to ADR reports as a basis for regulatory action. In 1982 the CSM suspended *Opren* from the market based partly on the justification that the Committee had received significantly more ADR reports about *Opren* than other NSAIDs. Yet by 1985 when similar concerns were raised about the safety of *Feldene* differences in the number of ADR reports between different NSAIDs were no longer considered a valid basis for regulatory intervention. Much more proof of drug injury was going to be required before the British regulators would act.

Nevertheless, it is an oversimplification to characterize the FDA, the CSM or the British Department of Health as "captured" in the sense used by Bernstein's life-cycle theory or other public interest theories of regulatory capture. As discussed in Chapter 2, one reason for this is that none of these regulatory organizations was established primarily to protect the public interest in the first place. A second reason is that they have exhibited some autonomy from the commercial interests of the pharmaceutical industry. For example, the CSM did not permit Lilly to characterize benoxaprofen as an exceptionally efficacious NSAID on the *Opren* data sheet, the FDA withheld approval of benoxaprofen until detailed phototesting provided clearer evidence of the nature of the drug's photo-sensitivity, and both the British and American regulators refused to re-market *Zomax* because of the risk of anaphylactoid reactions. Moreover, individual scientists within the FDA have demonstrated some autonomy from the agency's management when the organization has adopted a commercially biased posture (e.g. Hein and Nestor). One important vir-tue of the historical evidence adduced in Chapter 2 together with the de-tailed analyses of the regulatory authorities' handling of scientific data in the chapters following, is that it demonstrates that corporate bias in regu-lation should not be equated with regulatory capture, and enables one to distinguish carefully the former from the latter.

Before turning to policy implications it is worth underlining that the research for this book has employed a methodology for identifying *specific* biases in scientific knowledge. Corporate bias, then, is an undesirable phenomenon that can be empirically specified and, *in principle*, removed, although that might be far more difficult in practice. This conclusion con-flicts sharply with the relativistic stance of Schwarz & Thompson who, in equating bias with the mere presence of values, believe that "all is bias",[15] and that:

> What we have is not the real risks versus a whole lot of mispercep-tions of those risks, but a clash of plural rationalities, each using impeccable logic to derive conclusions from different premises.[16]

Empirical investigation of regulatory controversies over the safety of NSAIDs reveals that scientists frequently recognize common aspects of re-ality, such as the existence of a tumour or a certain number of clinical re-ports of ADRs. On the basis of that commonly shared reality, it is often possible to demonstrate that some scientists' claims are more consistent and truthful than others. The present research implies that scientists' risk assessments cannot be adequately characterized as a "clash of plural rationalities" using "impeccable logic". On the contrary, some of the sci-entists involved held views which could be discussed within a common rationality of agreed standards. Yet those views were derived from many inconsistencies and self-contradictions that defy the most liberal defini-tion of "logic". These are further reasons for rejecting relativism in favour of a realist sociology of science. Such realism presupposes some com-monly shared standards of truth that are informed by a bridgehead of shared human experiences of a mind-independent reality.

Policy implications

Since the declared purpose of drug regulation is to provide patients with safe and effective medicines, and since corporate bias in drug testing and regulation is generally against the best interests of patients, it follows that the removal of such bias should be a goal for any regulatory organization. The foregoing analysis of the testing and regulation of NSAIDs clearly demonstrates that government and industrial scientists could have acted in ways less biased towards the commercial interests of manufacturers and more committed to patients' interests. The relevant policy question is: what kind of organizational changes could militate in favour of bringing about such alternative actions by scientists?

Pharmaceutical firms' complete control of drug testing in animals and clinical trials does not provide adequate safeguards against corporate bias. Given the burden of proof of harm which falls on the regulatory authorities after a new drug has been approved, and the gross uncertainties surrounding post-marketing spontaneous ADR reports, regulators need to be extremely rigorous and vigilant in their pre-approval risk-benefit assessments. For this reason regulatory authorities should be involved much more directly in the pre-approval testing of new drugs. This would allow regulators as well as industrial scientists to be sufficiently close to the data to make decisions about which results to highlight.

Some carcinogenicity testing could be undertaken by scientists employed by the regulatory authorities rather than by companies with a commercial interest in the results. The Government could charge companies for the cost of such testing. In this institutional context scientists would be less inclined to embrace the commercial values of the drug manufacturers and, therefore, less inclined to prioritize commercial interests over patient protection. Regarding clinical trials, the regulatory authorities could be responsible for the organization and selection of clinical investigators so that manufacturers might be prevented from choosing solely clinicians sympathetic to the commercial interests of the industry. Moreover, consultant clinical investigators could be required to declare any financial links with manufacturers, and to state publicly whether a company has been permitted to comment on, re-write or editorialize any publication prior to distribution.

A most remarkable feature of the responses of the British and American regulators to the risk controversies discussed here is the extent to which they consistently trusted the manufacturers' evaluations. But that trust

251

derives partly from a position of weakness, that is, on regulators' substantial dependence on the industry for expertise. In order to reduce such dependence the regulatory authorities could develop a more autonomous sector of scientific expertise by training toxicologists and clinical pharmacologists in government institutions separate from industry. These policies should be implemented in a context where the responsibilities of the drug regulatory authority are entirely separate from any government sponsoring role for the pharmaceutical industry in order to avoid institutional conflicts of interest. Acknowledgement of conflicts of interests (of individual government scientists or expert scientific advisers) as possible contributors to corporate bias is also necessary. Conflict of interest laws preventing scientists from moving easily from the regulatory authorities to the pharmaceutical industry, and from having personal financial interests in drug companies while involved in regulatory activities could help to reduce the possiblilty of such bias. In exceptional circumstances where the need for certain expertise demands scientists who have substantial commercial interests in a drug company, then those scientists could provide technical advice, but be denied the opportunity to vote on any regulatory decisions.

The more rigorous regulatory approach in the US suggests that freedom of information laws discourage regulatory bias towards commercial interests to some degree, as compared with the official secrecy which characterizes the British approach. However, American freedom of information tends to be confined to the period after regulatory approval has been granted. These laws could be extended to permit public scrutiny of animal and clinical tests *during* regulatory review so that regulatory decisions themselves could be made subject to public debate. Furthermore, the regulatory authorities should include patient/consumer representatives with sufficient scientific knowledge and voting power to ensure that when patients' interests and those of industry conflict, the benefit of the scientific doubt is awarded to the former rather than to the latter. Regulators could be charged explicitly with the statutory responsibility of protecting patients' interests in safe and effective medicines over and above the commercial interests of industry.

Whatever the final decision of the regulators, a comprehensive transcript of their proceedings together with a summary justification for their decision should be publicly available within ten days so that the wider medical community and patient population are given the opportunity to assess its validity for themselves. Rather like Congressional Committees in the US my proposed regulatory authority could have the power to scrutinize any aspect of a sponsor's application. In the US these policy measures should be implemented in addition to the fairly active legislative and judicial review of the drug regulatory authorities that already obtains. In the UK an increase in the existing sparse legislative oversight of drug regulation would be desirable as a supplementary check on the activities of the new regulatory regime that I am advocating.

A frequent objection to the extensive public access to information proposed above is that it would fail to provide pharmaceutical companies' commercial discoveries and designs with adequate protection from competitors. Consequently, so it might be argued, "fair competition" would suffer. The irony of this argument, as a defence of Government secrecy, however, is that because firms in the pharmaceutical industry do not trust each other, patients are expected to trust the entire industry and Government together. Moreover, if companies' trade secrets were narrowly enough defined it might be possible for patients and doctors to obtain adequate information with only minimal impact on the confidentiality of the industry's discoveries and designs. In so far as industrial drug testing affects patients' interests in an effective and safe supply of medicines, however, it should be the role of the regulatory authorities to make that knowledge available to the public. A pharmaceutical product worthy of being put on the market should be able to withstand such public exposure and any ensuing investigations into its therapeutic value. Thus, greater freedom of information could actually direct competition towards higher standards of drug testing thereby improving, not damaging, "fair competition". Of course, steps should be taken to safeguard the privacy of individual doctors and patients.

Finally, the existing regulatory systems in both the UK and the US provide few incentives to reduce the scientific uncertainties of toxicology and clinical pharmacology. Under current institutional arrangements industrial and government scientists tend to use uncertainty to serve their own strategic purpose with the result that interpretive flexibility about scientific standards tends to be encouraged rather than constrained. A further problem is that there are insufficient incentives to direct pharmaceutical research towards medicines that are genuinely needed by patients as distinct from those for which there is a large market. Sometimes needs and market demands coincide, but not always. An improved regulatory system could direct scientific efforts towards reducing uncertainty in risk-benefit assessment and towards increasing the proportion of drugs developed to satisfy medical needs. To achieve this, regulators should first ensure that data from clinical trials and ADRs during clinical practice are collected systematically in order to ascertain the safest drugs for patients, rather than collected defensively to protect the reputation of the drug product in question. And secondly, regulators should be required to take account of comparative effectiveness and medical need as factors in assessing whether the pharmaceutical product ought to be put on the market.

Unfortunately in the UK, where the aforementioned policy changes are most needed, there is little evidence of such developments – in some respects quite the reverse. The *Opren* controversy in the UK led to a review of the efficiency of British regulation of ADRs, and to the establishment of a Working Party chaired by Graham-Smith. The terms of reference of that Working Party were:

> To consider how best the CSM should fulfil its statutory functions of promoting the collection and investigation of information relating to adverse reactions for the purpose of enabling it to give advice on safety, quality or efficacy of medicinal products; and to make recommendations.[17]

In June 1983 the Working Party reported and made 29 recommendations. Later it was reconvened and published a second report with 13 recommendations in January 1986.[18]

The two reports concentrated on how communications about ADRs between doctors, the pharmaceutical industry, patients and the CSM could be improved. The fundamental weakness of these reports is that they construed this task as a problem of technical efficiency rather than as a political issue. Consequently, no significant institutional or legislative changes were recommended. Instead various research training and publication schemes were proposed to raise the awareness of the medical and pharmacy professions about ADR reporting to the CSM. The pharmaceutical industry was to be provided with guidance clarifying the extent of its legal obligation to report ADRs, but there was no mention of how the industry would be forced to comply, perhaps by more frequent and extensive regulatory inspections of manufacturers' databases.

The second Working Party concluded that "patients should be given more information about the drugs they use, including possible ADRs". Yet neither Working Party discussed the desirability of freedom of information laws in the UK and, as is evident from the case studies in this book, the CSM continued to provide doctors and patients with no information on the product data sheets about the carcinogenicity testing of some mar-

keted drugs. That Working Party also suggested more formalized arrangements for post-marketing surveillance studies between industry and
the CSM apparently in order to provide reassurance that regulatory action
against a pharmaceutical product might be unnecessary. While extended
post-marketing surveillance may be given a cautious welcome, there is a
danger that they might either become promotion exercises for manufacturers or be seen as substitutes for improved pre-market clinical trials.
Notably there was no mention of more rigorous controls on the conduct
of pre-market drug testing such as stricter controls on the selection of
clinical investigators. Problems of corporate bias and conflicts of interest
in drug development were entirely ignored.

In 1993 a Private Member's Medicines Information Bill was put before
the British Parliament. In its original form this Bill would have: (a) required the regulatory authorities to keep an index identifying the drugs
subject to licences under the Medicines Act; (b) established rights of access
to data on the regulatory basis for approval, revocation or withdrawal of a
licence, on CSM advice and on regulatory inspection reports; and (c) established wider rights of access to regulatory information about the safety
and efficacy of medicines, subject to restrictions designed to protect patient confidentiality and manufacturing secrets.

The British pharmaceutical industry strongly opposed the wider rights
of access to information under (c) above. To appease industrial objections
Giles Radice, the MP who was the prime mover of the Bill, revised it to
exclude such wider rights of access. However, even in its compromised
form the Bill was not supported by either the British Government's Department of Health or the pharmaceutical industry. Although the Bill got
two readings in Parliament, it failed to complete its report stage on 30
April amid allegations of obstructive delaying tactics by hostile MPs encouraged by Government collusion with the industry. Those allegations
were denied by the Government and the ABPI, but clearly the Government had not been sympathetic to the Bill. Thus, a major effort to increase freedom of information about drug regulation in the UK was
defeated.

It is deeply ironic that that defeat occurred in the same year as the British Government's white paper on *Open Government*. It stated the following
general principles:

> Open government is part of an effective democracy. Citizens must
> have adequate access to the information and analysis on which
> government business is based. Ministers and public servants have a

duty to explain their policies and actions to the public. . . . The Government believes that people should have the freedom to make their own choices on the important matters which affect their lives. Information is a condition of choice and provides a measure of quality. Even where there is little effective alternative to a public service, information enables citizens to demand the quality of service to deliver high standards. The provision of full, accurate information in plain language about public services, what they cost, who is in charge and what standards they offer is a fundamental principle of the Citizen's Charter.[19]

As regards medicines in particular, the Government's main excuse in *Open Government* for not reforming the 1968 Medicines Act in order to permit greater access to safety information was that new European-wide procedures were forthcoming in 1995. The Government claimed that it was "seeking to ensure that the European procedures are as open as possible".[20] However, such overtures are not convincing because if the British Government really was trying to encourage European procedures to be as open as possible we would expect it to have supported the Medicines Information Bill as a way of taking a lead among the European nation states. By contrast, the Government reiterated in the White Paper its unswerving commitment to the commercial interests of the pharmaceutical industry as follows:

medicines must be licensed by the Government. Industry has to provide full details of manufacture, and the results of safety and efficacy tests. Included among this information are trade secrets of great commercial amd market sensitivity, which need to be protected if the pharmaceutical industry is to continue to invest here and to make new medicines available here.[21]

A few months later the British National Consumer Council (NCC) produced a major report on conflicts of interest arising from the Department of Health's role as both promoter and regulator of the pharmaceutical industry, and from the consultancy contracts with the industry held by individual members of regulatory committees.[22] The response of the regulatory authorities was extremely defensive. For example, Rosalinde Hurley, chairperson of the Medicines Commission, justified the members of the Commission holding consultancies with pharmaceutical companies on the grounds that the 1968 Medicines Act stipulates that the Commission must include at least one member with a wide and recent experience of activity in the pharmaceutical industry. But that response does not explain why the Commission regularly contains far more than one member with financial interests in the industry. Nor does it consider the possibility that the Medicines Act might be in need of substantial reform.

Hurley challenged "any allegation, suggestion or implication of partiality and improper conduct on the part of members of the Medicines Commission and of the expert committees established under the Act".[23] As such, she seems to deny that conflicts of interest are a problem within British regulatory committees and reduces the issue to one of personal integrity. My research suggests that corporate bias in regulation is a problem, but it should not be reduced to matters of personal integrity. To do so misses the major point made by the NCC report, namely, that a different *political system* of drug regulation is required in the UK.

Yet Hurley's response needs to be seen as part of a broader political conviction in the UK that is reluctant to acknowledge conflicts of interest between industry and the wider public. The year 1993 also saw the publication of the British Government's White Paper *Realising our potential* on Science, Engineering and Technology, which stated:

> The central thesis of this White Paper is that we could and should improve our performance by making the science and engineering base more aware of and responsive to the needs of industry. . . . the Government recognizes that the key to success is frequent and productive informal contacts between scientists and firms.[24]

Underlying this goal of making science "more responsive" to industrial interests is the assumption that improving the commercial performance of industry never conflicts with, nor diverges from, the public interest. Evidently such an assumption overlooks conflicts of interest in drug testing and regulation; and it encourages the complacent view that above all regulation should be minimal in order to ensure that the commercial enterprise of industry is not hampered.

Consistent with this political philosophy, there was a policy shift in 1989 allowing the Medicines Control Agency (MCA) to be almost entirely funded by licencing application fees from the pharmaceutical industry. Previously the Medicines Division (the regulatory predecessor of the MCA) was funded 65 per cent by industry fees and 35 per cent via taxes.[25] The MCA is now essentially run as a business selling its "regulatory services" to the industry and promoting itself as one of the fastest licencing authorities in the world for new drugs.[26]

Thus, corporate bias in drug testing and regulation shows little sign of being properly tackled by the British Government. However, there is increasing public dissatisfaction with the existing regulatory arrangements in the UK and the US. It remains to be seen whether intelligent policies will be forthcoming. In the meantime it is important that such corporate bias continues to be systematically identified, monitored and revealed by researchers so that policy proposals can be well informed.

Notes

Preface

1. C. Medawar 1992. *Power and dependence: social Audit on the safety of medicines.* London: Social Audit. S. Wolfe & C. M. Coley 1981. *Pills that don't work.* New York: Farrar Straus Giroux.
2. H. G. Grabowski 1976. *Drug regulation and innovation: empirical evidence and policy options.* Washington DC: American Institute for Public Policy Research; W. D. Reekie 1975. *The economics of the pharmaceutical industry.* London: Macmillan; M. Statman 1983. *Competition in the pharmaceutical industry: the declining profitability of drug innovation.* Washington and London: American Enterprise Institute for Public Policy Research; D. Schwartzmann 1976. *Innovation in the pharmaceutical industry.* Baltimore: The Johns Hopkins University Press.
3. J. Braithwaite 1984. *Corporate crime in the pharmaceutical industry.* London: Routledge & Kegan Paul; J. Collier 1989. *The health conspiracy.* London: Century; C. Medawar 1984. *The wrong kind of medicine?* London: Consumers Association/Hodder & Stoughton; S. M. Wolfe & C. M. Coley 1981. *Pills that don't work.* New York: Farrar Straus Giroux; M. Mintz 1965. *The therapeutic nightmare.* Boston: Houghton Miflin & Riverside Press.
4. S. Jasanoff 1990. *The fifth branch: science advisers as policy makers.* Cambridge, Mass.: Harvard University Press; E. Richards 1991. *Vitamin C and cancer: medicine or politics?* London: Macmillan; R. Vos 1990. *Drugs looking for diseases.* Dordrecht: Kluwer.
5. G. Dukes 1985. *The effects of drug regulation,* 47. Lancaster: MTP Press.
6. World Health Organisation (WHO) 1991. Letter to J. Abraham from I. Lunde, Pharmaceuticals Consultant, WHO, Regional Office of Europe, 3 December.
7. G. Dukes 1985. op. cit. 107. (**n.5**)
8. L. Hancher 1989. *Regulating for competition: government, law and the pharmaceutical industry in the United Kingdom and France,* 4. PhD thesis, University of Amsterdam.
9. W. M. Wardell & L. Lasagna 1975. *Regulation and drug development,* pp.51–123, Washington DC: American Enterprise Institute for Public Policy Research. J. P. Griffin & G. E. Diggle 1981. A survey of products licenced in the United Kingdom from 1971–1981, *British Journal of Clinical Pharmacology* **12**, 453–563; F. Steward & G. Wibberley 1980. Drug innovation – what's slowing it down? *Nature* **284**, 119.
10. A. Irwin 1985. *Risk and the control of technology: public policies for road traffic safety in Britain and the United States,* 258. Manchester: Manchester University Press.
11. Committee on the Safety of Medicines (CSM) 1988. Letter to J. Abraham from Secretary of CSM, 20 May; CSM 1988. Letter to J. Abraham from the Chairman of CSM, May 1988.

259

NOTES

Chapter One

1. Pharmaceutical Society of Great Britain (PSGB) 1962. Testing of new drugs. *Pharmaceutical Journal* **188**, 552–3.
2. US Court 1983. Deposition of F. B. Peck, *Clarence Borom vs Eli Lilly and Company*, 127. District Court for the Middle District of Georgia, Columbus Division, 12 May.
3. D. Jack 1979. The work of a company research department. In *Pharmaceutical medicine*, N. MacLeod (ed.), 16–22. London: Churchill Livingstone.
4. J. Erlichman 1990. Deaths from ICI heart drug raise questions on testing. *Guardian*, 13 June.
5. PSGB 1963. The industry and the health service. *Pharmaceutical Journal*, **190**, 417–18.
6. K. Clarke 1985. Written answers. *Hansard*, 3 June, 669.
7. J. Erlichman 1990. Safety experts linked to firms. *Guardian*, 14 June.
8. Joint Hearings before the Subcommittee on Health of the Committee on Labour and Public Welfare and the Subcommittee on Administrative Practice and Procedure of the Senate Committee on the Judiciary 1974. *Examination of the pharmaceutical industry (part 7)*, 2953–4. Washington DC: US GPO.
9. R. K. Merton 1938. Science and the social order. In *The sociology of science: theoretical and empirical investigations*, N. W. Storer (ed.), 254–78. Chicago: University of Chicago Press.
10. R. Keat 1981. *The politics of social theory: Habermas, Freud and the critique of positivism*, 11–37. Oxford: Basil Blackwell.
11. R. K. Merton 1938. op. cit., 258–9 (**n.9**).
12. M. Bunge 1991. A critical examination of the new sociology of science: part 1. *Philosophy of Social Sciences* **21**, 524–60; M. Hammersley 1992. On feminist methodology. *Sociology* **26**, 187–206.
13. T. S. Kuhn 1962. *The structure of scientific revolutions*. Chicago: University of Chicago.
14. K. D. Knorr-Cetina & M. Mulkay 1983. Introduction: emerging principles in social studies of science. In *Science observed: perspectives on the social study of science*, K. D. Knorr-Cetina & M. Mulkay (eds), 2–6. London: Sage.
15. T. S. Kuhn 1962. op. cit., 78. (**n.13**)
16. Ibid. 121.
17. For example M. Mulkay 1979. *Science and the sociology of knowledge*, 41, 73. London: Allen & Unwin; A. F. Chalmers 1982. *What is this thing called science?*, 97. Milton Keynes: Open University Press.
18. D. Bloor 1973. Wittgenstein and Mannheim on the sociology of mathematics. *Studies in the History and Philosophy of Science* **4**, 173–191.
19. D. Mackenzie 1981. Notes on the science and social relations debate. *Capital and Class* **14**, 49; S. Shapin 1982. History of science and its sociological reconstructions. *History of Science* **20**, 187.
20. B. Barnes & S. Shapin 1979. Introduction. In *Natural order: historical studies of scientific culture*, B. Barnes & S. Shapin (eds), 10. London: Sage.
21. D. Mackenzie 1981. op. cit., 55. (**n.19**)
22. K. D. Knorr-Cetina 1983. The ethnographic study of scientific work: towards a constructivist interpretation of science. See Knorr-Cetina & Mulkay (1983), 116. (**n.14**)
23. D. Mackenzie 1981. *Statistics in Britain 1865–1930: the social construction of scientific knowledge*. Edinburgh: Edinburgh University Press.
24. S. Shapin 1979. Homo phrenologicus: anthropological perspectives on an historical problem. See Barnes & Shapin (1979), 54. (**n.20**)
25. A. Webster 1991. *Science, technology and society: new directions*. London: Macmillan.
26. D. Bloor 1973. op. cit. (**n.18**); D. Bloor 1976. *Knowledge and social imagery*. London: Routledge & Kegan Paul.

27. D. Bloor 1984. The sociology of reasons: or why epistemic factors are really "social factors". In *Scientific rationality: the sociological turn*, T. R. Brown (ed.), 298. Dordrecht: Reidel.
28. H. M. Collins 1983. The sociology of scientific knowledge: studies of contemporary science. *Annual Review of Sociology* **9**, 269–76; H. M. Collins 1985. *Changing order: replication and induction in scientific practice*, 3. London: Sage.
29. E. R. Fuhrman & K. Oehler 1986. Discourse analysis and reflexivity. *Social Studies of Science* **16**, 302.
30. H. M. Collins 1975. The seven sexes: a study in the sociology of a phenomenon, or the replication of experiments in physics. *Sociology* **9**, 208, 220.
31. M. Hollis & S. Lukes 1982. Introduction. In *Rationality and relativism*, M. Hollis & S. Lukes (eds), 1–20. Oxford: Basil Blackwell.
32. H. M. Collins 1983. op. cit., 273. (**n.28**)
33. H. M. Collins 1985. op. cit., 18. (**n.28**)
34. Ibid. 19.
35. Ibid. 169.
36. H. M. Collins 1981. Stages in the empirical programme of relativism. *Social Studies of Science* **11**, 4.
37. H. M. Collins 1983. An empirical relativist programme in the sociology of scientific knowledge. See Knorr-Cetina & Mulkay (1983), 94–5. (**n.14**)
38. H. M. Collins 1983. op. cit., 275. (**n.28**)
39. Ibid. 99.
40. H. M. Collins 1985. op. cit., 159–60. (**n.28**); H. M. Collins 1983. op. cit., 99. (**n.28**)
41. K. D. Knorr-Cetina 1983. op. cit., 118–19. (**n.22**); K. Knorr-Cetina & K. Amann 1990. Image dissection in natural scientific inquiry. *Science, Technology and Human Values* **15**, 259–83.
42. S. Restivo 1981. Commentary: some perspectives in contemporary sociology of science. *Science, Technology and Human Values* **6**, 25–6; R. Hagendijk 1990. Structuration theory, constructivism and scientific change. In *Theories of Science in Society*, S. E. Cozzens & T. F. Gieryn (eds), 44–51. Bloomington: Indiana University Press.
43. R. N. Keat & J. R. Urry 1975. *Social theory as science*. London: Routledge & Kegan Paul.
44. B. Latour & S. Woolgar 1979. *Laboratory life: the social construction of scientific facts*. London: Sage; B. Latour & S. Woolgar 1986. *Laboratory life: the construction of scientific facts*. Princeton, New Jersey: Princeton University Press.
45. K. D. Knorr-Cetina 1983. op. cit., 120. (**n.22**)
46. Ibid. 126–7.
47. B. Latour 1983. Give me a laboratory and I will raise the world. See Knorr-Cetina & Mulkay (1983), 161. (**n.14**)
48. K. D. Knorr-Cetina 1983. op. cit., 122, 124. (**n.22**)
49. J. Law 1986. Laboratories and texts. In *Mapping the dynamics of science and technology: sociology of science in the real world*, M. Callon, J. Law, A. Rip (eds), 49. London: Macmillan.
50. S. Woolgar 1982. Laboratory studies: a comment on the state of the art. *Social Studies of Science* **12**, 482.
51. Ibid. 484–5; Restivo, S. 1987. Science studies – what is to be done. *Science, Technology and Human Values* **12**, 17; B. Latour 1983. op. cit., 157. (**n.47**)
52. K. D. Knorr-Cetina 1983. op. cit., 117. (**n.22**)
53. B. Latour 1987. *Science in action: how to follow scientists and engineers through society*, 175. Milton Keynes: Open University Press.
54. Ibid. 99.
55. B. Latour & F. Bastide 1986. Writing science – fact and fiction: the analysis of the process of reality construction through the application of socio-semiotic methods to scientific texts. See Callon et al. (1986), 65. (**n.49**)
56. M. Mulkay, J. Potter, S. Yearley 1983. Why an analysis of scientific discourse is needed.

See Knorr-Cetina & Mulkay (1983), 196. (**n.14**)

57. G. N. Gilbert & M. Mulkay 1984. *Opening Pandora's box: a sociological analysis of scientists' discourse*, 1–2. Cambridge: Cambridge University Press.

58. S. Woolgar 1982. op. cit., 488. (**n.50**)

59. M. Mulkay, J. Potter, S. Yearley 1983. op. cit., 195–7. (**n.56**)

60. Ibid. 199.

61. Ibid. 198–200; J. Potter & A. McKinlay 1989. Discourse – philosophy – reflexivity: comment on Halfpenny. *Social Studies of Science* **19**, 137–45.

62. G. N. Gilbert & M. Mulkay 1984. op. cit., 14. (**n.57**)

63. M. Mulkay 1981. *Sociology of science: a sociological pilgrimage*, 19–20. Milton Keynes: Open University Press.

64. S. Woolgar 1988. *Science: the very idea*, 73, 89. London: Tavistock.

65. S. Woolgar (ed.) 1988. *Knowledge and reflexivity: new frontiers in the sociology of knowledge*. London: Sage; M. Mulkay 1991. op. cit. 25–30. (**n.63**); S. Woolgar 1989. Response to Slezak *Social Studies of Science* **19**, 658–68.

66. B. Barnes 1982. On the implication of a body of knowledge. *Knowledge* **4**, 108–9.

67. H. M. Collins 1983. op. cit., 101–2. (**n.37**); H. M. Collins 1983. op. cit., 280. (**n.28**)

68. M. Mulkay, J. Potter, S. Yearley 1983. op. cit., 199. (**n.56**)

69. H. M. Collins 1983. op. cit., 102–3. (**n.32**); E. R. Fuhrman & K. Oehler 1986. op. cit., 293–307. (**n.24**); P. Halfpenny 1989. Reply to Potter and McKinlay. *Social Studies of Science* **19**, 145–52.

70. B. Barnes 1974. *Scientific knowledge and sociological theory*, 154. London: Routledge & Kegan Paul.

71. C. Doran 1989. Jumping frames: reflexivity and recursion in the sociology of science. *Social Studies of Science* **19**, 517.

72. T. F. Gieryn 1982. Relativist/constructivist programmes in the sociology of science: redundance and retreat. *Social Studies of Science* **12**, 291.

73. K. D. Knorr-Cetina & M. Mulkay 1983. op. cit., 6. (**n.14**)

74. R. Bhaskar 1979. *The possibility of naturalism*, 73. Sussex: Harvester.

75. S. E. Cozzens 1990. Autonomy and power in science. See Cozzens & Gieryn (1990), 181. (**n.42**)

76. B. Latour 1987. op. cit., p195. (**n.53**)

77. S. Sismondo 1993. Some social constructions. *Social Studies of Science* **23**, 515–53; S. Sismondo 1993. Response to Knorr-Cetina. *Social Studies of Science* **23**, 563–9.

78. D. Bloor 1976. *Knowledge and social imagery*, 9–10, 144. London: Routledge & Kegan Paul; S. Restivo 1981. op. cit., 26. (**n.42**); E. Millstone 1978. A framework for the sociology of knowledge. *Social Studies of Science* **8**, 115; D. E. Chubin & S. Restivo 1983. The "mooting" of science studies: research programmes and science policy. See Knorr-Cetina & Mulkay (1983), 69. (**n.14**)

79. E. Millstone 1978. op. cit., 115. (**n.78**)

80. S. Woolgar 1982. op. cit., 489, 494. (**n.50**)

81. K. D. Knorr-Cetina & M. Mulkay 1983. op. cit., 1–14. (**n.14**); J. Potter & A. McKinlay 1989. op. cit., 137–45. (**n.61**)

82. M. Mulkay, J. Potter, S. Yearley, 1983. op. cit., 199. (**n.56**); E. R. Fuhrman & K. Oehler 1986. op. cit., 296. (**n.29**)

83. M. Mulkay 1984. The scientist talks back: a one-act play with a moral about replication in science and reflexivity in sociology. *Social Studies of Science* **14**, 278.

84. S. Woolgar 1991. The turn to technology in social studies of science. *Science, Technology and Human Values* **16**, 29, 43.

85. M. Mulkay 1991. op. cit., xix. (**n.63**)

86. H. Rose & S. Rose 1976. The incorporation of science. In *The political economy of science: ideology of/in the natural sciences*, H. Rose & S. Rose (eds), 20–21. London: Macmillan; R.

Collins & S. Restivo 1983. Development, diversity and conflict in the sociology of science. *The Sociological Quarterly* **24**, 190–91.

87. S. Restivo 1987. op. cit., 13–14. (**n.51**)

88. R. Johnston & D. Robbins 1977. The development of specialties in industrialised science. *Sociological Review* **25**, 88.

89. N. D. Ellis 1969. The occupation of science. In *Sociology of science*, B. Barnes (ed.), 188–206. Harmondsworth: Penguin.

90. W. O. Hagstrom 1965. *The scientific community*. London: Basic Books.

91. S. B. Blume 1974. *Toward a political sociology of science*. London: The Free Press; L. Sklair 1973. *Organised knowledge*. London: Hart-Davis, MacGibbon; R. Johnston & D. Robbins 1977. op. cit., 101. (**n.72**); D. Robbins & R. Johnston 1976. The role of cognitive and occupational differentiation in scientific controversies. *Social Studies of Science* **6**, 352.

92. K. W. McCain 1991. Communication, competition and secrecy: the production and dissemination of research-related information in genetics. *Science, Technology and Human Values* **16**, 494–516.

93. K. D. Knorr-Cetina & M. Mulkay 1983. op. cit., 6. (**n.14**)

94. K. D. Knorr-Cetina 1983. op. cit., 131–2 (**n.22**); S. E. Cozzens & T. F. Gieryn 1990. Introduction: putting science back in society. See Cozzens & Gieryn (1990) op. cit., 1. (**n.42**); B. Martin 1993. The critique of science becomes academic. *Science, Technology and Human Values* **18**, 247–59.

95. E. Richards 1988. The politics of therapeutic evaluation: the vitamin C and cancer controversy. *Social Studies of Science* **18**, 655.

96. E. R. Fuhrman & K. Oehler 1986. op. cit., 304. (**n.29**)

97. T. F. Gieryn 1982. op. cit., 281. (**n.72**); B. Latour 1988. The politics of explanation. In *Knowledge and reflexivity*, S. Woolgar (ed.), 173. London: Sage; S. E. Cozzens & T. F. Gieryn, 1990. op. cit., 9. (**n.94**)

98. H. M. Collins 1983. op. cit., 275. (**n.28**)

99. D. Chubin 1981. Values, controversy and the sociology of science. *Bulletin of Science, Technology and Society* **1**, 428.

100. F. B. McCrea & G. E. Markle 1984. The estrogen replacement controversy in the USA and UK: different answers to the same question? *Social Studies of Science*, **14**, 1–26; E. Richards 1988. op. cit., 653–701. (**n.95**).

101. D. Nelkin 1989. Science studies in the 1990s. *Science, Technology and Human Values*, **14**, 305.

102. B. Hessen 1931. The social and economic roots of Newton's "Principia". In *Science at the crossroads*, N. I. Bukharin (ed.), 155–92. London: Frank Cross.

103. A. Sohn-Rethel 1976. Science as alienated consciousness. *Radical Science Journal* **3**, 97.

104. J. Slack 1972. Class struggle among the molecules. In *Counter course*, T. Pateman (ed.), 203. London: Penguin.

105. D. Fisher 1990. *Boundary work and science: the relation between power and knowledge*. In S. E. Cozzens & T. F. Gieryn (eds) op. cit., 98 (**n.42**); T. F. Gieryn 1983. Boundary-work and the demarcation of science from non-science: strains and interests in professional ideologies of scientists. *American Sociological Review* **48**, 781–95.

106. Ibid. 101–14.

107. E. Yoxen 1981. Life as a productive force. In *Science, technology and the labour process*, L. Levidow & B. Young (eds), 66–122. London: CSE Books.

108. B. Young 1976. Science is social relations. *Radical Science Journal* **5**, 65–117.

109. T. Shallice 1979. Science is not just social relations. *Science for People* **43/44**, 37–40.

110. S. Restivo 1981. op. cit., 27. (**n.42**)

111. J. Stewart 1982. Facts as commodities? *Radical Science Journal* **12**, 135.

112. G. Lukacs 1971. *History and class consciousness*. London: Merlin Press.

113. K. Marx 1973. *Grundrisse*. London: Penguin (translation and foreword by M. Nicolous).

NOTES

114. K. Marx 1965. *The German ideology.* London: Lawrence & Wishart.
115. J. D. Bernal 1939. *The social function of science.* London: Routledge & Kegan Paul.
116. T. Shallice 1979. op. cit. (**n.109**)
117. R. Keat 1981. op. cit. (**n.10**)
118. A. Mazur 1985. Bias in risk-benefit analysis. *Technology in Society* **7**, 25–30.
119. S. S. Jasanoff 1987. Contested boundaries in policy-relevant science. *Social Studies of Science* **17**, 195–230.
120. A. Weinberg 1972. Science and trans-science. *Minerva* **10**, 209.
121. Ibid. 209, 218.
122. H. Kunreuther & E. Ley 1982. Overview. In *The risk analysis controversy: an institutional perspective,* H. Kunreuther & E. Ley (eds), 3–12. Berlin: Springer; F. M. Lynn 1986. The interplay of science and values in assessing and regulating environmental risks. *Science, Technology and Human Values,* **11**, 40–50; D. Collingridge 1980. *The social control of technology.* London: Francis Pinter; H. Nowotny 1977. Scientific purity and nuclear danger: the case of risk assessment. In *The social production of scientific knowledge,* E. Mendelsohn, P. Weingart, R. Whitley (eds), 243–64. Dordrecht-Holland: Reidel; J. Conway (ed.) 1980. *Society, technology and risk assessment.* London: Academic Press; H. C. Kunreuther et al. 1983. *Risk analysis and decision processes: the story of liquefied energy and gas facilities in four countries.* Berlin: Springer.
123. W. M. Lowrance 1976. *Of acceptable risk: science and the determination of safety.* Los Altos, California: Kaufmann.
124. A. Mazur 1973. Disputes between experts. *Minerva* **11**, 243–62; A. Mazur 1975. Opposition of technological innovation. *Minerva* **13**, 58–81.
125. J. R. Ravetz 1987. Uncertainty, ignorance and policy. In *Science for public policy,* H. Brooks & C. L. Cooper (eds), 77–94. Oxford: Pergamon.
126. R. Johnston 1980. The characteristics of risk assessment research. In J. Conway (ed.). op. cit., 105–22. (**n.122**); B. Wynne 1987. Uncertainty – technical and social. In H. Brooks & C. L. Cooper (eds), op. cit., 95–114. (**n.125**)
127. J. Linnerooth 1984. The political processing of uncertainty. *Acta Psychologica* **56**, 222.
128. J. Brown (ed.) 1989. *Environmental threats: perception, analysis and management.* London: Bellhaven Press.
129. U. Beck 1992. *Risk society: towards a new modernity,* 55. London: Sage.
130. M. Schwarz & M. Thompson 1990. *Divided we stand: redefining politics, technology and social choice.* Hemel Hempstead, Herts: Harvester-Wheatsheaf.
131. Ibid. 61.
132. M. Douglas & A. Wildavsky 1982. *Risk and culture: an essay on the selection of technical and environmental dangers.* Berkeley, CA: University of California Press; A. Irwin & K. Green 1983. The control of chemical carcinogens in Britain. *Policy and Politics* **11**, 439–59; A. Irwin 1985. *Risk and the control of technology: public policies for road traffic safety in Britain and the United States.* Manchester: Manchester University Press.
133. D. Hattis & D. Kennedy 1986. Assessing risks from health hazards: an imperfect science. *Technology Review* **89**, 71.
134. B. Wynne 1983. Redefining the issues of risk and public acceptance: the social viability of technology. *Futures* **20**, 13.
135. D. J. Fiorino 1990. Citizen participation and environmental risk: a survey of institutional mechanisms. *Science, Technology and Human Values* **15**, 239.
136. U. Beck 1992. op. cit., 62. (**n.129**)
137. Ibid. 161.
138. M. Schwarz & M. Thompson 1990. op. cit., 13. (**n.130**)
139. A. Irwin 1985. op. cit. (**n.132**)
140. M. Bernstein 1955. *Regulating business by independent commission.* Princeton, New Jersey: Princeton University Press.

141. Judge Lee Loevinger cited in R. Harris 1964. *The real voice*, 145. New York: Macmillan.
142. B. M. Mitnick 1980. *The political economy of regulation*, 95–109. New York: Columbia University Press.
143. C. Offe 1983. The capitalist state. *Political Studies* **31**, 669.
144. R. Miliband 1983. State power and class interests. *New Left Review* **138**, 57–68.
145. B. Jessop 1979. Corporatism, parliamentarism and social democracy. In *Trends toward corporatist intermediation*, P. C. Schmitter & G. Lehmbruch (eds), 185–212. London: Sage.
146. For a brief summary of the work of these other "early" private interest theorists see P. Sabatier 1975. op. cit., 303–4. (**n.149**)
147. G. Stigler 1971. The theory of economic regulation. *Bell Journal of Economics and Managerial Science* **2**, 21–45.
148. B. M. Mitnick 1980. op. cit., 111–15. (**n.126**)
149. P. Sabatier 1975. Social movements and regulatory agencies: toward a more adequate – and less pessimistic – theory of "clientele capture". *Policy Sciences* **6**, 301–42.
150. D. P. McGaffrey 1982. Corporate resources and regulatory pressures: toward explaining a discrepancy. *Administrative Science Quarterly* **27**, 398–419.
151. Ibid.
152. J. Q. Wilson 1980. The politics of regulation. In *The politics of regulation*, J. Q. Wilson (ed.), 357–94. USA: Basic Books.
153. A. Cawson 1986. *Corporatism and political theory*. Oxford: Basil Blackwell.
154. A. Cawson 1985. Introduction: varieties of corporatism: the importance of the meso-level of interest intermediation. In *Organised interests and the state: studies in meso-corporatism*, A. Cawson (ed.), 1–21. London: Sage.
155. K. Middlemas 1979. *Politics in industrial society: the experience of the British system since 1911*. London: Andre Deutsch.
156. Ibid. 373.
157. W. Streek & P. C. Schmitter 1985. Community, market, state – and associations? The prospective contribution of interest governance to social order. In *Private interest government: beyond market and state*, W. Streeck & P. C. Schmitter (eds), 16. London: Sage.
158. A. Cawson 1985. op. cit. (**n.154**).
159. H. Meynell 1977. On the limits of the sociology of knowledge. *Social Studies of Science* **7**, 498.
160. S. Lukes 1982. Relativism in its place. See Hollis & Lukes (1982), 262. (**n.31**)
161. M. Hollis 1982. The social destruction of reality. See Hollis & Lukes (1982), 67–86. (**n.31**)
162. R. Bhaskar 1986. *Scientific realism and human emancipation*, 898–9. London: Verso.
163. A. F. Chalmers 1982. op. cit. (**n.17**)
164. E. Nagel 1962. *The structure of science*. New York: Routledge & Kegan Paul.
165. R. Bhaskar 1978. *Realist theory of science*. Sussex: Harvester Press.
166. B. Latour & S. Woolgar 1979. op. cit. (**n.44**)
167. I. Hacking 1982. Language, truth and reason. See Hollis & Lukes (1982), 62–3. (**n.31**)
168. R. Bhaskar 1986. op. cit., 90. (**n.162**)
169. P. F. Strawson 1959. *Individuals*, 10. London: Methuen.
170. R. Bhaskar 1986. op. cit., 91. (**n.162**)
171. H. Meynell 1977. op. cit., 492. (**n.159**)
172. S. Russell 1986. The social construction of artefacts: a response to Pinch and Bijker. *Social Studies of Science* **16**, 331–46.
173. D. E. Chubin & S. Restivo 1983. op. cit., 63, 70. (**n.78**)
174. P. Scott, E. Richards, B. Martin 1990. Captives of controversy: the myth of the neutral social researcher in contemporary scientific controversies. *Science, Technology and Human Values*, **15**, 474–94.
175. E. Millstone 1978. op. cit., 115, 121. (**n.78**)

176. D. Bartels 1985. Commentary: it's good enough for science, but is it good enough for social action. *Science, Technology and Human Values*, **10**, 69–74.
177. D. Mackenzie 1981. op. cit., 47–60. (**n.21**)
178. H. M. Collins 1983. op. cit., 280. (**n.28**)
179. S. Sismondo 1993. op. cit. (**n.77**)
180. B. Barnes 1974. op. cit., 41–2, 136. (**n.70**)
181. Ibid. 138.
182. Ibid. 137.
183. D. Chubin 1981. op. cit., 432. (**n.99**)
184. B. Wynne 1984. The institutional context of science, models and policy: the IIASA energy study. *Policy Sciences* **17**, 277–320.
185. B. Martin 1979. *The bias of science*. Marrickville, Australia: Society for Social Responsibility in Science.
186. B. Martin 1978. The selective usefulness of game theory. *Social Studies of Science* **8**, 85–110.
187. T. H. Engelhardt & A. L. Caplan 1987. Introduction: patterns of controversy and closure: the interplay of knowledge, values and political forces. In *Scientific controversies*, T. H. Engelhardt & A. L. Caplan (eds), 1–4. Cambridge: Cambridge University Press; R. N. Giere 1987. Controversies involving science and technology: a theoretical perspective. In H. T. Engelhardt & A. L. Caplan (eds), ibid. 126.
188. T. Brante & A. Elzinga 1990. Toward a theory of scientific controversies. *Science Studies* **2**, 35, 43.
189. E. Richards 1988. op. cit., 654. (**n.95**); T. J. Pinch & W. E. Bijker 1984. The social construction of facts and artefacts: or how the sociology of science and the sociology of technology might benefit each other. *Social Studies of Science* **14**, 429.
190. H. M. Collins 1975. op. cit. (**n.30.**)
191. B. Martin 1988. Analyzing the fluoridation controversy: resources and structures. *Social Studies of Science* **18**, 352.
192. R. Keat 1981. op. cit. (**n.10**)
193. M. Hollis 1977. *Models of man: philosophical thoughts on social action*, 124. Cambridge: Cambridge University Press.
194. R. Brubaker 1984. *The limits of rationality: an essay on the social and moral thought of Max Weber*. London: Allen & Unwin.
195. A. Cawson (ed.) 1985. op. cit., 4. (**n.154**)
196. A. Cawson 1986. op. cit., 14, 22. (**n.154**)
197. S. Wilks & M. Wright 1987. Conclusion: comparing government–industry relations: states, sectors and network. In *Comparative government–industry relations*, S. Wilks & M. Wright (eds), 275. Oxford: Clarendon Press.
198. M. Schwarz & M. Thompson 1990. op. cit., 49. (**n.130**)
199. V. Ronge 1980. Theoretical concepts of political decision-making processes. In J. Conrad (ed.) op. cit., 209–38. (**n.112**)
200. M. Schwarz & M. Thompson 1990. op. cit., 39–56. (**n.130**)
201. Ibid. 49.
202. Ibid. 40–41.
203. M. A. Crenson 1971. *The unpolitics of air pollution: a study of non-decisionmaking in the cities*. New York: The Johns Hopkins University Press.
204. S. Lukes 1974. *Power: a radical view*. London: Macmillan.
205. Ibid.
206. L. Hancher 1989. *Regulating for competition: government, law and the pharmaceutical industry in the United Kingdom and France*, 4. PhD thesis, University of Amsterdam.
207. A. Cawson (ed.) 1985. op. cit., 4. (**n.154**); L. Hancher 1989. op. cit., 12–13. (**n.206**)

Chapter Two

1. J. Liebenau 1981. *Medical science and medical industry 1890–1929: a study of pharmaceutical manufacturing in Philadelphia.* PhD thesis, University of Pennsylvania.

2. J. H. Young 1961. *The toadstool millionaires: a social history of patent medicines in America before federal regulation.* Princeton, New Jersey: Princeton University Press; J. H. Young 1967. *The medical messiahs: a social history of health quackery in twentieth century America.* Princeton, New Jersey: Princeton University Press.

3. R. G. Marks 1974. Pharmaceuticals. In *The legislation of product safety, vol. 2,* S. S. Epstein & R. D. Grundy (eds). Cambridge, Mass.: MIT Press.

4. P. Temin 1980. *Taking your medicine: drug regulation in the United States.* Cambridge, Mass.: Harvard University Press.

5. M. Jenkins 1987. A history of the UK's drug controls. *Mims Magazine,* 56–7; M. Hodges 1987. Control of the safety of drugs, 1868–1968. *Pharmaceutical Journal* **240**, 119–22; R. D. Mann 1984. *Modern drug use: an enquiry based on historical principles.* Lancaster: MTP Press; R. D. Mann 1988. From mithridatium to modern medicine: the management of drug safety. *Journal of the Royal Society of Medicine* **81**, 725–8; R. G. Penn 1979. The state control of medicines: the first 3000 years. *British Journal of Clinical Pharmacology* **8**, 293–305.

6. R. G. Penn 1982. *The development of the regulatory control of the safety, quality and supply of medicines.* MD thesis, Welsh National School of Medicine.

7. T. D. Whittet 1970. Drug control in Britain: from World War I to the Medicines Bill of 1968. In *Safeguarding the public: historical aspects of medicinal drug control,* J. B. Blake (ed.), 27–37. Baltimore: The Johns Hopkins University Press.

8. E. W. Stieb 1966. *Drug adulteration: detection and control in nineteenth century Britain.* Madison, Milwaukee: University of Wisconsin Press.

9. E. W. Stieb 1970. Drug control in Britain, 1850–1914. In J. B. Blake (ed.) op. cit. (**n.7**)

10. J. H. Young 1961. op. cit., 16–17. (**n.2**)

11. R. G. Penn 1979. op. cit., 295–9. (**n.5**); E. W. Stieb 1966. op. cit., 105–13. (**n.8**); J. Burnett 1966. *Plenty and want: a social history of diet in England from 1815 to the present day.* London: Nelson.

12. R. G. Penn, ibid; E. W. Stieb, ibid; J. Burnett, ibid.

13. E. W. Stieb 1966. op. cit., 114. (**n.8**)

14. J. G. Burrow 1963. *AMA voice of American medicine,* 72. Baltimore: The Johns Hopkins University Press.

15. J. H. Young 1961. op. cit., 8, 24–5. (**n.2**); J. Liebenau 1981. op. cit., 37. (**n.1**)

16. R. D. Mann 1984. op. cit., 390–485. (**n.5**)

17. J. H. Young 1961. op. cit., 38. (**n.2**)

18. G. Tweedale 1990. *At the sign of the plough: 275 years of Allen and Hanbury's and the British pharmaceutical industry 1715–1990.* London: John Murray.

19. T. Mahoney 1959. *The merchants of life: an account of the American pharmaceutical industry.* New York: Harper & Brothers; W. Haynes 1943. *American chemical industry: background and beginnings,* 210–21. Toronto: D. Van Nostrand.

20. J. Liebenau 1981. op. cit., 29. (**n.1**)

21. E. W. Stieb 1966. op. cit., 27–97. (**n.8**)

22. D. C. Somervell 1929. *English thought in the nineteenth century,* 3–16. London: Methuen; L. Woodward 1962. *The age of reform: 1815-1870,* 19–20. Oxford: Oxford University Press.

23. M. Bruce 1961. *The coming of the welfare state.* London: Batsford; D. C. Somervell 1929. op. cit., 42–55. (**n.22**)

24. G. Sonnedecker 1982. Drug standards become official. In *The early years of federal food and drug control,* J. H. Young (ed.), 28–9. Madison, Wisconsin: American Institute of the His-

tory of Pharmacy.

25. D. C. Somervell 1929. op. cit., 84–8. (**n.22**)
26. F. Bedarida 1976. *A social history of England 1851–1975*, 3–35. London: Methuen; J. Burnett 1966. op. cit., 91–112. London: Nelson.
27. D. C. Somervell 1929. op. cit., 88. (**n.22**)
28. M. Bruce 1961. op. cit., 89–153. (**n.23**)
29. E. W. Stieb 1966. op. cit., 68–9. (**n.8**)
30. Ibid. 51–68.
31. J. Forrester 1978. The *Lancet*'s analytical sanitary commission. *Lancet* 2, 1360–62.
32. E. W. Stieb 1970. op. cit., 21–2. (**n.9**)
33. House of Commons Select Committee on Adulteration of Food, Drinks and Drugs 1856. *Minutes of evidence*, 56–7, 253. London: HMSO.
34. Ibid. 63–5, 91–100, 142–9.
35. Ibid. 69, 288–94.
36. House of Commons Select Committee on Adulteration of Food, Drinks and Drugs 1856. *Report*, iii. London: HMSO.
37. Ibid. v.
38. House of Commons 1856. op. cit., 253. (**n.33**)
39. House of Commons 1856 op. cit., v. (**n.36**)
40. Ibid. vii
41. E. W. Stieb 1970. op. cit., 20–22. (**n.9**)
42. E. W. Stieb 1966. op. cit., 143–54. (**n.8**)
43. M. Hodges 1987. op. cit., 119. (**n.5**)
44. E. W. Stieb 1966. op. cit., 156–7. (**n.8**)
45. Ibid. 204–9.
46. J. H. Young 1961. op. cit., 94–5, 100 (**n.2**); J. Liebenau 1981. op. cit. 49. (**n.1**)
47. J. Liebenau 1981. op. cit., 45. (**n.1**)
48. M. Silverman & P. R. Lee 1974. *Pills, profits and politics*, 258. Berkeley: University of California Press.
49. R. G. Penn 1979. op. cit., 299. (**n.5**)
50. E. W. Stieb 1966. op. cit., 121–2. (**n.8**)
51. Ibid. 204–9.
52. E. W. Stieb 1966. op. cit., 129–31. (**n.8**); E. W. Stieb 1970. op. cit., 23–5. (**n.9**); W. J. Bell 1910. *The Sale of Food and Drugs Acts 1875 to 1910*, 26–7. London: Butterworth.
53. G. Tweedale 1990. op. cit., 120. (**n.18**)
54. J. H. Young 1961. op. cit., 165. (**n.2**)
55. J. Liebenau 1981. op. cit., 10–11. (**n.1**); J. J. Beer 1958. Coal tar dye manufacture and the origins of the modern industrial research laboratory. *Isis*, **49**, 123–31.
56. R. H. Wiebe 1967. *The search for order: 1877–1920*, 154. London: Macmillan.
57. J. Liebenau 1981. op. cit., 13, 53–5. (**n.1**)
58. Ibid. 15–17.
59. A. D. Chandler 1977. *The visible hand: the managerial revolution in American business.* Cambridge, Mass.: Harvard University Press.
60. I. D. Barkan 1985. Industry invites regulation: the passage of the Pure Food and Drug Act of 1906. *American Journal of Public Health*, **75**, 18–26; A. D. Chandler 1977. op. cit. (**n.59**)
61. G. Porter 1973. *The rise of big business: 1860–1910*, 56. Arlington Heights, Illinois: AHM Publishing Corporation; J. H. Young 1961. op. cit., 106–7. (**n.2**); I. D. Barkan 1985. op. cit., 18–26. (**n.60**)
62. J. H. Young 1961. op. cit., 205–25. (**n.2**)
63. R. H. Wiebe 1967. op. cit., 133–63. (**n.56**); J. H. Young 1961. op. cit., 209–10. (**n.2**)
64. J. H. Young 1961. op. cit., 211. (**n.2**)

65. T. A. Bailey 1930. Congressional opposition to pure food legislation 1879–1906. *American Journal of Sociology* **36**, 52.
66. J. H. Young, op. cit, 236. (**n.2**)
67. J. G. Burrow 1963. op. cit., 78–9. (**n.14**)
68. Ibid. 238–42.
69. H. W. Wiley 1976. *The history of a crime against the food law*, 276. Washington DC: Arno Press; G. Sonnedecker 1982. op. cit., 28–39. (**n.24**)
70. J. H. Young 1961. op. cit., 243. (**n.2**)
71. H. W. Wiley 1976. op. cit., 276. (**n,69**); G. Sonnedecker 1982. op. cit., 28–39. (**n.24**); W. J. Bell 1910. op. cit., 27. (**n.51**)
72. E. W. Stieb 1966. op. cit., 204–17. (**n.8**)
73. G. Sonnedecker 1982. op. cit., 35. (**n.24**)
74. E. W. Stieb 1966. op. cit., 204–17. (**n.8**)
75. H. W. Wiley 1976. op. cit. (**n.69**); R. H. Wiebe 1967. op. cit. (**n.56**)
76. E. W. Stieb 1966. op. cit. (**n.8**)
77. S. Hall 1984. The rise of the representative/interventionist state 1880s–1920s. In *State and society in contemporary Britain*, G. McLennan, D. Held, S. Hall (eds), 7–49. Cambridge: Polity Press.
78. J. R. Hay 1975. *The origin of the liberal welfare reforms 1906–1914*. London: Macmillan.
79. M. Bruce 1966. op. cit., 5. (**n.23**)
80. Ibid. 133–95.
81. Public Record Office (PRO) 1921. MH58/241B. *Committee on the supply of drugs for insured persons (CSDIP) report*.
82. Pharmaceutical Society of Great Britain (PSGB) 1939. Drugs in war time. *Pharmaceutical Journal* **142**, 404.
83. PSGB 1920. Manchester section. *Pharmaceutical Journal*, **104**, 308–9; PSGB 1920. Ministry of Health: first annual report. *Pharmaceutical Journal* **105**, 288–9.
84. PSGB 1920. The first year of the Ministry of Health. *Pharmaceutical Journal* **105**, 454.
85. N. A. Wynn 1986. *From progressivism to prosperity: World War I and American society*, 6. New York: Holmes & Meier.
86. Ibid. 1–25.
87. M. Plesur 1969. Introduction. In *The 1920s problems and paradoxes: selected readings*, M. Plesur (ed.), 1–13. Boston: Allyn & Bacon; M. Heald 1969. Business thought in the twenties: social responsibility. In M. Plesur (ed.), 113–27.
88. M. Silverman & P. R. Lee 1974. op. cit. 1–47. (**n.48**)
89. G. Tweedale 1990. op. cit., 116–25. (**n.18**)
90. R. K. Murray 1969. Labour and Bolshevism. In M. Plesur (ed.) op. cit., 129–44. (**n.87**); N. A. Wynn 1986. op. cit., 196–225. (**n.85**)
91. E. W. Hawley 1979. *The Great War and the search for modern order: a history of the American people and their institutions 1917–1933*, 1–7, 26–7, 80–85. New York: St Martins Press.
92. J. K. Galbraith 1969. Cause and consequence. In M. Plesur (ed.) op. cit., 153–62. (**n.87**)
93. E. W. Hawley 1979. op. cit., 81. (**n.90**)
94. Ibid. 86.
95. N. A. Wynn 1986. op. cit. 196–225. (**n.85**)
96. D. H. Aldcroft 1986. *The British economy: vol.1 the years of turmoil 1920–51*, 1–43. Sussex: Harvester.
97. PRO 1921 op. cit. (**n.81**)
98. Ibid.
99. Ibid.
100. Ibid.
101. PRO 1921. MH58/241B. *Minister of Health Minute Sheet*, 18 February.

102. PRO 1921. MH58/241B. Letter from Rolf Harris, on behalf of the CSDIP, to the Ministry of Health, 10 June.

103. PSGB 1925. Testing drugs and appliances for insured persons. *Pharmaceutical Journal* **114**, 286; PSGB 1925. Scheme for testing drugs and appliances supplied to insured persons. *Pharmaceutical Journal* **114**, 275; T. D. Whittet 1970. op. cit., 30–31. (**n.7**); PSGB 1923. National Association of Clerks to insurance committees – "the testing of drugs supplied to insured persons". *Pharmaceutical Journal* **111**, 443; PSGB 1925. Blackburn – testing dispensed medicine. *Pharmaceutical Journal* **111**, 505.

104. Dr Saleeby 1916. Sale of cocaine to soldiers on leave. *Daily Chronicle,* 19 July; R. G. Penn 1979. op. cit., 301. (**n.5**)

105. PSGB 1920. The Dangerous Drugs Act. *Pharmaceutical Journal* **104**, 33–5; PSGB 1920. The wholesalers' view. *Pharmaceutical Journal* **106**, 36–7; PSGB 1921. The retail pharmacists' view. *Pharmaceutical Journal* **106**, 37; PSGB 1921. Bureaucratic legislation. *Pharmaceutical Journal* **107**, 47–8.

106. PSGB 1921. The Dangerous Drugs Act: report of committee appointed by the Home Secretary to consider objections to the draft regulations. *Pharmaceutical Journal* **106**, 431.

107. PSGB 1922. Administration of the Dangerous Drugs Act. *Pharmaceutical Journal* **108**, 211.

108. PSGB 1921. The Dangerous Drugs Act: report of the committee appointed by the Home Secretary to consider objections to the draft regulations. *Pharmacedutical Journal* **106**, 431–2.

109. J. K. Galbraith 1969. Vision and boundless hope and optimism. In M. Plesur (ed.) op. cit., 151. (**n.87**)

110. PSGB 1928. Extravagant prescribing. *Pharmaceutical Journal* **121**, 412–13; PSGB 1933. The insurance medical benefit services. *Pharmaceutical Journal* **130**, 21.

111. PSGB 1930. Definition of drugs for medical benefit: reports of advisory committee. *Pharmaceutical Journal* **124**, 211–13.

112. R. L. Heilbroner 1968. *The making of economic society,* 6. Engelwood Cliffs, New Jersey: Prentice Hall.

113. F. D. Roosevelt 1937. The philosophy of the new deal. In *The new deal at home and abroad: 1929–1945,* C. A. Chambers (ed.), 73. New York: Free Press.

114. T. Ziporyn 1985. The food and drug administration: how "those regulations" came to be. *Journal of the American Medical Association* **254**, 2043.

115. N. Swachev 1990. The rise of statism in 1930s America: a Soviet view of the social and political effects of the new deal. In *The Great Depression and the New Deal,* M. Dubofsky & S. Burwood (eds), 105. New York: Garland; T. Ferguson 1990. From normalcy to New Deal: industrial structure, party competition and American public policy in the Great Depression. In M. Dubofsky & S. Burwood (eds) op. cit., 184–237. (**n.114**)

116. W. E. Leuchtenberg (ed.) 1968. *The new deal: a documentary history.* Columbia: University of South Carolina Press; M. Dubofsky & S. Burwood (eds) 1990. op. cit. (**n.115**)

117. B. Sternsher 1964. *Rexford Tugwell and the New Deal.* New Jersey: Rutgers University Press.

118. J. H. Young 1967. op. cit., 158–80. (**n.2**)

119. J. G. Burrow 1963. op. cit., 270–71. (**n.14**)

120. P. Temin 1980. op. cit., 34. (**n.4**); R. H. Wiebe 1967. op. cit., 298. (**n.56**)

121. M. Mintz 1964. *The therapeutic nightmare,* 46. Boston/Cambridge: Houghton/Mifflin/Riverside Press.

122. Ibid. 44–7.

123. Ibid. 45.

124. J. H. Young 1967. op. cit., 163. (**n.2**)

125. Ibid. 175-82.

126. D. F. Cavers 1970. The evolution of the contemporary system of drug regulation under the 1938 Act. In J. B. Blake (ed.) op. cit., 160. (**n.7**)

127. D. H. Aldcroft 1986. op. cit., 56–78. (**n.95**); A. C. Hill 1935. The changing foundations of pharmaceutical manufacture. *Pharmaceutical Journal* **134**, 533–4; G. Tweedale 1990. op. cit., 128–30. (**n.18**)

128. G. Tweedale 1990. op. cit., 127. (**n.18**)

129. PSGB 1929. The trade outlook II. *Pharmaceutical Journal* **122**, 23–4.

130. PSGB 1929. The wholesale drug trade association. *Pharmaceutical Journal* **123**, 486; PSGB 1945. The WDTA. *Pharmaceutical Journal* **155**, 223.

131. Anon. 1934. The other side of the medal. *Pharmaceutical Journal* **133**, 335.

132. PSGB 1934. Control of drug distribution. *Pharmaceutical Journal* **133**, 117; PSGB 1939. An onlooker's notebook: drug adulteration. *Pharmaceutical Journal* **143**, 291; PSGB 1937. Ministry of Health annual report. *Pharmaceutical Journal* **139**, 168.

133. PSGB 1934. Control of drug distribution. op. cit., 118. (**n.132**)

134. H. E. Chapman 1935. Twenty-five years of patent medicines. *Pharmaceutical Journal* **134**, 544; G. A. Mallinson 1935. National health insurance 1911–1935 *Pharmaceutical Journal* **134**, 535–7.

135. BMA 1909. *Secret remedies: what they are and what they contain.* London: BMA.

136. W. S. Howells 1941. The Pharmacy and Medicines Act 1941: pitfalls for pharmacists. *Pharmaceutical Journal* **147**, 140–41.

137. Quoted in H. E. Chapman 1935. op. cit., 543. (**n.134**)

138. R. G. Penn 1979. op. cit., 302. (**n.5**)

139. PRO 1940. MH80/21.

140. PRO 1940. MH80/21. Letter from M. J. Hewitt, Ministry of Health to De Montmorency, 9 November.

141. PRO 1941. MH80/21. Customs and Excise Department, *Report to the Chancellor of the Exchequer and the Minister of Health on the medicine stamp duties and the control of proprietary medicines.*

142. D. H. Aldcroft 1986. op. cit., 182–3. (**n.95**); PSGB 1939. The drug market in war time. *Pharmaceutical Journal* **143**, 325-6.

143. PRO 1941. MH80/21. Customs and Excise Department op. cit. (**n.141**); PSGB 1941. The Pharmacy and Medicines Bill. *Pharmaceutical Journal* **147**, 1.

144. PRO 1941. MH80/21. Letter from Sir Ian Fraser MP to Sir Kingsley Wood, Chancellor of the Exchequer, 24 January 1941.

145. PRO 1941. MH80/21. Customs and Excise op. cit. (**n.141**)

146. PRO 1941. MH80/21. *Minute Sheet,* 13 February; PRO 1941. MH80/21. *Medicine Stamp Acts.*

147. PSGB 1941. The Pharmacy and Medicines Act 1941: The Society and the NPU. *Pharmaceutical Journal* **147**, 86.

148. PRO 1941. MH80/21. Letter from W. Eady, Customs and Excise to Sir John Maude, Secretary of Health, 26 February.

149. PRO 1941. MH80/21. Letter from J. N. Beckett, Ministry of Health to H. N. Linstead, PSGB, 17 April.

150. R. D. Mann 1984. op. cit. (**n.5**); G. Tweedale 1990. op. cit. (**n.18**); P. R. Silverman M. and Lee, 1974. op. cit. (**n.88**)

151. M. Silverman & P. R. Lee 1974. op. cit., 1–6. (**n.88**)

152. P. Temin 1980. op. cit., 4. (**n.4**)

153. P. Temin 1980. op. cit., 58–87. (**n.4**); M. Silverman & P. R. Lee 1974. op. cit., 48–80. (**n.88**); R. Harris 1964. *The real voice,* 31, 64. New York: Macmillan.

154. PSGB 1970. Scottish drug testing 1969. *Pharmaceutical Journal* **204**, 199.

155. PRO 1951. MH58/688. *Review of drug legislation.*

156. Ministry of Health/Department of Health for Scotland and Central Health Services

Council 1950 *The second interim report of the joint committee on prescribing*, 4. London: HMSO.

157. PSGB 1957. The classification of proprietaries. *Pharmaceutical Journal* **178**, 239.

158. Ministry of Health 1950 op. cit., 7. (**n.156**)

159. PRO 1951. op. cit. (**n.155**)

160. Ibid.

161. Ibid.

162. Ibid.

163. PSGB 1948. The ABPI. *Pharmaceutical Journal* **160**, 387–8; PSGB 1948. The WDTA: change of name. *Pharmaceutical Journal* **160**, 402.

164. PSGB 1950. Anxiety for the future. *Pharmaceutical Journal* **164**, 294; R. W. Lang 1974. *The politics of drugs: a comparative pressure-group study of the Canadian pharmaceutical manufacturers association and the association of the British pharmaceutical industry 1930–1970*, 63. Farnborough, England: Saxon House; PSGB 1950. Pharmaceutical industry and export drive. *Pharmaceutical Journal* **164**, 11; PSGB 1956. Recruitment by the industry. *Pharmaceutical Journal* **176**, 1.

165. PSGB 1950. Annual report of the ABPI. *Pharmaceutical Journal* **164**, 11.

166. D. H. Aldcroft 1986. op. cit., 201–49. (**n.96**)

167. G. Thompson 1984. Economic intervention in the post-war economy. In *State and society in contemporary Britain*, G. McLennan, D. Held, S. Hall (eds), 77–118. Cambridge: Polity Press.

168. PSGB 1956. Recruitment by the industry. *Pharmaceutical Journal* **176**, 1.

169. PRO 1946–53. MH58/687. Draft memorandum (undated) on a long-term policy for securing the availability of supplies of drugs and medical products.

170. PRO 1950. MH133/76. Note of discussion on 8 June between representatives of the Ministry of Health and the ABPI; PRO 1950. MH133/76. Memorandum from J. S. Walmsley, Secretary of the Proprietry Association of Great Britain (PAGB) to the Ministry of Health on 14 June, regarding the second interim report of the JCP.

171. PRO 1950. MH133/76. Letter from Sir J. H. Woods, Board of Trade, to Sir William Douglas, Ministry of Health, 20 July.

172. PRO 1950. MH133/76. Letter from Sir William Douglas to Sir J. Woods, Board of Trade, 28 July.

173. For example, in 1954 the Parliamentary Secretary to the Ministry of Health told the ABPI: "I wish well to the export trade without which there will be no welfare service and we shall be the poorer to pay the country". See PSGB 1954. ABPI annual dinner: speech by Miss Hornsby-Smith MP. *Pharmaceutical Journal* **172**, 312. Also see PSGB 1956. British pharmaceutical industry: speech by Minister of Health. *Pharmaceutical Journal* **176**, 239.

174. PSGB 1957. VPRS: arrangement between the ABPI and the Health Departments. *Pharmaceutical Journal* **178**, 441.

175. PSGB 1959. Trade association news. *Pharmaceutical Journal* **182**, 348–9.

176. PSGB 1960. The industry reviews 1959–60. *Pharmaceutical Industry* **184**, 401–2.

177. J. H. Young 1967. op. cit., 408–22. (**n.2**)

178. R. Harris 1964. op. cit., 1–50. (**n.153**)

179. Ibid. 90.

180. Ibid. 78–9.

181. Ibid. 89.

182. M. Silverman & P. R. Lee 1974. op. cit., 49. (**n.88**)

183. W. Dameshek 1960. Chloramphenicol: a new warning. *Journal of the American Medical Association* **174**, 1853; R. Harris 1964. op. cit., 96–104. (**n.153**)

184. R. Harris 1964. op. cit., 121–2. (**n.153**)

185. Ibid. 124–6.

186. Ibid. 124.

187. Ibid. 141.
188. Ibid. 162–6.
189. Ibid. 221.
190. PSGB 1959. Testing of new drugs. *Pharmaceutical Journal* **183**, 1; PSGB 1960. Testing of new drugs. *Pharmaceutical Journal* **184**, 148; PSGB 1960. The industry reviews 1959–60. *Pharmaceutical Journal* **184**, 401–2.
191. PSGB 1961. Evidence by Advertising Inquiry Council. *Pharmaceutical Journal* **186**, 155; PSGB 1962. Hot milk at bedtime? *Pharmaceutical Journal* **189**, 174.
192. L. Hancher 1989. *Regulating for competition: government, law and the pharmaceutical industry in the United Kingdom and France*. PhD thesis, University of Amsterdam.
193. P. I. Folb 1977. *The thalidomide disaster and its impact on modern medicine*. University of Capetown inaugural lecture 8 September, 2–4; *Sunday Times* 1973. *The thalidomide children and the law*, 7, 11. London: Andre Deutsch.
194. H. Taussig 1962. The thalidomide syndrome. *Scientific American* **207**, 29.
195. PSGB 1962. Toxic hazards of new drugs. *Pharmaceutical Journal* **188**, 112.
196. PSGB 1962. Clinical trials of drugs. *Pharmaceutical Journal* **188**, 429; PSGB 1962. Drug toxicity: debate on drug control. *Pharmaceutical Journal* **189**, 523–4.
197. PSGB 1962. Testing of new drugs. *Pharmaceutical Journal* **188**, 552–3; PSGB 1962. Testing of new drugs. *Pharmaceutical Journal* **189**, 83.
198. Association of the British Pharmaceutical Industry (ABPI) 1963. Safety testing and clinical trials. *ABPI annual report 1962–63*, 10.
199. P. Temin 1980. op. cit., 123. (**n.4**); R. Harris 1964. op. cit., 182–94. (**n.153**)
200. R. Harris 1964. op. cit., 204–5. (**n.153**)
201. Ibid. 220.
202. Ibid. 206.
203. P. Temin 1980. op. cit., 125. (**n.4**); M. Silverman & P. R. Lee 1974. op. cit., 121. (**n.88**)
204. R. G. Marks 1974. Pharmaceuticals. In S. S. Epstein & R. D. Grundy (eds) op. cit., 175–7. (**n.3**)
205. H. F. Dowling 1970. *Medicines for man*, 255. New York: Knopf.
206. M. Silverman & P. R. Lee 1974. op. cit., 122. (**n.88**)
207. Division of Medical Sciences, National Research Council (NRC) 1969. *Drug efficacy study: final report to commissioner of FDA*, 9. Washington DC: National Academy of Sciences; M. Silverman & P. R. Lee 1974. op. cit., 131. (**n.87**)
208. M. Silverman & P. R. Lee 1974. op. cit., 124. (**n.88**)
209. Ibid. 125. '
210. P. Temin 1980. op. cit., 133–7. (**n.4**)
211. Hearings Before a Subcommittee of the Committee on Government Operations, House of Representatives 1969. *Drug efficacy* (Part 2), 199, 201. Washington DC: US Government Publications Office.
212. Review Panel on New Drug Regulation (Special Counsel) 1977. *Investigation of allegations relating to the Bureau of Drugs, Food and Drug Administration*, 47–64. Washington DC: US Government Publications Office.
213. R. G. Marks 1974. op. cit., 157. (**n.3**)
214. S. M. Wolfe, C. M. Coley and Health Research Group 1980. *Pills that don't work: a consumers' and doctors' guide to over 600 prescription drugs that lack evidence of effectiveness*. New York: Farrar Straus Giroux.
215. PSGB 1962. Testing of new drugs. *Pharmaceutical Journal* **188**, 552–3; PSGB 1963. The industry and the health service. *Pharmaceutical Journal* **150**, 417–18.
216. ABPI 1963. op. cit., 10. (**n.198**); PSGB 1962. Ministry of Health: interim advice on testing of new drugs. *Pharmaceutical Journal* **189**, 450–51.
217. PSGB 1962. op. cit., 451. (**n.216**)
218. PSGB 1962. "Magnificent" export performance. *Pharmaceutical Journal* **189**, 445.

219. D. E. Wheeler 1963. President's statement. *ABPI annual report 1962–1963*, 5–6; D. E. Wheeler 1964. President's statement. *ABPI annual report 1963–64*, 2.

220. PSGB 1962. Drug toxicity: industry's proposals to Joint Subcommittee. *Pharmaceutical Journal* **189**, 522; PSGB 1963. Drug toxicity: industry's memo to Joint Subcommittee *Pharmaceutical Journal* **190**, 86; ABPI 1963. op. cit., 10. (**n.197**)

221. Ministry of Health/Scottish Home and Health Department 1963. *Safety of drugs: final report of the Joint Sub-Committee of the Standing Medical Advisory Committees*, 12–14. London: HMSO; PSGB 1963. Safety of drugs. *Pharmaceutical Journal* **190**, 311–12.

222. Ministry of Health/Scottish Home and Health Department 1963. op. cit., 5–11. (**n.221**); PSGB 1963. Safety of drugs: Joint Subcommittee's final report. *Pharmaceutical Journal* **190**, 317–21; PSGB 1963. op. cit. (**n.221**)

223. PSGB 1963, The industry and the health service. *Pharmaceutical Journal* **190**, 417–18.

224. G. M. Wilson 1962. Assessing new drugs. *New Scientist* **297**, 196.

225. PSGB 1963. Committee on safety of drugs: members and terms of reference. *Pharmaceutical Journal* **190**, 534.

226. PSGB 1975. Eraldin: limited to hospitals. *Pharmaceutical Journal* **215**, 140.

227. F. Lesser 1977. Drug warnings. *New Scientist* **78**, 442.

228. PSGB 1963. Committee on Safety of Drugs: assessment of reports to begin on Jan. 1st. *Pharmaceutical Journal* **191**, 313.

229. PSGB 1963. Committee on Safety of Drugs: memo to manufacturers and importers. *Pharmaceutical Journal* **191**, 433.

230. D. E. Wheeler 1964. op. cit., 3. (**n.219**)

231. Committee on Safety of Drugs (CSD) 1965. *Annual report for the year ending 1964*, 6–8. London: HMSO.

232. PSGB 1966. Safety of drugs: Dunlop Committee Second Report. *Pharmaceutical Journal* **197**, 86–7.

233. PSGB 1967. Safety of drugs: Committee's Annual Report. *Pharmaceutical Journal* **199**, 59–60.

234. ABPI 1966. Safety of medicines. *ABPI annual report 1965–66*, 13. London: ABPI.

235. ABPI 1965. Safety of medicines. *ABPI annual report 1964–65*, 9–10. London: ABPI.

236. ABPI 1966. The industry and the NHS. *ABPI annual report 1965–66*, 7–8. London: ABPI; ABPI 1967 efficacy of medicines. *ABPI annual report 1966–1967*, 10. London: ABPI.

237. Cited in Cmnd 3410 1967. *Report of the committee of enquiry into the relationship of the pharmaceutical industry with the National Health Service 1965–1967*, 68. London: HMSO.

238. ABPI 1964. Trade marks and sales promotion. *ABPI annual report 1963–64*, 10; Cmnd 3410 1967. op. cit., 63. (**n.237**)

239. Cmnd 3410 1967. op. cit., 63–71. (**n.237**)

240. Ibid. 75–98.

241. PSGB 1967. New ABPI code of practice. *Pharmaceutical Journal* **198**, 692–3; ABPI 1967. Marketing. *ABPI annual report 1966–67*, 16. London: ABPI.

242. ABPI 1967. Review of the year: code of practice. *ABPI annual report 1966–67*, 8. London: ABPI.

243. ABPI 1968. Review of the year: the Sainsbury report. *ABPI annual report 1967–68*, 6–7; ABPI 1968. Legislation: Medicines Bill. *ABPI annual report 1967–68*, 9.

244. Cmnd 3395 1967. *Forthcoming legislation on the safety, quality and description of drugs and medicines*. London: HMSO.

245. PSGB 1968. Industry, safety, Sainsbury and the Bill. *Pharmaceutical Journal* **200**, 274–5.

246. D. Dunlop 1971. *The problem of modern medicines and their control*, 20. 11 February, Twelfth Maurice Bloch lecture, University of Glasgow.

247. Twenty-second Report Committee on Government Operations 1970. *The British drug safety system*, 37. 91st Congress, 2nd Session. Washington DC: US Government Publications Office.

248. O. L. Wade 1983. Achievements, problems and limitations of regulatory bodies. In *Medicines review worldwide – a patient benefit or a regulatory burden? Proceedings of the fifth annual symposium of the British Institute of Regulatory Affairs*, D. Farrell (ed.), 3. London: BIRA.

249. PSGB 1968. op. cit. (**n.245**)

250. PSGB 1968. The Medicines Bill in committee. *Pharmaceutical Journal* **200**, 334–5; PSGB 1968. Medicines Bill: committee stage. *Pharmaceutical Journal* **200**, 368–9.

251. PSGB 1968. Medicines Bill: committee stage. *Pharmaceutical Journal* **200**, 457–8.

252. Anon. 1962. Open meeting statutes: the press fights for the "right to know". *Harvard Law Review*, **75**, 1199–203; E. Campbell 1967. Public access to government documents. *The Australian Law Journal* **41**, 73–89; R. Nader 1970. Freedom from information: the act and the agencies. *Harvard Civil Liberties Law Review*, **5**, 1; M. Elengold 1980. Freedom of information policy at the FDA. *Food, Drug and Cosmetic Law Journal*, **35**, 631; R. M. Halperin 1979. FDA disclosure of safety and effectiveness data: a legal and policy analysis. *Duke Law Journal*, **286**, 286–326.

253. PSGB 1968. Medicines Bill receives cautious approval. *Pharmaceutical Journal* **286**, 215–18.

254. ABPI 1970. Legislation: Medicines Commission. *ABPI annual report 1969-1970*, 9. London: ABPI.

255. ABPI 1971. Annual dinner. *ABPI annual report 1970–71*, 15. London: ABPI.

256. PSGB 1970. Medicines Act reassurance for manufacturers. *Pharmaceutical Journal* **204**, 48.

257. ABPI 1971. The Medicines Act: committees. *ABPI annual report 1970–71*, 10. London: ABPI.

258. Ibid.

259. D. Gould 1972. Sir Derrick Dunlop – noblesse oblige? *New Scientist* **53**, 626.

260. *Medicines Act 1968*, 2. London: HMSO.

261. J. Collier 1985. Licencing and provision of medicine in the UK: an appraisal. *Lancet* **2**, 377–80.

262. ABPI 1984. Dr John Griffin takes over as ABPI Chief. *ABPI News* **198**, 1; ABPI 1984. New ABPI director stresses importance of two-way flow between medicines division and industry. *ABPI News* **198**, 3.

263. Ibid.

264. Ibid.

265. ABPI 1972. Review of the year: Medicines Act 1968. *ABPI annual report 1971–72*, 5. London: ABPI.

266. J. Collier 1989. *The health conspiracy*. London: Century.

267. J. Liebenau 1987. *Medical science and medical industry*, 89. London: Macmillan; J. Braithwaite 1986. *Corporate crime in the pharmaceutical industry*, 298. London: Routledge & Kegan Paul.

268. United States Office of Government Ethics 1979. *Summary of the post-employment restrictions of the Ethics in Government Act of 1978 and important interpretations in the regulations*. Washington DC: US Government Publications Office.

269. ABPI 1972. Review of the year: Medicines Act 1968. *ABPI annual report 1971–72*, 5. London: ABPI.

270. Committee on Safety of Medicines (CSM) 1978. *Annual report 1977*, 28. London: HMSO; CSD 1972. *Report for year ending 1971*, 12. London: HMSO.

271. B. J. Cromie 1980. Testing new drugs in the UK. *Journal of the Royal Society of Medicine* **73**, 379–80.

272. J. P. Griffin & G. E. Diggle 1981. A survey of products licenced in the UK from 1971–81. British *Journal of Clinical Pharmacology* **12**, 461; ABPI 1977. Lessons of a decade. *ABPI News* **164**, 6.

273. F. Lesser 1977. op. cit., 442. (**n.226**)

274. PSGB 1976. MPs call for official inquiry into Eraldin. *Pharmaceutical Journal* **217**, 427.
275. British Medical Association (BMA) 1978. New proposals on surveillance of drugs. *British Medical Journal* **1**, 588; ABPI 1977. Sir Eric calls for restricted release. *ABPI News* **166**, 3.
276. T. B. Binns 1980. The Committee on the Review of Medicines. *British Medical Journal* **281**, 1614–15; BMA 1977 Committee on the Review of Medicines: testing the golden oldies. *British Medical Journal* **279**, 716.
277. R. Hurley 1983. The Medicines Act – is it working? *Journal of the British Institute of Regulatory Affairs (BIRA)* **2**, 3.
278. L. Hancher 1989. op. cit. (**n.192**)
279. Ibid.
280. ABPI 1974. Review of the year: nationalization or public ownership. *ABPI annual report 1973–74*, 6; ABPI 1974. Information and services and public relations: nationalization. *ABPI annual report 1973–74*, 17.
281. G. Thompson 1984. "Rolling Back" the state? Economic intervention 1975–82. In G. McLennan, D. Held, S. Hall (eds) op. cit, 286. (**n.167**)
282. Cited in G. Thompson 1984. op. cit., 274. (**n.281**)
283. ABPI 1977. *ABPI annual report 1976–77*, 9.
284. Ibid. 17.
285. R. D. Smart 1981. Foreword. *ABPI annual report 1980–81*, 3.
286. BMA 1976. Pharmaceutical industry. *British Medical Journal* **278**, 1397. PSGB 1976. CSM asked to speed up procedures. *Pharmaceutical Journal* **217**, 46.
287. PSGB 1976. op. cit. (**n.286**)
288. ABPI 1980. Annual dinner 1980. *ABPI annual report 1979–80*, 24.
289. Ibid; ABPI 1981 medical and scientific affairs. *ABPI annual report 1980–81*, 6; DHSS 1981. MLX 130 Medicines Act 1968: data requirements for clinical trial certificates. London: DHSS; L. Hancher 1989. op. cit., 99. (**n.192**)
290. R. D. Smart 1981. op. cit., 3. (**n.285**)
291. J. P. Griffin & J. R. Long 1981. New procedures affecting the conduct of clinical trials in the United Kingdom. *British Medical Journal* **283**, 477.
292. PSGB 1976. Unsatisfactory Advertisements. *Pharmaceutical Journal* **217**, 106.
293. PSGB 1979. ABPI Produces New Code of Advertising Practice. *Pharmaceutical Journal* 3 March, 78; ABPI 1978. Advertising Regs: Government pushes them through. *ABPI News* **172**, 1.
294. Joint Hearings Before the Subcommittee on Health of the Committee on Labor and Public Welfare and the Subcommitee on Administrative Practice and Procedure of the Senate Committee on the Judiciary 1974. Examination of the Pharmaceutical Industry (Part 7), 2830. Washington DC: US Government Publications Office.
295. Joint Hearings op. cit., 2834, 2839. (**n.294**)
296. Ibid. 2953–4.
297. A. M. Schmidt 1975. *The commissioner's report of investigation of charges from Joint Hearings*, 901. Washington DC: US Government Publications Office.
298. Review Panel on New Drug Regulation 1976. *Assessment of the commissioner's report of October 1975*, (summary), 2. Washington DC: US Government Publications Office.
299. Review Panel on New Drug Regulation 1976 op. cit. (main report), 20–21. (**n.298**)
300. Review Panel on New Drug Regulation 1976 op. cit., 16. (**n.298**)
301. Review Panel on New Drug Regulation 1977 Summary of Special Counsel's Conclusions, 2. Washington DC: US Government Publications Office.
302. Ibid. 2.
303. Special Counsel to Review Panel on New Drug Regulation 1977. *Investigation of allegations relating to the bureau of drugs, food and drug administration*, 720. Washington DC: Dept of Health, Education and Welfare.
304. Ibid. 720.

305. J. Collier 1989. op. cit., 74. (**n.266**)
306. US Department of Health and Human Services 1987. *All about FDA: an orientation handbook*, 47–9. Rockville, Maryland: FDA.
307. R. G. Penn 1980. The drug industry. *British Medical Journal* **281**, 1563–4.
308. J. Braithwaite 1986. op. cit., 382. (**n.267**)
309. J. Liebenau 1981. op. cit., 265. (**n.1**)
310. J. Smith 1980. Drug famine: possible solutions. *British Medical Journal* **281**, 1476.

Chapter Three

1. E. C. Huskisson 1983. Classification of anti-rheumatic drugs. In *Anti-rheumatic drugs*, E. C. Huskisson (ed.), 1–4. New York: Praeger.
2. J. A. Mills 1974. Non-steroidal anti-inflammatory drugs. *New England Journal of Medicine* **288**, 781.
3. A. R. Cooke 1973. The role of acid in the pathogenesis of aspirin-induced gastro-intestinal erosions and haemorrhage. *American Journal of Digestive Diseases* **18**, 225–37.
4. H. K. Von Rechenberg 1962. *Phenylbutazone*. London: Edward Arnold.
5. J. M. Bland, D. R. Jones, S. Bennett, D. G. Cook, A. P. Haines, A. J. MacFarlane 1985. Is the clinical trial evidence about new drugs statistically adequate? *British Journal of Clinical Pharmacology* **19**, 156.
6. R. T. Woods & P. G. Britton 1985. *Clinical psychology with the elderly*, 2–6. Kent: Croom Helm.
7. S. J. Hopkins 1986. *Drugs and pharmacology for nurses*, 75. Edinburgh: Churchill Livingstone.
8. P. J. Piper & J. R. Vane 1971. The release of prostaglandins from lung and other tissues. *Annals of the New York Academy of Sciences* **180**, 363.
9. J. R. Vane 1971. Inhibition of prostaglandin synthesis as a mechanism for aspirin-like drugs. *Nature New Biology* **231**, 232–5.
10. G. A. Higgs, S. Moncada, J. R. Vane 1983. The mode of action of anti-inflammatory drugs which prevent peroxidation of arachidonic acid. In E. C. Huskisson (ed.), op. cit, 11–36. (**n.1**)
11. G. Weissman 1967. The role of lysosomes in inflammation and disease. *Annual Review of Medicine* **18**, 97–112.
12. M. Di Rosa, J. M. Papadimitriou, D. A. Willoughby 1971. A histopathological and pharmacological analysis of the mode of action of nonsteroidal anti-inflammatory drugs. *Journal of Pathology* **105**, 239.
13. G. A. Higgs, J. R. Vane, F. D. Hart, J. A. Wojtulewski 1974. Effects of anti-inflammatory drugs on prostaglandins in rheumatoid arthritis. In *Prostaglandin synthetase inhibitors – their effects on physiological functions and pathological states*, H. J. Robinson & J. R. Vane (eds), 172. New York: Raven Press.
14. E. Millstone 1986. *Food additives: taking the lid off what we really eat*, 74–86. London: Penguin.
15. T. H. Maugh 1978. Chemical carcinogens: the scientific basis for regulation. *Science* **201**, 1200–1205.
16. Ibid. 1200.
17. World Health Organisation (WHO) 1974. Assessment of the carcinogenicity and mutagenicity of chemicals. *Technical Report Series* **546**, 8–9.
18. Ibid. 6–8.
19. Ibid. 9.
20. J. M. Barnes & F. A. Denz 1954. Experimental methods used in determining chronic

toxcity: critical review. *Pharmacological Reviews* **6**, 191–242.

21. D. E. Stevenson 1979. Current problems in the choice of animals for toxicity testing. *Journal of Toxicology and Environmental Health* **5**, 9.

22. D. Salsburg 1983. The lifetime feeding study in mice and rats – an examination of its validity as a bioassay for human carcinogens. *Fundamental and Applied Toxicology* **3**, 63–7.

23. FDA 1976. "IBT study carried out for Syntex". Memo by M. Hein & A. Gross, 10 August.

24. FDA 1976. "Naproxen chronic toxicity/carcinogenesis study by IBT". Memo by C. King, 15 July, 3.

25. US Congress Hearings before the Subcommittee on Health and Scientific Research of the Senate Committee on Human Resources. *Preclinical and Clinical Testing by the Pharmaceutical Industry 1977, Part IV*, 10 March 1977, 4. Hereafter referred to as "Naprosyn Hearings".

26. FDA 1976. "Summary of inspectional findings made in connection with 22-month oral administration study conducted in rats by IBT on naproxen". Memo by A. Gross & M. Hein.

27. FDA 1976. "IBT study on naproxen". Memo by M. Hein & A. Gross, 10 August.

28. Ibid. 19–21.

29. FDA 1976. "Naproxen chronic toxicity/carcinogenesis study by IBT". Memo by C. King, 15 July, 2–3.

30. FDA 1976. "Naproxen chronic toxicity/carcinogenesis study by IBT". Memo by C. King, 15 July, 3.

31. FDA 1976, op. cit. (**n.26**)

32. FDA 1976. "Inspection of IBT/naprosyn". Memo, 6 July.

33. FDA 1976. "Naproxen". Memo by F. Kelsey, 20 July. Letter from R. Crout, Director of Bureau of Drugs, FDA to H. Anderson, Syntex Corporation, 5 August 1976, 4.

34. Letter from R. Crout, Director of Bureau of Drugs, FDA to H. Anderson, Syntex Corporation, 5 August 1976, 4.

35. FDA 1976. Memo of meeting with Syntex, 20 August.

36. FDA 1976. "Syntex meeting – naproxen". Memo, 2 September.

37. FDA 1976. "Syntex – naprosyn". Memo, 30 August.

38. FDA 1976. Pharmacology review of naproxen, 30 August, 14.

39. Ibid. 15.

40. FDA 1977. "Review and evaluation of the Syntex submission in response to our notice of hearing (NOH) to withdraw the NDA on naprosyn". Memo by A. Gross, 14 January. FDA 1977. "Review of data submitted in relation to NOH for naproxen. Memo by M. Hein, 14 January.

41. Naprosyn Hearings, 7.

42. Ibid. 9.

43. Ibid.

44. Ibid.

45. Interview with Dr Kerausitis, FDA Medical Officer, 3 November 1988.

46. *Naprosyn Data Sheets*, 1975–81.

47. Ibid.

Chapter Four

1. Dista Products Ltd (Dista) 1981. Opren advertisement, "A brand new way of working". *British Medical Journal* **282**, 10 and 24 January.

2. Dista 1981. Opren advertisement. "Why is the tide turning in the treatment of arthri-

tis?" *British Medical Journal* **282**, 21 February, 21 March, 18 April, 2 May, 16 May, 30 May; Dista 1981. Opren advertisement. "Here's the news in black and white and here it is in colour". *British Medical Journal* **283**, 5 September, 12 September, 19 September, 10 October.

3. Oraflex Press Kit, 1–4.

4. US Congress 1982 Hearings before a Subcommittee of the Committee on Government Operations House of Representatives 97th Congress. *The regulation of new drugs by the Food and Drug Administration: the new drug review process*, 3 and 4 August, 485–6. Washington DC: US Government Publications Office. (Hereafter referred to as "Hearings 1982")

5. W. E. Brocklehurst & W. Dawson 1974. New data concerning the inhibition of prostaglandin formation by anti-inflammatory drugs. In *Future trends in inflammation*, G. P. Velo, D. A. Willoughby, J. P. Giroud (eds), 40. London: Piccin Medical Books.

6. Ibid. 43.

7. C. H. Cashin, W. Dawson, E. A. Kitchen 1977. The pharmacology of benoxaprofen (2-[4-chlorophenyl]-a-methyl–5-benzoxazole acetic acid), LRCL 3794, a new compound with anti-inflammatory activity apparently unrelated to inhibition of prostaglandin synthesis. *Journal of Pharmacy and Pharmacology* **29**, 335–6.

8. Ibid. 336.

9. A. W. Ford-Hutchinson, J. R. Walker, N. S. Connor, A. M. Oliver, M. J. H. Smith 1977. Separate anti-inflammatory effects of indomethacin, flurbiprofen and benoxaprofen. *Journal of Pharmacy and Pharmacology* **29**, 372.

10. J. A. Salmon, G. A. Higgs, L. Tilling, S. Moncada, J. R. Vane 1984. Mode of action of benoxaprofen. *Lancet* **1**, 848.

11. G. A. Higgs, K. E. Eakins, K. G. Mugridge, S. Moncada, J. R. Vane 1980. The effects of non-steroid anti-inflammatory drugs on leucocyte migration in carrageenan-induced inflammation. *European Journal of Pharmacology* **66**, 81–6.

12. J. E. Smolen & G. Weissman 1980. Effects of indomethacin, 5,8,11,14-eicosatetracynoic acid, and p-bromphenacyl bormide on lysosomal enzyme release and superoxide anion generation by human polymorphonuclear leukocytes. *Biochemical Pharmacology* **29**, 533–8.

13. W. Dawson 1979. Mediators of inflammation, particularly prostaglandins and their relative importance. *European Journal of Rheumatology and Inflammation* **3**, 21–2.

14. E. C. Huskisson 1979. Clinical studies with benoxaprofen. *European Journal of Rheumatology and Inflammation* **3**, 29.

15. S. C. R. Meacock, E. A. Kitchen, W. Dawson 1979. Effects of benoxaprofen and some other non-steroidal anti-inflammatory drugs on leucocyte migration. *European Journal of Rheumatology and Inflammation* **3**, 23.

16. Ibid. 369–70.

17. W. Dawson 1980. The comparative pharmacology of benoxaprofen. *Journal of Rheumatology Supplement* **7**, 5; S. C. R. Meacock, E. A. Kitchen, W. Dawson 1979. op. cit., 28. (**n.15**)

18. W. Dawson 1980. op. cit., (**n.17**)

19. S. S. Adam, C. A. Burrows, N. Skeldon, D. Yates 1977. Inhibition of prostaglandin synthesis and leukocyte migration by flurbiprofen. *Current Medical Research and Opinion* **5**, 11–16; A. Blackman & R. T. Owen 1975. Prostaglandin synthetase inhibitors and leucocyte emigration. *Journal of Pharmacy and Pharmacology* **27**, 201–2; M. Di Rosa, J. P. Papadimitriou, D. A. Willoughby 1971. Histopathological and pharmacological analysis of the mode of action of non-steroid anti-inflammatory drugs. *Journal of Pathology* **105**, 239–56; A. W. Ford-Hutchinson et al. 1975 Effects of a human plasma fraction on leucocyte migration into inflammatory exudates. *Journal of Pharmacy and Pharmacology* **27**, 106–12; I. Rivkin, G. Foschi, C. H. Rosen 1976. Inhibition of in vitro neutrophil

chemotaxis and spontaneous motility by anti-inflammatory agents. *Proceedings of the Society of Experimental Biology and Medicine* **153**, 236–40; M. Sato, K. Furuta, A. Yamaguchi 1980. Inhibitory effect of non-steroidal anti-inflammatory drugs on neutrophil chemotaxis by casein. *Japanese Journal of Pharmacology* **30**, 919–22; S. Spisani, G. Vanzini, S. Traniello 1979. Inhibition of human leukocyte locomotion by anti-inflammatory drugs. *Experimentia* **35**, 803–4; J. R. Walker, M. J. H. Smith, A. W. Ford-Hutchinson 1976. Anti-inflammatory drugs, prostaglandins and leukocyte migration. *Agents and Actions* **6**, 602–6.

20. US Court 1983. Deposition of W. O'Brien *Clarence Borom vs Eli Lilly and Company*, District Court for the Middle District of Georgia, Columbus Division, 28 September. (Hereafter referred to as O'Brien depo). W. M. O'Brien 1983. Selective immobilization of monocytes by benoxaprofen. Unpublished letter submitted to *Arthritis and Rheumatism*, 17 February, 1–2.

21. W. Dawson 1980. op. cit., 10–11. (**n.17**)

22. M. Di Rosa et al. 1971. op. cit., 255. (**n.19**)

23. A. Blackman & R. T. Owen 1975. op. cit., 201–2 (**n.19**); J. R. Walker et al. 1976. op. cit., 602–6. (**n.19**)

24. R. J. Smith & S. S. Iden 1980. Pharmacological modulation of chemotactic factor-elicited release of granule-associated enzymes from human neutrophils. *Biochemical Pharmacology* **29**, 2392.

25. M. W. Ropes & W. Bauer 1953. *Synovial fluid changes in joint disease*, 150. Cambridge, Mass.: Harvard University Press.

26. W. Dawson, J. R. Boot, J. Harvey, J. R. Walker 1982. The pharmacology of benoxaprofen with particular reference to effects on lipoxygenase product formation. *European Journal of Rheumatology and Inflammation*. **5**, 61.

27. Ibid. 61.

28. Dista 1980. *Opren Data Sheet*. April.

29. W. Dawson et al. 1982. op. cit., 67. (**n.26**)

30. Ibid. 61.

31. W. Dawson 1980. op. cit., 9 & 11. (**n.17**)

32. G. A. Higgs & K. G. Mugridge 1982. The effects on carrageenan-induced inflammation of compounds which interfere with arachidonic acid metabolism. *British Journal of Pharmacology* **76**, 284P.

33. D. J. Masters & M. McMillan 1984. 5-lipoxygenase from human leucocytes. *British Journal of Pharmacology* **81**, 70P.

34. J. R. Walker & W. Dawson 1979. Inhibition of rabbit PMN lipoxygenase activity by benoxaprofen. *Journal of Pharmacy and Pharmacology*. **31**, 779.

35. W. Dawson et al. 1982. op. cit. (**n.26**)

36. J. A. Salmon et al. 1984. op. cit., 848. (**n.10**)

37. R. Anderson & H. A. Eftychis 1986. Potentiation of the generation of reactive oxidants by human phagocytes during exposure to benoxaprofen and ultraviolet radiation in vitro. *British Journal of Dermatology*, **115**, 292; K. A. Brown, J. Ferrie, B. Wilbourn, D. C. Dumonde 1984. Benoxaprofen, a potent inhibitor of monocyte/endothelial-cell interaction. *Lancet* **2**, 643; R. D. R. Camp et al. 1985. The role of chemo-attractant lipoxygenase products in the pathogenesis of psoriasis. *British Journal of Dermatology* **113**, Suppl., 100; M. Forrest & P. M. Brooks 1988. Mechanism of action of non-steroidal anti-rheumatic drugs. *Balliere's Clinical Rheumatology* **2**, 282; M. W. Greaves 1987. Pharmacology and significance of non-steroidal anti-inflammatory drugs in the treatment of skin diseases. *Journal of the American Academy of Dermatology* **16**, 759; M. Greaves, R. Barr, R. Camp 1984. Leukotriene-B$_4$-like immunoreactivity and skin disease. *Lancet*, **2**, 160; G. A. Higgs & S. Moncada 1985. Leukotrienes in disease implications for drug development. *Drugs* **30**, 4; K. Kragballe, S. Ternowitz, T. Herlin 1985. Normalization of monocyte chemotaxis precedes clinical resolution of psoriasis treated with

benoxaprofen. *Acta Dermatologica Venereologica* **65**, 319; P. T. Lukey, R. Anderson, U. H. Dippenaar 1988. Benoxaprofen activates membrane-associated oxidative metabolism in human polymorphonuclear leucocytes by apparent modulation of protein kiase C. *British Journal of Pharmacology* **93**, 289; P. D. L. Maurice, P. C. Bather, B. R. Allen 1986. Arachidonic acid metabolism by polymorhonuclear leukocytes in psoriasis. *British Journal of Dermatology,* **114**, 58; P. D. L. Maurice, B. R. Allen, S. Heptinstall, P. C. Bather 1986. Arachidonic acid metabolism by peripheral blood cells in psoriasis. *British Journal of Dermatology* **114**, 554; S. Moncada & E. A. Higgs 1988. Metabolism of arachidonic acid. *Annals of the New York Academy Science* **522**, 460; J. A. Salmon, L. C. Tilling, S. Moncada 1984. Benoxaprofen does not inhibit formation of leukotriene B$_4$ in a model of acute inflammation. *Biochemical Pharmacology* **33**, 2930; J. A. Salmon, L. C. Tilling, S. Moncada 1985. Evaluation of inhibitors of eicosanoid synthesis in leukocytes: possible pitfalls of using the calcium ionophore A23187 to stimulate 5' lipoxygenase. *Prostaglandins* **29**, 383; H. K. E. Schaffer 1989. Essential fatty acids and eicosanoids in cutaneous inflammation. *International Journal of Dermatology.* **28**, 285; A. Szczeklik 1986. Analgesics, allergy and asthma. *Drugs* **32** Suppl., 155; H. B. Yaacob & P. J. Piper 1988. Inhibition of leukotriene release in anaphylactic guinea-pig hearts by a 5-lipoxygenase inhibitor, CGS 8515. *British Journal of Pharmacology.* **95**, 1327.

38. M. W. Greaves & R. D. R. Camp 1988. Prostaglandins, leukotrienes, phospholipase, platelet activating factor, and cytokines: an integrated approach to inflammation of human skin. *Archives of Dermatological Research* **280** Suppl., pS37.

39. D. N. Benslay & R. Nickander 1982. Radiographic studies of the effect of benoxaprofen on bone damage in the adjuvant arthritic rat. *European Journal of Rheumatology and Inflammation* **5**, 175.

40. Ibid. 182

41. Ibid. 175.

42. M. E. J. Billingham 1983. Models of arthritis and the search for anti-arthritic drugs. *Pharmacology and Therapeutics.* **21**, 391.

43. Ibid. 392.

44. Ibid. 399.

45. Ibid. 415.

46. FDA 1982. "Oraflex Brand of benoxaprofen NDA 18–250". Memo, 29 March.

47. US Court 1983. Deposition of F. B. Peck *Clarence Borom* vs *Eli Lilly and Company*. District Court for the Middle District of Georgia, Columbus Division, 12 May 196–201. (Hereafter referred to as Peck depo).

48. US Court 1983. Deposition of B. Gennery *Clarence Borom* vs *Eli Lilly and Company*. District Court for the Middle District of Georgia, Columbus Division 19 October, 163. (Hereafter referred to as Gennery depo).

49. G. B. Bluhm, D. W. Smith, W. M. Mikulaschek 1982. Radiologic assessment of benoxaprofen therapy in rheumatoid arthritis. *European Journal of Rheumatology and Inflammation* **5**, 186.

50. US Court 1983. Deposition of G. Bluhm *Clarence Borom* vs *Eli Lilly*. District Court for the Middle District of Georgia, Columbus Division, 27 October, 21. (Hereafter referred to as Bluhm depo).

51. G. B. Bluhm et al. 1982. op. cit., 186. (**n.49**)

52. Ibid. 190.

53. O'Brien depo, 44; W. M. O'Brien 1986. Radiological evaluation of erosions: a quantitative method for assessing long-term remittive therapy in rheumatoid arthritis. *British Journal of Clinical Pharmacology* **22**, 1795.

54. BBC1 1983. "The Opren scandal (part 2)". *Panorama*, 17 January.

55. Ibid.

56. Ibid.

57. E. C. Huskisson 1982. Editorial. *European Journal of Rheumatology and Inflammation* **5**, 50.
58. W. Dawson et al. 1982. op. cit., 61. (**n.26**)
59. Bluhm depo, 48–9.
60. V. C. H. Tyson & A. Glynne 1980. A comparative study of benoxaprofen and ibuprofen in osteoarthritis in general practice. *Journal of Rheumatology Supplement* **7**, 132–8.
61. E. C. Huskisson 1976. Trials of anti-rheumatic drugs. In *The principles and practice of clinical trials*, C. S. Good & C. Clarke (eds), 192. Edinburgh: Churchill Livingstone.
62. Ibid. 196.
63. Ibid. 192.
64. FDA 1982. "Medical Officer's Review, 27 October 1980", 3. In *Summary basis of approval (benoxaprofen)*.
65. O. B. Gum 1980. Long-term efficacy and safety of benoxaprofen: comparison with aspirin and ibuprofen in patients with active rheumatoid arthritis. *Journal of Rheumatology Supplement* **7**, 82.
66. D. Alarcon-Segovia 1980. Long-term treatment of symptomatic osteoarthritis with benoxaprofen: double-blind comparison with aspirin and ibuprofen. *Journal of Rheumatology Supplement* **7**, 98.
67. O. B. Gum 1980. op. cit., 82–7. (**n.65**)
68. Ibid. 82–3.
69. Gennery depo, 163–5.
70. FDA 1982. op. cit. (**n.46**)
71. DHSS 1976. MAL 2. *Notes on applications for product licences and clinical trial certificates*, section 21.3.2., 49. London: HMSO
72. FDA 1977. *General considerations for the clinical evaluation of drugs*, 3. Washington DC: US Government Publications Office.
73. R. H. Gifford & A. R. Feinstein 1969. A critique of methodology in studies of anticoagulant therapy for acute myocardial infarction. *New England Journal of Medicine* **280**, 351–7; N. D. W. Lionel & A. Herxheimer 1970. Assessing reports of therapeutic trials. *British Medical Journal* **3**, 637–40; A. W. Mahon & E. E. Daniel 1964. A method for the assessment of reports on drug trials. *Canadian Medical Association Journal* **90**, 565–9; J. A. Freiman, T. C. Chalmers, H. Smith, R. R. Kuebler 1978. The importance of beta, the type ii error and sample size in design and interpretation of the randomised control trial: a survey of 71 "negative" trials. *New England Journal of Medicine* **299**, 690–94; T. C. Chalmers et al. 1981. A method for assessing the quality of a randomised clinical trial. *Controlled Clinical Trials* **2**, 31–49; C. L. Meinert, S. Tonascia, K. Higgins 1984. Content of reports on clinical trials: a critical review. *Controlled Clinical Trials* **5**, 328–47; J. M. Bland et al. 1985. Is the clinical trial evidence about new drugs statistically adequate? *British Journal of Clinical Pharamcology* **19**, 155–60; H. A. Smythe 1980. Editorial: prostaglandins and benoxaprofen. *Journal of Rheumatology Supplement* **7**, 2.
74. Dista 1980. *Opren Data Sheet*, April
75. Dista 1980. *Opren Data Sheet*, August.
76. FDA 1981. Certified mail letter of non-approval for benoxaprofen from M. Finkel, Associate Director, New Drug Evaluation, Bureau of Drugs, to Lilly, 25 February, 1.
77. FDA 1982. op. cit. (**n.46**)
78. Ibid.
79. Hearings 1982, 486.
80. FDA 1979. Supplemental Pharmacology Review No. 7 by M. Hein, 10 April.
81. G. B. Bluhm, D. W. Smith, W. M. Mikulaschek 1982. Radiological assessment of benoxaprofen therapy in rheumatoid arthritis. *European Journal of Rheumatology and Inflammation* **5**, 187; W. M. Mikulaschek 1980. Long-term safety of benoxaprofen. *Journal of Rheumatology Supplement* **7**, 100.

82. Pharmaceutical Manufacturers' Association (PMA) 1977. Guidelines for the assessment of drug and medical device safety in animals, 58. Washington DC: PMA; DHSS 1979. MAIL 24. *Notes for guidance on carcinogenicity testing on medicinal products*, i. London: DHSS.
83. A. N. Worden 1974. Toxicological methods. *Toxicology* 2, 362.
84. FDA 1979. op. cit. (**n.80**)
85. Eli Lilly (Lilly) 1984. *General commentary on the long-term rat study on benoxaprofen*. Lilly Research Laboratories, Toxicology Division, 22 February.
86. Ibid. 6.
87. WHO 1969. Principles for the testing and evaluation of drugs for carcinogenicity. *Technical Report Series* **426**, 15.
88. ABPI 1977. *Guidelines for preclinical and clinical testing of new medicinal products part I – laboratory investigations*, 25. London: ABPI.
89. PMA 1977. op. cit., 58. (**n.82**)
90. DHSS 1979. MAIL 24. op. cit. (**n.82**)
91. US Court 1983. Deposition of W. I. Shedden *Clarence Borom* vs *Eli Lilly* District Court for the Middle District of Georgia, Columbus Division, 21 June, 18. (Hereafter referred to as Shedden depo). ABPI *Annual Reports 1973/74–1976/77.*
92. ABPI *Annual Report 1973/74*, 4; ABPI *Annual Report 1975/76*, 4.
93. FDA 1982. Pharmacology Review No. 10 by Sydney Stolzenberg, 1 March.
94. Lilly 1984. op. cit., 3. (**n.85**)
95. WHO 1969. op. cit., 14–15. (**n.87**)
96. A. N. Worden 1974. op. cit., 362 (**n.83**); DHSS 1979. MAIL 24. op. cit. (**n.82**); PMA 1977. op. cit. ref 82, 59.
97. FDA 1979 Supplemental Pharmacology Review No. 7, 10 April.
98. Ibid.
99. WHO 1969. op. cit., 14. (**n.87**)
100. PMA 1977. op. cit., 57. (**n.82**)
101. ABPI 1977. op. cit., 24. (**n.88**)
102. DHSS 1979. MAIL 24. op. cit., i. (**n.82**)
103. D. E. Stevenson 1979. Current problems in the choice of animals for toxicity testing. *Journal of Toxicology and Environmental Health* **5**, 12.
104. DHSS 1978. MLX 108. Consultation document – notes for guidance on carcinogenicity testing of medicinal products. London: DHSS.
105. Dista 1980. *Opren Data Sheet*, April; Dista 1980. *Opren Data Sheet*, August.
106. FDA 1980. Pharmacology Review No. 8 by M. Hein, 20 March.
107. FDA 1982. Pharmacology Review No.10 by S. Stolzenberg, 1 March.
108. Ibid.
109. Lilly Research Laboratories, Toxicology Division 1984 op. cit. (**n.85**)
110. Lilly 1984. op. cit. (**n.85**)
111. Ibid.
112. PMA 1977. op. cit., 54. (**n.82**)
113. WHO 1969. op. cit., 12. (**n.87**)
114. FDA 1984. Pharmacology Review No. 14, 10 April.
115. FDA 1982. Certified letter to Lilly of approval for benoxaprofen by Finkel, April 19.
116. Report of the Interagency Regulatory Liaison Group 1979. Scientific Basis for Identification of Potential Carcinogens and Estimation of Risks. *Journal of the National Cancer Institute* **63**, 251.
117. FDA 1982. op. cit. (**n.115**)
118. Ibid.
119. Lilly 1982. Oraflex package insert, May. Oraflex brochure for US Physicians.
120. FDA 1982. "Summary Basis Of Approval (Benoxaprofen)", 3.
121. US Congress 1983. Hearings of the Intergovernmental Relations and Human Re-

sources Subcommittee of the House of Representatives 1983, *FDA's Regulation of Zomax*, 26 and 27 April 1983, 412 (hereafter referred to as "Zomax Hearings").

122. FDA 1983. Memo of meeting with Lilly on 21 December.
123. Ibid.
124. Lilly 1983. "Dear Doctor". Letter of 22 December.
125. FDA 1984. Memo of meeting with Lilly on 27 January.
126. Lilly Research Laboratories 1984. Preliminary analysis of pathological findings in B6C3F1 mice given benoxaprofen in the diet for two years, 28 February.
127. Ibid.
128. Interagency Regulatory Liaison Group, Work Group on Risk Assessment 1979. op. cit., 241–68. (**n.116**)
129. FDA 1984. Pharmacology Review No. 14 by S. Stolzenberg, 10 April.
130. Ibid.
131. FDA 1984. Pharmacology Review No. 14, 10 April.
132. FDA 1983. Memorandum of Meeting with Lilly on 21 December.
133. FDA 1985. Memo of Meeting between J. Harter and D. Pease of the FDA with Max Talbott of Lilly, 18 July.
134. Zomax Hearings, 88, 189.
135. Hearings 1982, 43.
136. M. Bigby & R. Stern 1985. Cutaneous reactions to non-steroidal anti-inflammatory drugs. *Journal of the American Academy of Dermatology* **12**, 871.
137. B. L. Diffey & S. Brown 1983. A method for predicting the phototoxicity of non-steroidal anti-inflammatory drugs. *British Journal of Clinical Pharmacology* **16**, 637.
138. B. L. Diffey, I. Oliver, A. Davis 1982. A personal dosemeter for quantifying the biologically effective sunlight exposure of patients receiving benoxaprofen. *Physical and Medical Biology* **27**, 1507.
139. B. A. Newman & H. Sharlit 1937. Sulfanilimide: a photosensitizing agent of the skin. *Journal of the American Medical Association* **109**, 1036–7.
140. S. Epstein 1939. Photoallergy and primary photosensitivity to sulfanilimide. *Journal of Investigative Dermatology* **2**, 43–51.
141. Ibid. 43.
142. O. F. Jillson & W. L. Curwen 1959. Phototoxicity, photoallergy and photoskin tests. *Archives of Dermatology* **80**, 78–9.
143. L. C. Harber & R. L. Baer 1972. Pathogenic mechanisms of drug-induced photosensitivity. *Journal of Investigative Dermatology* **58**, 327–42.
144. Ibid; J. M. Knox 1961. Clinical aspects and types of drug-induced photosensitivity. *Annals of Allergy* **19**, 750–51.
145. L. C. Harber & D. R. Bickers 1981. *Photosensitivity diseases: principles of diagnosis and treatment*, 138–9. Philadelphia & London: W. B. Saunders.
146. E. Sidi, M. Hinky, A. Gervais 1955. Allergic sensitization and photosensitization to phenergan cream. *Journal of Investigative Dermatology* **24**, 345–52; L. C. Harber & D. R. Bickers 1981. op. cit., 138–9. (**n.145**)
147. O. F. Jillson & R. D. Baughman 1963. Contact photodermatitis from bithionol. *Archives of Dermatology* **88**, 409–18.
148. J. M. Knox 1961. op. cit., 751. (**n.144**)
149. L. C. Harber & D. R. Bickers 1981. op. cit., 126. (**n.145**)
150. E. C. Huskisson 1976. Trials of anti-rheumatic drugs. In *The principles and practice of clinical trials: based on a symposium organised by the association of medical advisors in the pharmaceutical industry*, C. S. Good and Sir Cyril Clark (eds), 192–3. Edinburgh: Churchill Livingstone.
151. E. C. Huskisson, J. Scott, P. Dieppe 1978. Benoxaprofen: a clinical trial with an unusual design. *Rheumatology and Rehabilitation* **17**, 257; E. C. Huskisson & J. Scott 1979. Treatment of rheumatoid arthritis with a single daily dose of benoxaprofen. *Rheumatology and*

Rehabilatation. **18**, 112; J. Highton & R. Grahame 1980. Benoxaprofen in the treatment of osteoarthritis – a comparison with ibuprofen. *Journal of Rheumatology Supplement* **7**, 131; P. A. Bacon, J. Davies, F. J. Ring 1980. op. cit., 48–53. (**n.28**); H. Berry et al. 1980. Dose-range studies of benoxaprofen compared with placebo in patients with active rheumatoid arthritis. *Journal of Rheumatology Supplement* **7**, 54–9.

152. J. Highton & R. Grahame 1980. op. cit., 131. (**n.151**)
153. US Court 1983. Deposition of W. H. Shedden *Clarence Borom vs Eli Lilly and Company* District Court for the Middle District of Georgia, Columbus Division 21 June 1983, 41. (Hereafter referred to as Shedden depo).
154. E. C. Huskisson 1976. op. cit., 191–2. (**n.150**)
155. O. B. Gum 1980. Long-term efficacy and safety of benoxaprofen: comparison with aspirin and ibuprofen in patients with active rheumatoid arthritis. *Journal of Rheumatology Supplement* **7**, 76–88; D. Alarcon-Segovia 1980. Long-term treatment of symptomatic osteoarthritis with benoxaprofen: double-blind comparison with aspirin and ibuprofen. *Journal of Rheumatology Supplement* **7**, 89–99.
156. O. B. Gum 1980. op. cit., 85–6. (**n.155**)
157. D. Alarcon-Segovia 1980. op. cit., 98. (**n.155**)
158. K. Clarke 1983. *Hansard,* 27 January, col. 1120.
159. Ibid.
160. Ibid.
161. Ibid.
162. W. M. Mikulaschek 1980. Long-term safety of benoxaprofen. *Journal of Rheumatology Supplement* **7**, 100–108.
163. J. M. Knox 1961. op. cit. (**n.144**)
164. L. C. Harbers & D. R. Bickers 1981. op. cit. (**n.145**)
165. V. C. H. Tyson & A. Glynne 1980. op. cit., 136. (**n.60**)
166. L. C. Harber & R. L. Baer 1972. op. cit., 331. (**n.143**)
167. J. Ferguson et al. 1982. A study of benoxaprofen-induced photosensitivity. *British Journal of Dermatology* **107**, 429.
168. W. M. Mikulaschek 1980. op. cit. (**n.162**); L. S. McCormack, M. L. Elgart, M. L. Turner 1982. Benoxaprofen-induced photo-onycholysis. *Journal of the American Academy of Dermatology* **7**, 679.
169. B. R. Allen 1983. Benoxaprofen and the skin. *British Journal of Dermatology* **109**, 363.
170. W. M. Mikulaschek 1980. op. cit., 103. (**n.162**)
171. K. Clarke 1983. op. cit., 1120. (**n.158**)
172. Dista 1980. *Opren Data Sheets,* April and August.
173. W. M. Mikulaschek 1980. op. cit., 104. (**n.162**)
174. FDA 1980. Statistical review and evaluation by J. P. Hsu, 20 October, 4–5.
175. FDA 1981. Certified mail letter of non-approval for benoxaprofen from M. Finkel, Associate Director, New Drug Evaluation, Bureau of Drugs, 25 February, 2–3.
176. Lilly 1980. Trip Report St Cloud by H. A. Barnett, 30 September, 3–4.
177. FDA 1981. Investigation of Eli Lilly (benoxaprofen adverse effects). Preliminary Report to Chief, Clinical Investigations Branch, Division of Scientific Investigations by M. J. Hensley, 16 September. Testimony of M. J. Hensley in US Court 1983 in *Clarence Borom vs Eli Lilly and Company.* Trial transcript. Vol.3, November, 535.
178. FDA 1981 op. cit., 1. (**n.177**)
179. Ibid, 2–4.
180. Hearings 1982, op. cit., 92.
181. Ibid. 92.
182. Ibid. 85.
183. Ibid. 85.
184. Ibid. 87, 93.

185. Ibid. 93.
186. Ibid. 86–7.
187. US Court 1983. Deposition of M. J. Hensley *Clarence Borom* vs *Eli Lilly and Company*, District Court for the Middle District of Georgia, Columbus Division, 90–120. (Hereafter referred to as Hensley depo); Lilly 1983. Letter from Edgar Davis, Vice President, Corporate Affairs, Lilly to Congressman Ted Weiss, 3 November.
188. Ibid. 154.
189. Ibid. 156, 159, 160.
190. US Court 1983. Deposition of R. G. Leventhal *Clarence Borom* vs *Eli Lilly and Company*, District Court for the Middle District of Georgia, Columbus Division, 18 August. (Hereafter referred to as Leventhal depo).
191. Ibid.
192. FDA 1982. Memorandum from J. Harter to F. Kelsey, Director of Division of Scientific Investigations, 24 March.
193. Testimony of M. J. Hensley op. cit., 563. (**n.177**)
194. Hearings 1982, op. cit., 92.
195. Hensley depo op. cit., 4–5.
196. Leventhal depo, op. cit., 47–8.
197. US Court 1983. Deposition of F. B. Peck *Clarence Borom* vs *Eli Lilly and Company* District Court for the Middle District of Georgia, Columbus Division, 12 May, 63–70. (Hereafter referred to as Peck depo); US Court 1983. Deposition of W. M. Mikulaschek *Clarence Borom* vs *Eli Lilly and Company* District Court for the Middle District of Georgia, Columbus Division, 20 June, 146–50. (Hereafter referred to as Mikulaschek depo).
198. US Court 1983. Deposition of H. A. Barnett *Clarence Borom* vs *Eli Lilly and Company* District Court for the Middle District of Georgia, Columbus Division, 9 May 1983. (Hereafter referred to as Barnett depo).
199. Ibid. 9–19.
200. "Judge's Summing Up". *Clarence Borom* vs *Eli Lilly and Company* Trial Transcript Vol. 9, 108.
201. "Closing Statements of Lawyers". *Clarence Borom* vs *Eli Lilly and Company* Trial Transcript Vol. 9, 84.
202. Hearings 1982. op. cit., 93.
203. Gennery depo, 66–71.
204. US Court 1983. Deposition of A. M. Kligman *Clarence Borom* vs *Eli Lilly and Company* District Court for the Middle District of Georgia, Columbus Division, 26 October, 7. (Hereafter referred to as Kligman depo).
205. Ibid. 7.
206. Ibid. 43–4.
207. Ibid. 9–10.
208. Ibid. 9.
209. A. M. Kligman & K. H. Kaidbey 1982. Phototoxicity to benoxaprofen. *European Journal of Rheumatology and Inflammation* **5**, 134.
210. Ibid. 125.
211. Kligman depo, 14.
212. A. M. Kligman & K. H. Kaidbey 1982. op. cit., 134. (**n.209**)
213. Ibid. 134.
214. Lilly 1984. Second general session, 27 April, 4–10.
215. A. M. Kligman & K. H. Kaidbey 1982. op. cit., 134. (**n.209**)
216. Kligman depo, 20–21.
217. Ibid. 21
218. Ibid. 24–5.
219. Ibid. 25.

220. Ibid. 24–5.
221. Ibid. 26.
222. Ibid. 29–30.
223. Ibid. 30.
224. Ibid. 32.
225. Ibid. 32.
226. Ibid. 33.
227. Ibid. 34.
228. Ibid. 53.
229. A. M. Kligman & K. H. Kaidbey 1982. op. cit., 137. (**n.209**)
230. Ibid. 124–37.
231. Kligman depo, 53.
232. Ibid. 37–40.
233. Lilly 1982. Day 1 "Second general session". 27 April, 25.
234. Ibid. 24.
235. W. M. Mikulaschek 1980. op. cit., 104. (**n.162**)
236. Dista 1980. "Dear Doctor" Letter, August.
237. R. D. Mann 1987. The yellow card data: the nature and scale of the adverse drug reactions problem. In *Adverse drug reactions: the scale and nature of the problem and the way forward*, R. D. Mann (ed.), 58. Carnforth, Lancashire/New Jersey: Parthenon; S. R. Walker & C. E. Lumley 1987. Reporting and under-reporting. In R. D. Mann (ed.), 124–5.
238. Gennery depo, 66–71.
239. FDA 1981. Statistical review and evaluation by J. P. Hsu, 13 August, 3.
240. FDA 1982. Dermatology review by W. Powell, 18 January, 1.
241. M. C. Greist, I. I. Ozols, A. S. Ridolfo, J. C. Muus 1982. The phototoxic effects of benoxaprofen and their management and prevention. *European Journal of Rheumatology and Inflammation* **5**, 146–7.
242. Ibid.
243. Ibid. 147.
244. FDA 1982 op. cit., 2. (**n.240**)
245. Ibid. 1.
246. FDA 1982. Memorandum of Meeting with Lilly by A. W. Yellin, 29 March.
247. D. P. Valenzeno & J. P. Pooler 1979. Phototoxicty: the neglected factor. *Journal of the American Medical Association* **242**, 453–4.
248. Hearings 1982, 370.
249. FDA 1982. Transcript of FDA Arthritis Advisory Committee Meeting, 21 January, 28.
250. Ibid. 8, 13–16.
251. FDA 1982. op. cit., 25. (**n.249**)
252. Kligman depo, 35–6.
253. Ibid. 37.
254. D. A. Fenton, J. D. Wilkinson, J. S. English 1981. Photosensitization to benoxaprofen not due to ultraviolet A alone. *Lancet*, **2**. 1231.
255. FDA 1982. op. cit., 31. (**n.249**)
256. Ibid. 31–3.
257. Dista 1980. *Opren Marketing Pack*; Dista 1981. Opren. A brand new anti-arthritic. A brand new way of working. *British Medical Journal* **282**, 10 and 24 January; Dista 1981. Why is there a wind of change in the treatment of arthritis? *British Medical Journal* **282**, 7 February, 7 March, 4 April, and 13 June; Dista 1981. Why is the tide turning in the treatment of arthritis? *British Medical Journal* **282**, 21 February, 21 March, 18 April, 2 May, 16 May, and 30 May 1981; Dista 1980. *Opren Data Sheet*, August op. cit. (**n.172**)
258. FDA 1982. op. cit., 8–16. (**n.249**)
259. V. C. H. Tyson & A. Glynne 1980. op. cit., 135–7. (**n.165**)

260. Gennery depo, 71–2.
261. FDA 1982. op. cit. (**n.246**); Lilly 1982. *Oraflex Package Insert*, May.
262. I. C. Stewart 1982. Gastrointestinal haemorrhage and benoxaprofen. *British Medical Journal* **284**, 163–4.
263. A. Du Vivier 1982. Bullous dermatitis associated with benoxaprofen. *Lancet* **1**, 27.
264. J. P. Halsey & N. Cardoe 1982. Gastrointestinal haemorrhage and benoxaprofen. *British Medical Journal* **284**, 508.
265. FDA 1982. Letter from M. J. Finkel, Associate Director for New Drug Evaluation, FDA, to R. Wood, Chairman of Board, Lilly, 12 March.
266. FDA 1982. Letter from M. J. Finkel, Associate Director for New Drug Evaluation, FDA to H. A. Barnett, Lilly Research Laboratories, Indianapolis 19 April.
267. Lilly 1982. *Oraflex Package Insert*, May. Cf. Dista 1980 *Opren Data Sheet*, August.
268. Lilly 1982. op. cit. (**n.267**)
269. H. E. Barber & J. C. Petrie 1981. Clinical pharmacology: elimination of drugs. *British Medical Journal* **282**, 809.
270. World Health Organisation (WHO) 1981. Health care in the elderly: report of the technical group on use of medicaments by the elderly. *Drugs* **22**, 279–94.
271. US Court 1983. Deposition of B. Gennery *Clarence Borom* vs *Eli Lilly and Company* District Court for the Middle District of Georgia, Columbus Division 19 October, 37. (Hereafter referred to as Gennery depo); US Court 1983. Deposition of R. Hamdy *Clarence Borom* vs *Eli Lilly and Company* District Court for the Middle District of Georgia, Columbus Division, 6 July, 17. (Hereafter referred to as Hamdy depo).
272. Hamdy depo, 21.
273. R. Hamdy, B. Murnane, N. Perera, K. Woodcock, I. M. Koch 1982. The pharmacokinetics of benoxaprofen in elderly subjects. *European Journal of Rheumatology and Inflammation* **5**, 69–75.
274. Gennery depo, 41–2.
275. R. Hamdy et al. 1982. op. cit., 69–70. (**n.273**)
276. A. Kamal & I. M. Koch 1982. Pharmacokinetic studies of benoxaprofen in geriatric patients. *European Journal of Rheumatology and Inflammation* **5**, 81, 76.
277. Gennery depo, 43; Hamdy depo, 23.
278. D. H. Chatfield, M. E. Tarrant, G. L. Smith, C. F. Spiers 1977. Pharmacokinetics studies with benoxaprofen in man: prediction of steady-state levels from single dose data. *British Journal of Clinical Pharmacology* **4**, 579.
279. G. R. Aronoff, T. Ozawa, A. S. Ridolfo, J. F. Nash, K. A. Desante 1982. Benoxaprofen elimination kinetics in renal impairment. *Clinical Research* **30**, 248A.
280. Ibid.
281. Hamdy depo, 23; R. Hamdy et al. 1982. op. cit., 69. (**n.273**)
282. Hamdy depo, 27. BBC1 1983 "The Opren Scandal", *Panorama*, 10 January. (Hereafter referred to as "Panorama Transcript").
283. Hamdy depo, 29.
284. Ibid. 29.
285. Gennery depo, 78.
286. US Court 1983. Deposition of C. B. Vaughan *Clarence Borom* vs *Eli Lilly and Company* District Court for the Middle District of Georgia, Columbus Division, 28 October, 56.
287. D. F. Davies & N. W. Shock 1950. Age changes in glomerular filtration rate, excretive renal plasma flow, and tubular excretory capacity in adult males. *Journal of Clinical Investigation* **29**, 496–507.
288. F. G. McMahon, A. Jain, A. Onel 1976. Controlled evaluation of fenoprofen in geriatric patients with osteoarthritis. *Journal of Rheumatology Supplement* **3**, 76, 82.
289. E. J. Triggs, R. L. Nation, A. Long, J. J. Ashley 1975. Pharmacokinetics in the elderly. *European Journal of Clinical Pharmacology* **8**, 55; E. J. Triggs & R. L. Nation 1975.

Pharmacokinetics in the aged: a review. *Journal of Pharmacokinetics and Biopharmacy* **3**, 387–413; R. E. Vestal 1978. Drug use in the elderly: a review of problems and special considerations. *Drugs* **16**, 358–82; J. Crooks, K. O'Malley, I. H. Stevenson 1976. Pharmacokinetics in the elderly. *Clinical Pharmacokinetics* **1**, 280; K. O'Malley, T. G. Judge, J. Crooks 1976. Geriatric clinical pharmacology and therapeutics. In *Drug treatment: principles and practice of clinical pharmacology and therapeutics*, G. S. Avery (ed.), 158–80. London: Adis Press; D. P. Richey & A. D. Bender 1977. Pharmacokinetic consequences of ageing. *Annals and Review of Pharmacological Toxicology* **17**, 49–65; C. M. Castleden & C. F. George 1979. The effect of ageing on the hepatic clearance of propanolol. *British Journal of Clinical Pharmacology* **7**, 49–54.

290. C. M. Castleden 1978. Prescribing for the elderly. *Prescribers' Journal* **18**, 90–91.
291. WHO 1981. op. cit., 280. (**n.270**)
292. Gennery depo, 50.
293. WHO 1981. op. cit., 285. (**n.270**)
294. Gennery depo, 50–55.
295. Ibid. 52.
296. US Court 1983. Deposition of K. Desante *Clarence Borom* vs *Eli Lilly and Company* District Court for the Middle District of Georgia, Columbus Division, 18 October, 81. (Hereafter referred to as Desante depo).
297. Ibid.
298. Ibid, 73, 81.
299. US Court 1983. Deposition of C. N. Christensen *Clarence Borom* vs *Eli Lilly and Company* District Court for the Middle District of Georgia, Columbus Division, 20 June, 59. (Hereafter referred to as Christensen depo).
300. Mikulaschek depo, 245.
301. Desante depo, 70–73.
302. Gennery depo, 65.
303. BBC1 1983 op. cit. (**n.282**)
304. Gennery depo, 130.
305. L. E. Ramsay & G. T. Tucker 1981. Clinical pharmacology: drugs and the elderly. *British Medical Journal* **282**, 126.
306. BBC1 1983 op. cit. (**n.282**)
307. Ibid. 78.
308. Ibid. 78.
309. Dista 1980. *Opren Data Sheet*, August.
310. Committee on the Safety of Medicines (CSM). *Annual Reports for 1979–85*. London: HMSO.
311. M. D. Rawlins 1981. Clinical pharmacology: adverse reactions to drugs. *British Medical Journal* **282**, 974–5.
312. BBC1 1983. op. cit. (**n.282**)
313. N. Christophilis & W. J. Louis 1983. Benoxaprofen. *The Medical Journal of Australia* **143**, 114–15; A. Darragh, A. J. Gordon, H. O'Byrne, D. Hobbs, E. Casey 1985. Single-dose and steady-state pharmacokinetics of non-steroidal anti-inflammatory drugs. *Balliere's Clinical Rheumatology* **2**, 281; A. Gallanosa & D. A. Spyker 1985. Sulindac hepato-toxicity: a case report and review. *Clinical Toxicology* **23**, 225; G. G. Graham 1987. Pharmacokinetics and metabolism of non-steroidal anti-inflammatory drugs. *The Medical Journal of Australia* **147**, 598; G. A. C. Hosie & J. Hosie 1987. The pharmacokinetics of sustained release tiaprofenic acid in elderly arthritic patients. *British Journal of Clinical Pharmacology* **24**, 93; M. J. Kendall, R. Jubb, H. A. Bird, P. le Gallez, J. Hill, A. J. Taggart, R. Rau 1990. A pharmacokinetic comparison of ibuprofen sustained release tablets given to young and elderly patients. *Journal of Clinical Pharmacy and Therapeutics* **15**, 35; J. J. McNeill, O. H. Drummer, E. L. Conway, B. S. Workman, W. J.

Louis 1987. Effect of age in pharmacokinetics of and blood pressure responses prazosin and terazosin. *Journal of Cardiovascular Pharmacology* **10**, 168; R. M. McVerry et al. 1986. Pharmacokinetics of naproxen in elderly patients. *European Journal of Clinical Pharmacology* **31**, 463. K. W. Woodhouse & H. Wynne 1987. The pharmacokinetics of non-steroidal anti-inflammatory drugs in the elderly. *Clinical Pharmacokinetics* **12**, 118.

314. Gennery depo, 86.
315. Dista 1982. *Opren Data Sheet,* May.
316. Hamdy depo, 115–16; BBC1 1983. op. cit. (**n.282**)
317. Mikulaschek depo, 244.
318. Mikulaschek depo, 133, 247–50
319. Ibid. 247–50.
320. FDA 1982. Arthritis Advisory Committee Meeting 3–4 June, II–44.
321. Ibid. II–147.
322. Lilly 1982. Telex from Oldfield, Erl Wood to Shedden, Indianapolis, 21 May.
323. Dista 1982. *Opren Data Sheet,* June.
324. B. M. Goudie et al. 1982. Jaundice associated with the use of benoxaprofen. *Lancet* **1**, 959.
325. Ibid.
326. US Court 1983. Deposition of H. McA. Taggart *Clarence Borom vs Eli Lilly and Company* District Court for the Middle District of Georgia, Columbus Division, 4 July, 151. (Hereafter referred to as Taggart depo).
327. H. McA Taggart & J. M. Alderdice 1982. Fatal cholestatic jaundice in elderly patients taking benoxaprofen. *British Medical Journal* **284**, 1372; Taggart depo, 117–43; US Congress 1982. Committee on Government Operation Memo by Dan Sigelman of telephone conversation with Hugh McA Taggart, 10 September.
328. Ibid.
329. Gennery depo, 188–9.
330. Taggart depo, 144–7.
331. Shedden depo, 127–9.
332. Taggart depo, 150; US Congress 1982. op. cit. (**n.327**); Dista Adverse Reaction Report Forms signed by H. Taggart, 9 February 1982.
333. CSM 1982. FO6 adverse reactions information service, "Opren: January 1964 to January 1982".
334. Gennery depo, 244.
335. Gennery depo, 244.
336. Shedden depo, 51–4, 77.
337. Taggart depo, 152; Gennery depo, 109.
338. Shedden depo, 131–2; US Congress 1982. op. cit. (**n.327**); Gennery depo, 215–16.
339. Taggart depo, 153–5.
340. Ibid. 179–80.
341. Gennery depo, 254–6.
342. Ibid. 270–75.
343. Ibid. 245–6.
344. Ibid. 222.
345. Taggart depo, 156.
346. BBC1 1983 op. cit. (**n.282**).
347. US Department of Justice 1985. District Court Southern District of Indiana, Indianapolis Division. *USA vs Lilly and W. I. H. Shedden,* factual basis for the pleas, 9–10. (Hereafter referred to as "Factual basis of the pleas").
348. FDA 1979. *Federal Register* **44**(65), 19435.
349. Ibid. 19435.
350. Ibid. 19435.

351. Hearings 1982, 111.
352. Ibid. 116, 122.
353. Lilly 1982. *Oraflex Package Insert*, May.
354. D. Pinns 1982. Florida hospital clinical resume, 10 April.
355. FDA. VRR adverse drug experience report form, initial report, undated.
356. FDA 1982. Letter from A. Lisook, Clinical Investigations Branch, Division of Scientific Investigations, FDA to D. Sigelman, Congressional Committee on Government Operations.
357. Lilly 1983. Letter from Richard Wood, Chairman of the Board, to Lilly Shareholders, 5 December, 3.
358. Mikulaschek depo, 92.
359. CSM 1982. F06 adverse reactions information service. "Opren January 1964 to 1982".
360. Drug Surveillance Research Unit 1983. *Prescription Event Monitoring News* **1**, 6.
361. Christensen depo, 50.
362. FDA 1982. Memo of telecon between Robert Temple, Acting Director of Office of New Drug Evaluation, FDA and C. Christensen, Lilly, 14 May.
363. W. I. H. Shedden 1982. Side effects of benoxaprofen. *British Medical Journal* **284**, 1630.
364. Mikulaschek depo, 93, 95.
365. Shedden depo. in *Clarence Borom vs Eli Lilly and Company Trial Transcript* Vol.3A, 765–8.
366. Ibid. 756–8.
367. FDA 1982. Memo of meeting with Lilly "Oraflex (benoxaprofen) NDA 18–250", 23 June.
368. Ibid.
369. Hearings 1982, 122.
370. Ibid. 126.
371. US Congress Intergovernmental Relations and Human Resources Subcommittee 1982. Memo of telecon between D. Sigelman and J. Harter, 16 July.
372. Hearings 1982, 119.
373. L. F. Prescott, P. J. Leslie, P. Padfield 1982. Side effects of benoxaprofen. *British Medical Journal* **284**, 1783; B. M. Fisher & J. D. McArthur 1982. Side effects of benoxaprofen. *British Medical Journal* **284**, 1783; H. Firth, G. K. Wilcock, M. Esiri 1982. Side effects of benoxaprofen. *British Medical Journal* **284**, 1784.
374. H. Firth et al. 1982. op. cit. (**n.373**)
375. Lilly 1982. Preliminary comment of Lilly to US Department of Health and Human Services and FDA on the Public Citizen Health Research Group's proposal to ban Oraflex, 2 July 1982, 2.
376. Ibid. 2.
377. BBC1 1983. op. cit. (**n.282**)
378. Dista 1982. *Opren Data Sheet*, June.
379. FDA 1982, op. cit. (**n.367**)
380. Ibid.
381. Gennery depo, 276–7.
382. Ibid. 190.
383. Ibid. 188–90, 205.
384. Ibid. 260–61.
385. FDA 1982. Inspection report by D. Duncan and L. Lanvermeyer 19 November.
386. Ibid. 13–14, 28–9.
387. Lilly 1982. Letter from G. Mallet, Director of Quality Assurance, Lilly to A. L. Hoeting, District Director FDA, 30 November, 2–3; Lilly 1983. Letter from E. Davis, Vice President of Lilly Corporate Affairs to Congressman Ted Weiss, November 5.
388. US Court 1983. Deposition of R. Wood *Chong Ho Kim vs Eli Lilly and Company* District Court of Virginia, Alexandria Division, 29 November, 18. (Hereafter referred to as

Wood depo *Kim* vs *Lilly*).
389. Lilly 1983. Letter from E. Davis, Vice President of Lilly Corporate Affairs to Congressman Ted Weiss, November, 5.
390. US Court Deposition of F. B. Peck, *Clarence Borom* vs *Eli Lilly and Company* District Court for the Middle District of Georgia, Columbus Division, 21 June, 128.
391. Ibid. 149.
392. Ibid. 155–6.
393. Mikulaschek depo, 107.
394. Christensen depo, 82.
395. Ibid. 50.
396. Ibid. 82–9.
397. Shedden depo, op. cit., 782–5. (**n.365**)
398. *Clarence Borom* vs *Eli Lilly and Company Trial Transcript*, 782–5.
399. Shedden depo, 40.
400. Ibid. 41.
401. Wood depo, *Kim* vs *Lilly*, 58–62.
402. Shedden depo, 90–92.
403. Mikulaschek depo, 138–42.
404. Lilly 1983. Letter from R. Wood, Chairman of the Board to Lilly Shareholders, 5 December, 3.
405. US Department of Justice 1985. District Court Southern District of Indiana, Indianapolis Division. *USA* vs *Lilly and W. I. H. Shedden* Information: Counts 1–10, 4. Factual basis for the pleas, 1–2. Press Release, 21 August.
406. Ibid. Factual basis for the pleas, 17.
407. Ibid. Factual basis for the pleas, 7.
408. US Department of Justice 1985. op. cit. Plea agreement. (**n.347**)
409. DHSS 1983. *On the state of the public health: the annual report of the chief medical officer for the year 1982*, 123. London: HMSO.
410. K. Clarke 1983. *Hansard*, 27 January, 582.

Chapter Five

1. Pfizer Ltd (Pfizer) 1980. *Feldene Data Sheet*.
2. US Congress 1982. Hearings Before a House Subcommittee of the Committee on Government Operations 1982. *The regulation of new drugs by the FDA: the new drug review process*, 4 August, 437. (Hereafter referred to as "Hearings 1982").
3. Ibid.
4. J. C. Steigerwald 1978. Piroxicam and rheumatoid arthritis: a double-blind 16-week study comparing piroxicam and indomethacin. *Royal Society of Medicine International Congress and Symposium Series* 1, 47–52; J. R. Ward, R. F. Willkens, J. S. Louie, L. P. McAdam 1978. Piroxicam and rheumatoid arthritis: a multicenter 14-week double-blind controlled study comparing piroxicam and aspirin. *Royal Society of Medicine International Congress and Symposium Series* 1, 31–40; T. M. Zizic, J. D. Sutton, M. B. Stevens 1978. Piroxicam and osteoarthritis: a controlled study. *Royal Society of Medicine International Congress and Symposium Series* 1, 71–82; FDA 1982. *Feldene summary basis of approval*.
5. FDA 1979. *Medical officer original review* by L. Ochota, 22 March, 70.
6. Ibid. 89.
7. FDA 1980. *Medical officer review* by L. Ochota, 21 January, 18.
8. FDA 1980. *Statistical review and evaluation* by H. Leung, 26 August, 4.
9. Ibid. 9.

10. Ibid. 11.
11. Letter from W. J. Gyarfus, Director of Division of Oncology and Radiopharmaceuticals, FDA to Pfizer, 2 June 1978.
12. Hearings 1982, 403.
13. FDA 1981. *Statistical review and evaluation* by H. Leung, 16 January.
14. FDA 1981. *Group leader's review* by J. Harter, 28 January.
15. Ibid.
16. Transcript of the FDA's Arthritis Advisory Committee Meeting, 3 June 1982, 64–5.
17. Ibid.
18. FDA 1981. Review by W. J. Gyarfus, Director of Division of Oncology and Radiopharmaceutical Products, 4 February 1981, 1.
19. Ibid. 2.
20. FDA 1981. Review by J. Harter, Group Leader, 14 April, 2.
21. Ibid. 5.
22. FDA 1981. *Group leader's review* J. Harter, 28 July, 5.
23. Ibid. 6.
24. FDA 1981. *Statistical review and evaluation* by H. M. Leung, 11 August.
25. FDA 1981. Review by M. Finkel, Associate Director for New Drug Evaluation, 17 September, 2.
26. Hearings 1982, 438.
27. FDA 1981 op. cit., 4–5. (**n.25**)
28. Hearings 1982, 368.
29. Ibid.
30. Ibid. 443–6.
31. Ibid.
32. Ibid. 441.
33. Letter from M. J. Finkel, Associate Director for New Drug Evaluation, FDA to Pfizer, 6 April 1982.
34. Hearings 1982, 370.
35. Ibid. 398.
36. Ibid. 368.
37. Pfizer 1982. *Feldene Package Insert*, April.
38. Hearings 1982. 478.
39. Letter from K. Feather, Acting Branch Chief, Division of Drug Advertising, FDA to J. Aterno, Pfizer, 13 July 1982.
40. FDA 1980. *Supplementary pharmacology review* by Manfred Hein, 21 February, 7.
41. Ibid.
42. Ibid. 8.
43. FDA 1980. *Statistical review and evaluation* by H. M. Leung, 26 August, 1.
44. Ibid. 1, 14.
45. FDA 1982. *Feldene Summary Basis of Approval*, 2.
46. Pfizer 1982. *Feldene Package Insert*, April.
47. ABPI 1977. *Guidelines for preclinical and clinical testing of new medicinal products: part 1 – laboratory investigations*, Appendix F, 40.
48. N. E. Pitts 1979. Review of clinical trial experience with piroxicam. *Piroxicam: a new non-steroidal anti-inflammatory agent*, 48–66. New York: Academy Professional Information Services; N. E. Pitts & R. R. Proctor 1978. Summary: efficacy and safety of piroxicam. *Piroxicam: Royal Society of Medicine International Congress and Symposium Series* **1**, 97–108. London: Academic Press & Royal Society of Medicine.
49. Pfizer 1980. *Feldene Product Data Sheet*.
50. D. C. Hobbs & T. M. Twomey 1979. Piroxicam pharmacokinetics in man: aspirin and antacid intereaction studies. *Journal of Clinical Pharmacology* **19**, 270–81; E. H. Wiseman

& D. C. Hobbs 1982. Review of pharmacokinetics studies with piroxicam. *American Journal of Medicine* **72**, 9–17.

51. Hearings 1982, 470–71.
52. *FDC Reports* 30 January 1984, 8.
53. K. Ward & D. G. Weir 1982. Piroxicam and upper gastrointestinal haemorrhage. *Irish Medical Journal* **75**, 10.
54. Letter from A. Scott, Medical Director, NDAB to Product Registration Officer, Pfizer, Kent, England 19 July 1982.
55. P. Emery & R. Grahame 1982. Gastrointestinal blood loss and piroxicam. *Lancet* **1**, 1302–3.
56. M. H. Gleeson 1982. A survey of peptic ulcers associated with NSAIDs. *European Journal of Rheumatology and Inflammation* **5**, 308–12.
57. Pfizer Notes of Meeting with CSM, 7 October 1981.
58. Pfizer 1983. *Feldene Product Data Sheet.*
59. Pfizer 1982. *Feldene Package Insert,* August.
60. A. del Favero 1986. Anti-inflammatory analgesic and drugs used in rheumatoid arthritis and gout. In *Side effects of drugs annual* **10**, M. N. G. Dukes (ed.), 94–5. Amsterdam: Elsevier.
61. Anon. 1983. Toxicity of non-steroidal anti-inflammatory drugs. *The Medical Letter* **25**, 16.
62. A. D. Woolf, H. J. Rogers, I. D. Bradbrook, D. Corless 1983. Pharmacokinetic observations on piroxicam in young, middle-aged and elderly patients. *British Journal of Clinical Pharmacology* **16**, 433–7.
63. Ontario Medical Association Committee on Drugs and Pharmacotherapy 1983. *The drug report* **10**.
64. K. Laake, L. Kjeldaas, C. F. Borchgrevink 1984. Side effects of piroxicam. *Acta Med Scand* **215**, 81–3.
65. K. Clarke 1984. Non-steroidal anti-inflammatory drugs. *Hansard (Written Answers)*, 28 March, 216.
66. Pfizer 1984. *Feldene Package Insert,* April.
67. Anon. 1984. NSAID adverse reaction report comparisons are not suitable as basis for therapeutic ranking of individual drugs, FDA Arthritis Advisory Committee agrees. *FDC Reports,* 29 October, 3.
68. Ibid. 4.
69. J. C. Richardson, K. L. N. Blocka, S. Ross, R. K. Verbeeck 1985. Effects of age and sex on piroxicam disposition. *Clinical Pharmacology and Therapeutics* **27**, 13.
70. K. H. Fok, P. J. M. George, F. R. Vicary 1985. Peptic ulcers induced by piroxicam. *British Medical Journal* **290**, 117.
71. B. Beerman 1985. Peptic ulcers induced by piroxicam. *British Medical Journal* **290**, 789.
72. P. Meyer & I. Thijs 1985. Peptic ulcers induced by piroxicam. *British Medical Journal* **290**, 789.
73. W. H. W. Inman & N. S. B. Rawson 1985. Peptic ulcer and piroxicam. *British Medical Journal* **290**, 932–3.
74. Transcript of FDA Arthritis Advisory Committee Meeting, 29 April 1985, 199–209.
75. J. Harter 1985. Modified summaries of 1984 adverse reaction reports associated with selected NSAIDs. FDA Division of Oncology and Radiopharmaceutical Drug Products, 9 April.
76. Ibid. 212–13.
77. D. St J. Collier & J. A. Pain 1985. Non-steroidal anti-inflammatory drugs and peptic ulcer perforation. *Gut* **26**, 359–63; D. St J. Collier & J. A. Pain 1985. Drug therapy and perforated ulcer: reply. *Gut* **26**, 981.
78. H. Jick, A. D. Feld, D. R. Perera 1985. Certain nonsteroidal antiinflammatory drugs

and hospitalisation for upper GI bleeding. *Pharmacotherapy* **5**, 283.

79. J. D. O'Brien & W. R. Burnham 1985. Bleeding from peptic ulcers and use of non-steroidal anti-inflammatory drugs in the Romford area. *British Medical Journal* **291**, 1609–10; W. R. Burnham & J. D. O'Brien 1986. GI bleeding in Romford. *British Medical Journal* **292**, 559.

80. A. Veitch 1985. Doctors get warning of drug hazard. *Guardian*, 23 December, 3; Hayhoe 1986. Feldene. *Hansard (Written Answers)*, 28 January, 896; Hayhoe 1986. arthritis drugs. *Hansard (Written Answers)*, 30 January, 956.

81. H. J. R. Evans 1986. Gastrointestinal bleeding in Romford. *British Medical Journal* **292**, 56; R. Swallow, H. Remington, V. Standing 1986. Gastrointestinal bleeding in Romford. *British Medical Journal* **292**, 56. D. St J. Collier & J. A. Pain 1986. Gastrointestinal bleeding in Romford. *British Medical Journal* **292**, 56; W. H. W. Inman 1986. Gastrointestinal bleeding in Romford. *British Medical Journal* **292**, 56–7.

82. W. R. Burnham & J. D. O'Brien 1986. GI bleeding in Romford. *British Medical Journal* **292**, 559.

83. Public Citizen 1986. *Feldene Petition*, 8 January, 1–3.

84. Ibid. 5.

85. Ibid. 3–4.

86. Ibid. 8–9.

87. Pfizer 1982. "Feldene blood levels" memo from N. E. Pitts, Medical Laboratories to G. Flouty 19 October, 2.

88. Ibid.

89. Ibid. 2–3.

90. Pfizer 1983. "Feldene (piroxicam) and GI ulceration" memo from N. E. Pitts, Medical Laboratories to G. Ando, 9 August, 1.

91. Ibid. 2–4.

92. FDA 1986 Feldene (piroxicam), a drug for human use; public hearing. *Federal Register* **51**(19), 3658–9.

93. D. H. Adams, J. Michael, P. A. Bacon, A. J. Howie, B. McConkey, D. Adu 1986. Non-steroidal anti-inflammatory drugs and renal failure. *Lancet* **1**, 59.

94. Ibid.

95. U. M. Moebius 1986. Adverse event profiles of some common NSAIDs. *Lancet* **1**, 384.

96. Transcript of FDA piroxicam public hearing 28 February 1986, 6–14. (Hereafter referred to as "Piroxicam Hearing").

97. Ibid. 14.

98. Ibid. 19–21. Public Citizen statement at FDA piroxicam public hearing 28 February 1986, 1. (Hereafter referred to as "Public Citizen Piroxicam Statement").

99. Piroxicam Hearing, 22–31. Also see R. K. Verbeeck, C. J. Richardson, K. L. N. Blocka 1986. Clinical pharmacokinetics of piroxicam. *Journal of Rheumatology* **13**, 789–96.

100. Ibid. 31–4.

101. Public Citizen Piroxicam Statement, 1, 7–8; Pfizer Feldene Australian Label 1986.

102. Piroxicam Hearing 48–56; Public Citizen Piroxicam Statement, 2–3.

103. R. Smith 1986. Medicine and the media. *British Medical Journal* **292**.

104. Piroxicam Hearing, 88.

105. Ibid. 72.

106. Ibid. 99.

107. Ibid. 93.

108. Ibid. 121.

109. Ibid. 117–21.

110. Ibid. 121–2.

111. Ibid. 124–34.

112. Ibid. 135.

113. Ibid. 190.
114. Ibid. 184.
115. Ibid. 177.
116. Ibid. 211.
117. CSM 1986. CSM Update: non-steroidal anti-inflammatory drugs and serious gastro-intestinal adverse reactions–1. *British Medical Journal* **292**, 614.
118. CSM 1986. Non-steroidal anti-inflammatory drugs and serious gastro-intestinal adverse reactions–2. *British Medical Journal* **292**, 1190–91.
119. FDA 1986. Review of Pfizer's 17 March 1986 submissions to NDA and docket related to the petition by HRG on piroxicam by J. Harter, 28 April, 1.
120. Ibid.
121. Ibid. 9.
122. Ibid. 13.
123. FDA 1986. Recommendation in piroxicam imminent hazard petition, 14 May, 14–16.
124. Ibid. 14.
125. Ibid. 19.
126. Ibid. 19–20.
127. Ibid. 31.
128. Ibid. 32–43.
129. Ibid. 43.
130. Ibid. 47.
131. FDA Memo for the Secretary of Health and Human Services for Commissioner Young 1986. FDA's recommendation regarding disposition of imminent hazard petition regarding feldene (piroxicam) – decision, 27 May, 3.
132. Pfizer Canada 1986. Start once-a-day feldene for full anti-arthritic action. *The Medical Post*, 8 July.
133. Novopharm 1986. *Novopharm Product Monograph*, March 1986, 5.
134. Pfizer 1986. *Feldene Data Sheet.*

Chapter Six

1. US Congress 1983. 31st Report. House Committee on Government Operations *FDA's regulation of Zomax*, 2. Washington DC: US Government Publications Office. (Hereafter referred to as "Zomax Report"); US Congress 1983. Hearings before a Subcommittee of the House Committee on Government Operations *FDA's regulation of Zomax*, 26 and 27 April, 86. Washington DC: US Government Publications Office. (Hereafter referred to as "Zomax Hearings")
2. Ibid. 140.
3. FDA 1979. *Supplemental pharmacology review no.2* by M. Hein, 25 October.
4. FDA 1980. *Statistical review and evaluation* by Richard Stein 19 September.
5. Zomax Hearings, 201. Also see letter from M. Novitch, Deputy Commissioner of FDA, to Congressman Ted Weiss, "FDA critique of Dr N. Adrian Gross: review of zomepirac chronic studies", 11, 21 July 1983.
6. FDA 1981. Memo of meeting between McNeil Laboratories and FDA, 23 November.
7. Transcript of FDA Arthritis Advisory Committee, 19 August 1983, 50. (Hereafter referred to as "Arthritis Advisory Committee").
8. Ibid.
9. Zomax Hearings, 458–9.
10. Arthritis Advisory Committee.
11. FDA 1980. *Supplemental pharmacology review* by M. Hein, 20 May.

12. FDA 1980. Memo of meeting between McNeil Laboratories and FDA, 16 October. Zomax Hearings, 161–2.
13. FDA 1980. Memo by M.J. Finkel, Associate Director of New Drug Evaluation, 7 October, 3.
14. McNeil 1980. *Zomax Package Insert*, October.
15. FDA 1981. *Pharmacological review no.9 (zomepirac)* by Sydney Stolzenberg, 21 September.
16. Zomax Hearings, 208.
17. Ibid. 69.
18. Arthritis Advisory Committee, 60.
19. Ortho-Cilag 1981. *Zomax Data sheet*, April.
20. Ibid.
21. Ibid.
22. Zomax Hearings, 163–4; Letter from FDA Deputy Commissioner, Mark Novitch to Congressman Ted Weiss, 21 July 1983.
23. Letter from W. Mulloy to Congressman Ted Weiss, 10 May 1983.
24. Letter from W. Mulloy to Congressman Ted Weiss, 31 May 1983.
25. McNeil 1981. *Zomax Package Insert*, October 1980.
26. Zomax Hearings, 114.
27. Ibid. 120.
28. FDA 1979. "Non-steroidal anti-inflammatory, analgesic agents", memo by J. Harter, 9 February 1979.
29. Zomax Hearing, 105–6.
30. McNeil 1983. Zomax advertisement, *New England Journal of Medicine*, 24 February.
31. FDA 1979. Memo by M.J. Finkel, Associate Director for New Drug Evaluation, 23 October.
32. Zomax Hearings, 97.
33. Report by A. Gross on Zomax carcinogenicity, 3.
34. Letter from FDA Deputy Commissioner, M. Novitch to Congressman Ted Weiss, 21 July 1983, 2.
35. Ibid. 2, 10.
36. Ibid. 2.
37. Zomax Report, 6.
38. Report by A. Gross on Zomax carcinogenicity, 13.
39. Ibid. 6.
40. Ibid. 6.
41. Ibid. 7–9.
42. Ibid. 9–11.
43. Zomax Hearings, 62–3.
44. Ibid. 115.
45. Ibid. 159.
46. Ibid. 115.
47. Ibid. 163.
48. Ibid. 140.
49. Ibid. 176–7.
50. Arthritis Advisory Committee, 60.
51. Zomax Hearings, 415.
52. FDA 1980. *Zomax summary basis of approval*, 23.
53. FDA 1982. "Adrenal tumour and combinations", memo of meeting with McNeil 5 February. Zomax Hearings, 197.
54. FDA 1979. *Supplemental pharmacology review* by M. Hein, 25 October, 13; FDA 1978. *Supplementary pharmacology review* by M. Hein, 7 December, 4.
55. Zomax Hearings 190–91.

56. FDA 1980. *Supplemental pharmacology review no.3* by M. Hein, 20 May, 3.
57. Zomax hearings, 88.
58. FDA 1983. Memo of meeting with McNeil, 4 March.
59. Ibid.
60. Zomax Hearings, 176.
61. FDA 1980. *Group leader's review* by J. Harter, 24 September.
62. FDA 1980. *Statistical review and evaluation* by J. Senturia, 4 February.
63. FDA 1980. *Statistical review and evaluation* by J. Senturia, 22 September.
64. Zomax Hearings, 177.
65. Ibid. 181.
66. Ibid. 189.
67. Ibid. 190. Zomax Report, 7–8.
68. Zomax Hearings, 189.
69. Zomax Hearings, 191.
70. Ibid. 191.
71. S. A. Samuel 1981. Apparent anaphylactoid reactions to zomepirac (*Zomax*). *New England Journal of Medicine* **304**, 978.
72. Zomax Hearings, 89.
73. FDA 1979. Tolectin (R) – tolmetin sodium anaphylactic reactions. *ADR Highlights*, 20 June. Zomax Hearings, 89.
74. Brown & Wier 1978. Drug fever from tolmetin administration. *Journal of the American Medical Association* **240**, 246; C. Restivo & H. E. Paulus 1978. Anaphylaxis from tolmetin. *Journal of the American Medical Association* **240**, 246.
75. Zomax Hearing, 99–100.
76. Ibid. 100–101.
77. Ibid. 101–2.
78. McNeil 1980. Pharmaceutical, *Zomax Package Insert*, 20 October. Zomax Hearings, 332.
79. Zomax Hearings, 284.
80. Zomax Hearing, 462. Arthritis Advisory Committee, 19 August 1983, 41.
81. Zomax Hearings, 342.
82. Ibid. 462.
83. Ibid.
84. McNeil 1982. Memo from T. W. Teal to J. E. O'Brien, 31 March.
85. McNeil 1981. *Zomax Data Sheet*.
86. McNeil 1982. *Zomax Data Sheet*.
87. Zomax Hearings, 297–326.
88. Letter from D. Ein to Congressman Weiss, 21 April 1983.
89. Zomax Hearings, 324, 327, 333–4.
90. FDA 1983. Responses to queries on Zomax asked by Chairman Weiss in his letter of 17 May 1983 to Dr Harter. Report to Congressman Weiss, 29 July.
91. Ibid.
92. McNeil 1985. Memo from J. A. Dale and E. F. Lemanowicz to R. S. Fine 19 February.
93. Zomax Hearings, 108–9.
94. Ibid. 108–9.
95. Ibid. 107–8.
96. McNeil 1982. "Dear Doctor" Letter, 9 April.
97. Zomax Hearings, 111.
98. FDA 1981. A comparison of anaphylactoid reactions associated with non-steroidal anti-inflammatory drugs. *ADR Highlights*, 26 May.
99. McNeil 1982. Memo from T. W. Teal to J. E. O'Brien, 31 March.
100. Zomax Hearings, 114; Zomax Report 19–20.
101. Zomax Hearings, 113–14.

102. McNeil 1982. Memo from J. Vaughan to J. Dale, 27 August.
103. FDA 1983. "Zomax anaphylactoid reactions". Memo, 11 February. FDA 1983. "Anaphylactoid reactions with Zomax". Memo, 28 February.
104. FDA 1983. "Zomax anaphylactoid reactions". Telecon between McNeil and J. Harter and D. Moore, FDA, 4 March.
105. Zomax Hearings, 102.
106. Arthritis Advisory Committee, 48.
107. Ibid. 21–2.
108. Arthritis Advisory Committee, 75.
109. Ibid. 76.
110. *Federal Register* **47**(101) (25 May 1982), 22550.
111. Zomax Hearings, 90.
112. Zomax Hearings, 90.
113. Arthritis Advisory Committee, 8.
114. Ibid. 30.
115. Letter from M. Novitch, Acting FDA Commissioner to Congressman Weiss, 6 October 1983.
116. Arthritis Advisory Committee, 141–2.
117. Zomax Report, 22.
118. Zomax Hearings, 112.
119. Ibid. 90.
120. Ibid. 90.
121. Ibid. 97.
122. Arthritis Advisory Committee Meeting, 109–18.
123. Zomax Hearings, 95–6.
124. Ibid. 98–9
125. Arthritis Advisory Committee Meeting, 25, 38.
126. Ibid.
127. FDA Zomax (zomepirac) discussion paper, 5–6.
128. Arthritis Advisory Committee, 173.
129. Zomax Hearings, 96.
130. Ibid. 97.
131. Letter from M. Novitch, Acting FDA Commissioner to Congressman Weiss, 6 October 1983. Transcript of Arthritis Advisory Committee Meeting 19 August 1983, 59–60.
132. Zomax Report, 26.
133. Arthritis Advisory Committee, 145.
134. Arthritis Advisory Committee, 203.
135. Draft FDA Letter from J. Harter to McNeil Laboratories "Suggestions for labeling revisions to the INDICATIONS AND PRECAUTIONS sections of Zomax for discussion", March 1985.
136. FDA Zomax (zomepirac) discussion paper.
137. Zomax Report, 27.
138. Department of Health and Human Services 1985. "Minutes of the General Staff Meeting", Memo, 13 May.

Chapter Seven

1. US Congress 1987. Hearings Before a Subcommittee of the House Committee on Government Operations *FDA's regulation of the new drug Suprol*, 27 May, 406. (Hereafter referred to as "Suprol Hearings").

2. Ortho-Cilag 1984–87. *Suprol data sheets,* ABPI Compendia.
3. A. Veitch 1986. Data faked to win drug licence. *Guardian,* 4 October.
4. FDA 1980. *Supplementary pharmacology review* by M. Hein, 7 July.
5. Addendum by D. J. Richman to FDA supplementary pharmacology review by M. Hein, 7 July 1980.
6. FDA 1985. *Review and evaluation of pharmacology and toxicology data* by Conrad Chen, 18 July.
7. FDA 1985. *Review and evaluation of pharmacology and toxicology data* by Conrad Chen, 20 March.
8. FDA 1982. op. cit. (**n.6**)
9. Addendum by D. J. Richman to FDA *Review and evaluation of pharmacology and toxicology data* by Conrad Chen, 18 July 1985.
10. Suprol Hearings, 375–6.
11. FDA 1985. *Group leader summary* by John Harter, 25 June.
12. Ibid.
13. McNeil 1986. *Suprol Package Insert,* 24 April.
14. Suprol Hearings, 68.
15. Ibid. 68.
16. Ibid. 68–9.
17. Ibid. 68–9.
18. Zomax Hearings, 159.
19. Suprol Hearings, 69.
20. A. Gross 1987. Report to Congress on Suprol, 3.
21. Ibid. 21–3, 26.
22. Ibid. 6–8.
23. Ibid. 14–17.
24. Ibid. 26.
25. A. Veitch 1987. Arthritis drug linked with cancer. *Guardian,* 22 June.
26. Suprol Hearings, 35.
27. FDA 1985. *Group leader summary* by J. Harter, 25 June.
28. FDA 1985. Memo of meeting with McNeil and Ortho, 25 November.
29. Letter from Congressman Weiss to FDA Commissioner Young, 26 February 1987.
30. Suprol Hearings, 257–8.
31. Ibid. 259.
32. FDA 1986. Memo of meeting with McNeil, 30 July. Letter from J. D. Siegfried, Executive Director, Regulatory Affairs, McNeil to J. F. Palmer, Director of Division of Oncology and Radiopharmaceutical Products, FDA, 29 July 1986.
33. Suprol Hearings, 46.
34. McNeil 1986. *Suprol Package Insert,* 24 April; McNeil 1986. "Dear Doctor" letter by C. L. Ellis, Director of Medical Services, 25 April.
35. Suprol Hearings, 37; McNeil 1986. "Dear Doctor" letter by C. L. Ellis, Director of Medical Services, 10 July.
36. McNeil 1986. "Dear Doctor" letter by C. L. Ellis, Director of Medical Services, 10 July.
37. Suprol Hearings, 48.
38. FDA 1986 Memo by J. Cobbs, 27 August.
39. Suprol Hearings, 52–3.
40. Ibid. 40.
41. Ibid. 41; McNeil 1986. "Dear Doctor" letter by C. L. Ellis, Director of Clinical Research, 10 October.
42. Suprol Hearings, 40.
43. Ibid. 58.
44. Ibid. 59.

45. Ibid. 41.
46. FDA Arthritis Advisory Committee Meeting, 2 December 1986, 107.
47. Suprol Hearings, 61.
48. FDA Arthritis Advisory Committee. op. cit., 114. (**n.46**)
49. *Federal Register* **47**(101) (25 May 1982), 225.
50. Suprol Hearings, 41.
51. Ibid. 41.
52. Ibid. 38.

Chapter Eight

1. M. Bunge 1991. A critical examination of the new sociology of science: part 1. *Philosophy of Social Sciences* **21**, 524–60; M. Hammersley 1992. On feminist methodology. *Sociology* **26**, 187–206.
2. N. D. Ellis 1972. The occupation of science. In *Sociology of science: selected readings*, B. Barnes (ed.), 196. London: Penguin.
3. B. Barnes 1971. Making out in industrial research. *Science Studies* **1**, 157–75.
4. M. Schwarz & M. Thompson 1990. *Divided we stand: redefining politics, technology and social choice*, 53–54. Hemel Hempstead, Herts: Harvester-Wheatsheaf.
5. F. M. Lynn 1986. The interplay of science and values in assessing and regulating environmental risks. *Science, Technology and Human Values* **11**, 40–50.
6. US Congress 1979. Senate Select Committee on Small Business *Competitive problems in the drug industry: drug testing*, 4. Washington DC: US Government Publications Office.
7. S. E. Cozzens & T. F. Gieryn 1990. Introduction: putting science back in society. In *Theories of science in society*, S. E. Cozzens & T. F. Gieryn (eds), 5. Bloomington, Indiana: Indiana University Press.
8. T. F. Gieryn 1983. Boundary-work and the demarcation of science from non-science: strains and interests in professional ideologies of scientists. *American Sociological Review* **48**, 7871–95.
9. S. S. Jasanoff 1987. Contested boundaries in policy-relevant science. *Social Studies of Science* **17**, 195–230; S. Jasanoff 1990. *The fifth branch: science advisers as policy makers*. Cambridge, Mass.: Harvard University Press.
10. E. Richards 1988. The politics of therapeutic evaluation: the vitamin C and cancer controversy. *Social Studies of Science* **18**, 653–701; E. Richards 1991. *Vitamin C and cancer: medicine or politics?* London: Macmillan.
11. J. Collier 1989. *The health conspiracy: how doctors, the drug industry and the government undermine our health*. London: Century.
12. B. Wynne 1983. Redefining the issues of risks and public acceptance: the social viability of technology. *Futures* **16**, 13–32; M. Schwarz & M. Thompson 1990. op. cit. (**n.4**)
13. J. van Eijndhoven & P. Groenewegan 1991. The construction of expert advice on health risks. *Social Studies of Science* **21**, 257–78.
14. US Office of Government Ethics 1979. *Summary of the post-employment restrictions of the ethics in Government Act of 1978 and important interpretations in the regulations*. Washington DC: US Government Publications Office.
15. M. Schwarz & M. Thompson 1990. op. cit., 61. (**n.4**)
16. Ibid. 57.
17. CSM 1983. *Adverse reaction working party report*, June.
18. CSM 1986. *Adverse reaction working party report*, January.
19. Cm 2290 1993. *Open Government*. London: HMSO.
20. Ibid. 49.

21. Ibid. 48–9.
22. National Consumer Council (NCC) 1993. *Balancing acts: conflicts of interest in the regulation of medicine.* London: NCC.
23. R. Hurley 1994. Conflicts of interest in drug regulation. *Lancet* **1**, 59.
24. Cm 2250 1993. *Realising our potential: a strategy for science, engineering and technology,* 14, 16–17. London: HMSO.
25. Scrip 1988. *World Pharmaceutical News* **1270**, 1–6 January, 24.
26. Scrip 1991. *World Pharmaceutical News* **1635**, 19 July, 2.

Index